Spinal Deformities in Adolescents, Adults and Older Adults

Edited by Josette Bettany-Saltikov and Gokulakannan Kandasamy

Published in London, United Kingdom

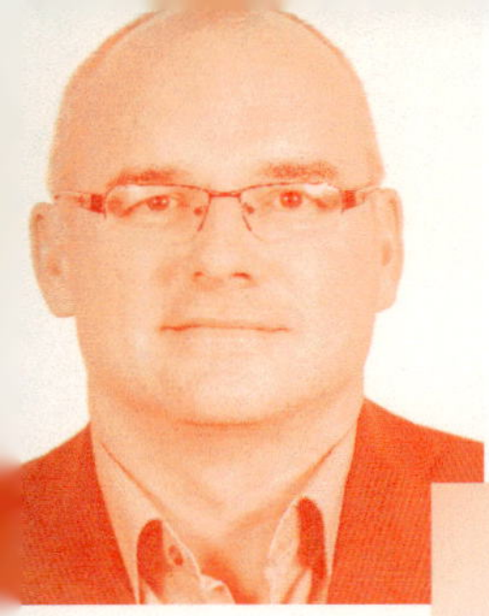
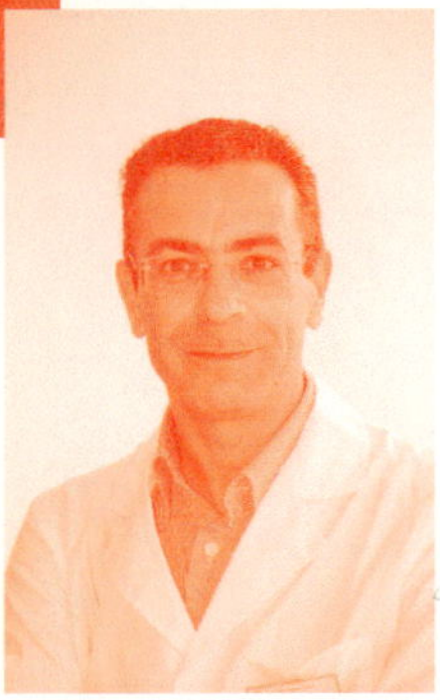
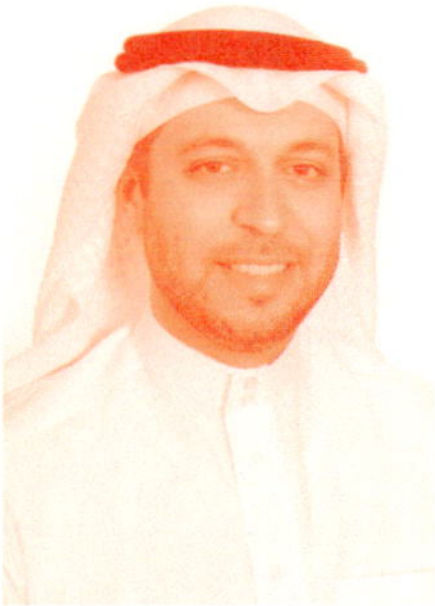
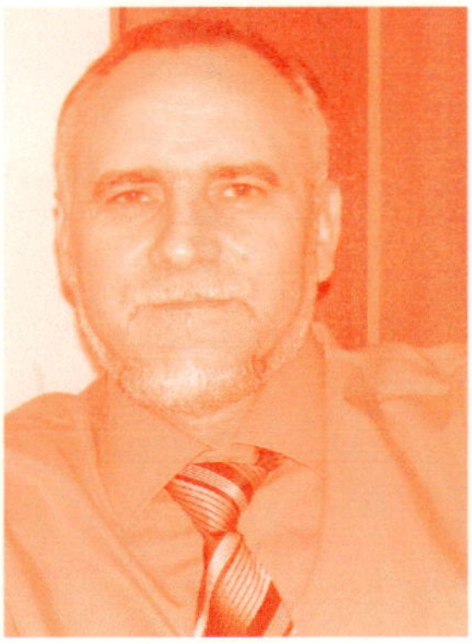
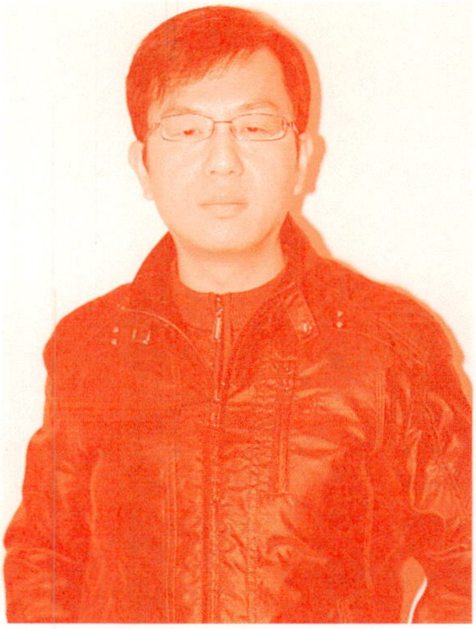
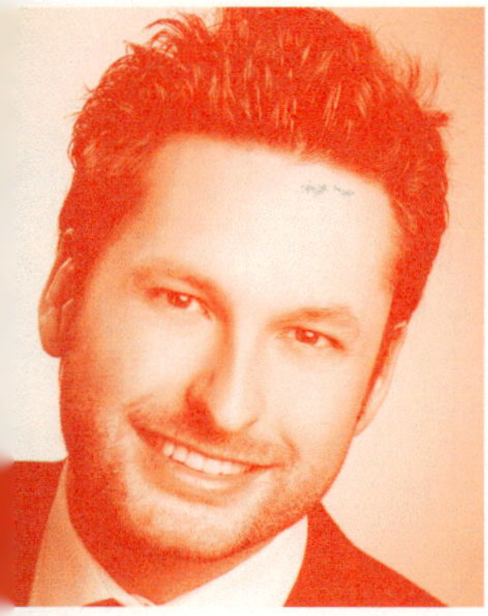
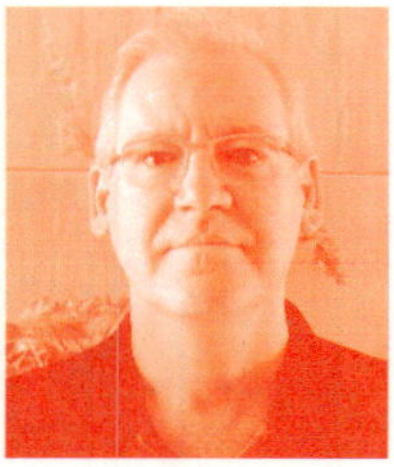

IntechOpen

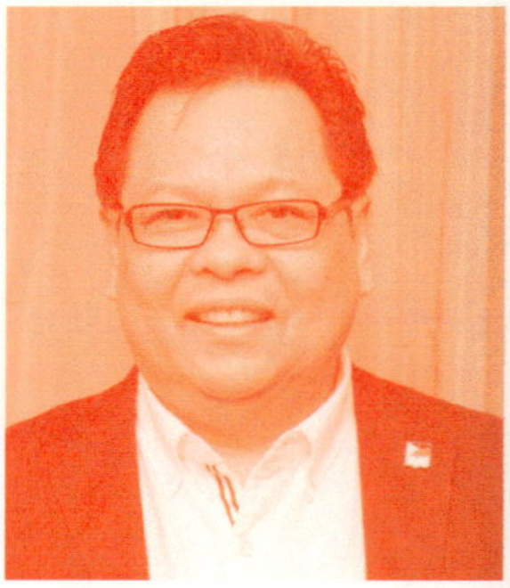
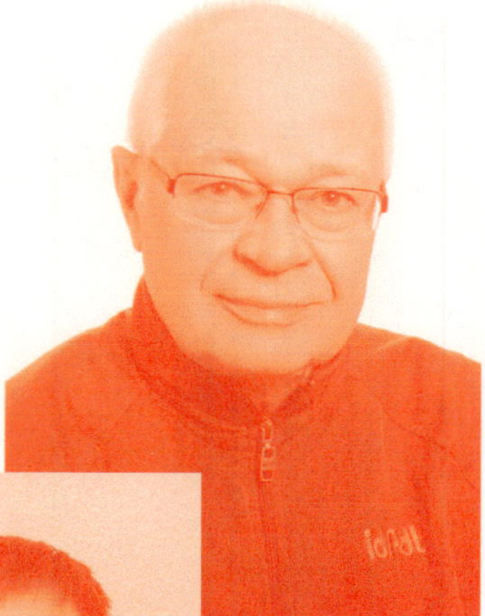
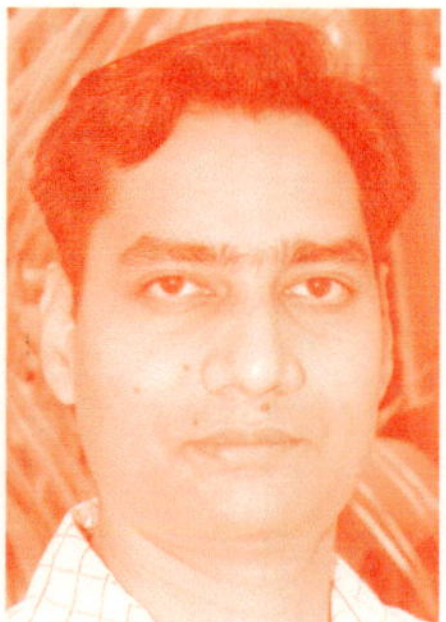
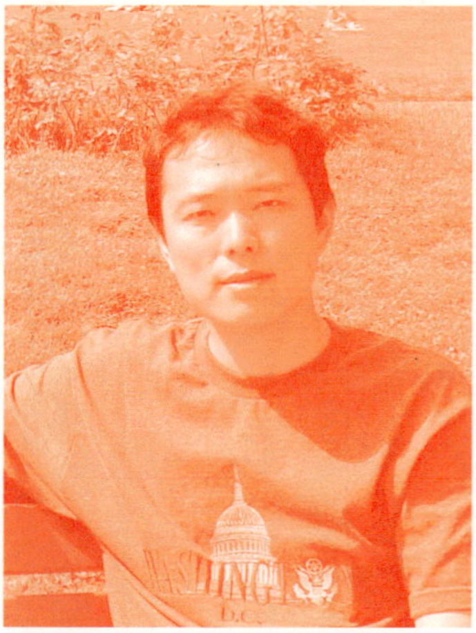
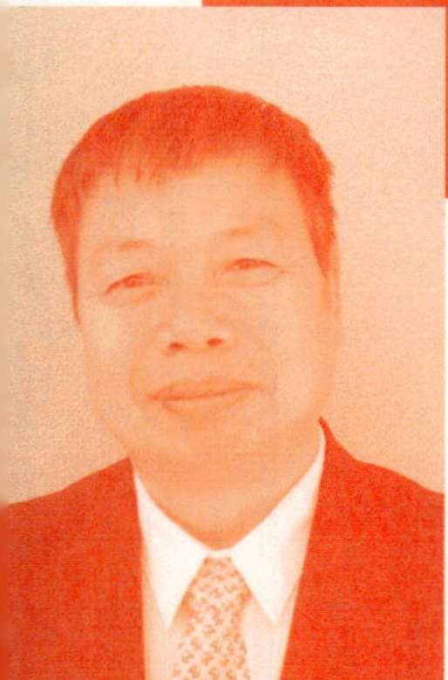
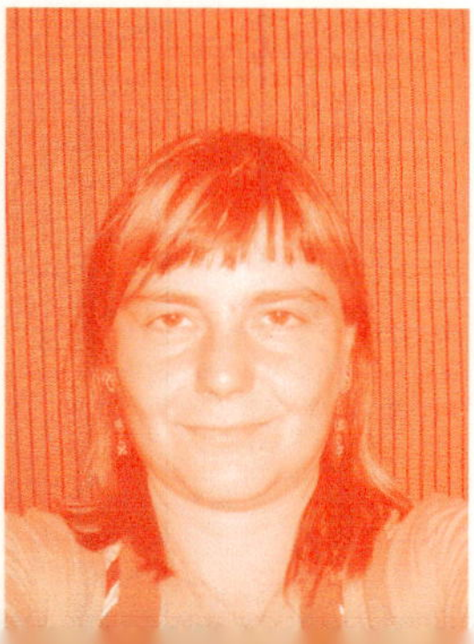

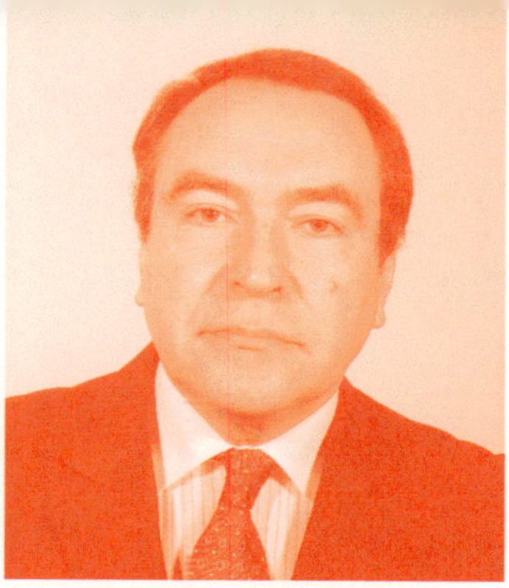
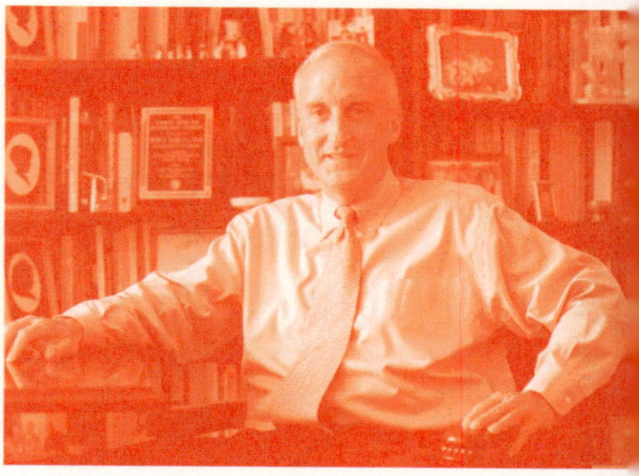
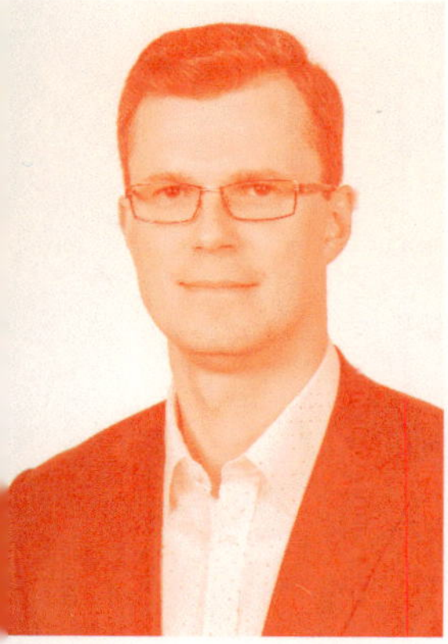
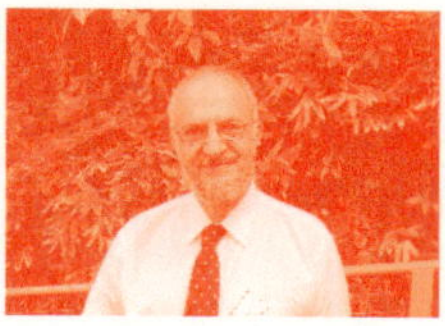
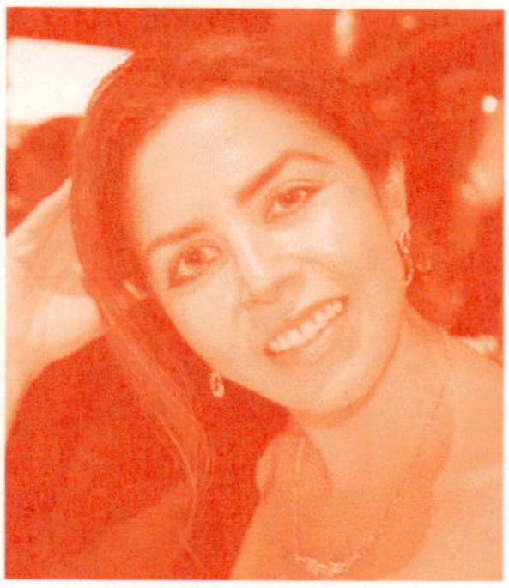

Supporting open minds since 2005

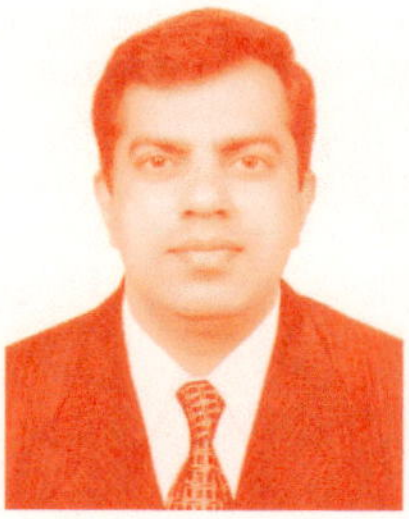
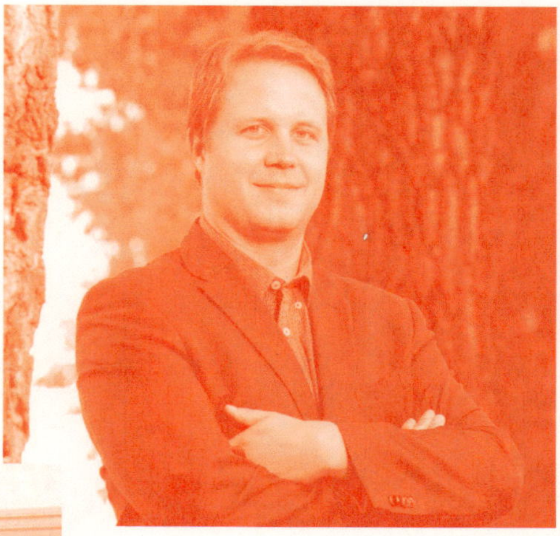
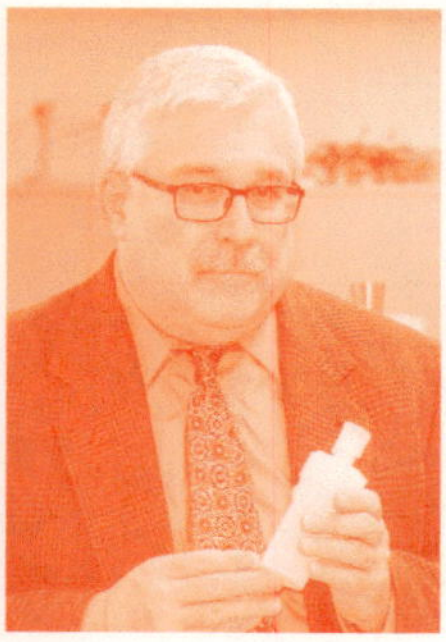
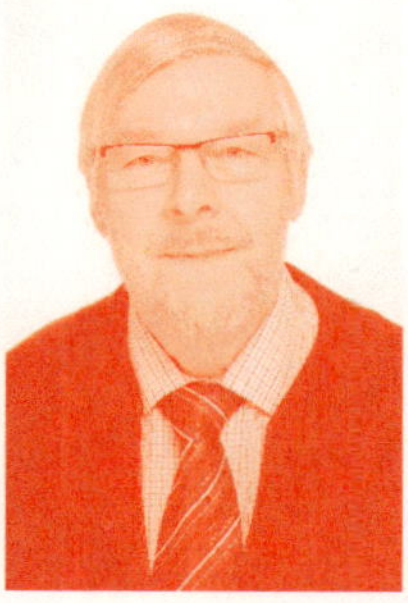
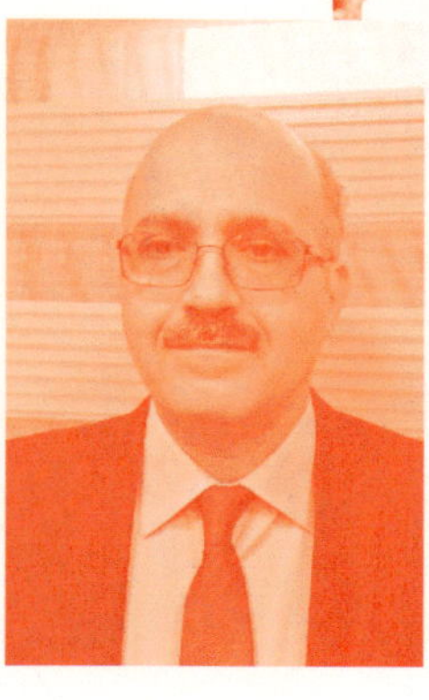
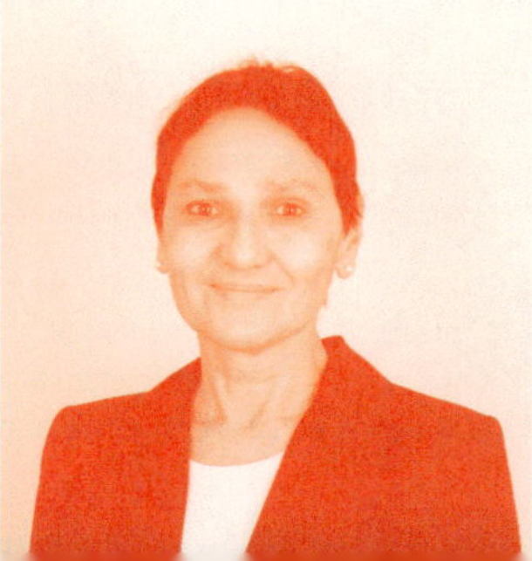
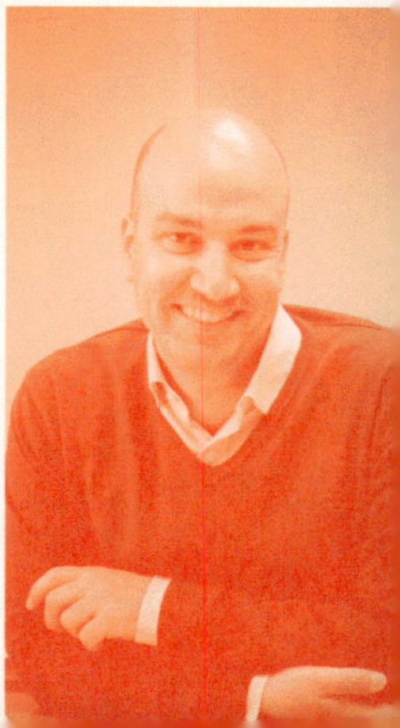

Spinal Deformities in Adolescents, Adults and Older Adults
http://dx.doi.org/10.5772/intechopen.83150
Edited by Josette Bettany-Saltikov and Gokulakannan Kandasamy

Assistant to the Editors: Deborah Turnbull

Contributors
David Christopher Kieser, Michael Wyatt, Jean Claude De Mauroy, Fabio Gagliano, Rosario Gagliano, Piera Lusenti, Niels Hammer, Josette Bettany-Saltikov, Jonathan Ling, Adam Park, Andrej Gogala, Shu Yan Ng, Paul A. Oakley, Deed E. Harrison, Ibrahim M. Moustafa, Hans-Rudolf Weiss, Deborah Turnbull, Gokulakannan Kandasamy, Paul Van Schaik, Martin John Matthews, James H. Wynne

First published in London, United Kingdom, 2021 by IntechOpen
IntechOpen is the global imprint of INTECHOPEN LIMITED, registered in England and Wales, registration number: 11086078, 5 Princes Gate Court, London, SW7 2QJ, United Kingdom
Printed in Croatia

British Library Cataloguing-in-Publication Data
A catalogue record for this book is available from the British Library

Additional hard and PDF copies can be obtained from orders@intechopen.com

Spinal Deformities in Adolescents, Adults and Older Adults
Edited by Josette Bettany-Saltikov and Gokulakannan Kandasamy
p. cm.
Print ISBN 978-1-83880-452-7
Online ISBN 978-1-83880-453-4
eBook (PDF) ISBN 978-1-83962-168-0

For EU product safety concerns:
IN TECH d.o.o., Prolaz Marije Krucifikse Kozulić 3, 51000 Rijeka, Croatia, info@intechopen.com or visit our website at intechopen.com.

Meet the editors

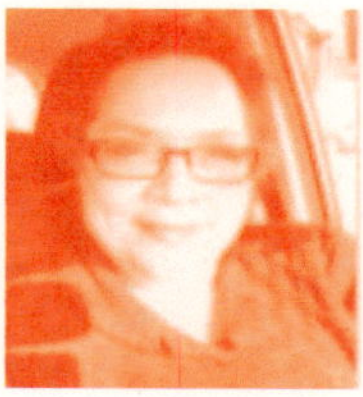

Josette-Bettany Saltikov, Ph.D., is a senior lecturer, researcher in scoliosis, and a chartered physiotherapist. She teaches and supervises numerous doctoral students and helps them to achieve their full potential. She has been conducting research into scoliosis for the last 30 years after having completed a Ph.D. in the area of back shape and posture, spinal mobility, and psychological factors before and after surgery in adolescent idiopathic scoliosis. Dr. Saltikov has published more than 130 papers to date including both Cochrane and Campbell systematic reviews. Additionally, she has served as both a grant and manuscript reviewer. She has also been invited to act as an external examiner to doctoral students in numerous countries. In the near future, Dr. Saltikov hopes to further her research into the perspectives and views of scoliosis patients and healthcare professionals who work with them to help scoliosis patients manage their own conditions.

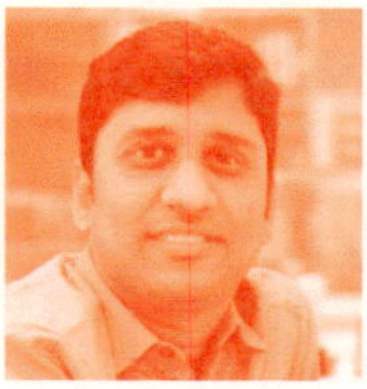

Gokulakannan Kandasamy, Ph.D., is a chartered physiotherapist and an associate professor at Teesside University, England. As a university teaching fellow and a HEA Senior Fellow. Dr. Kandasamy teaches and supports students at all levels. His research areas of focus are back shape, posture, spinal pain, and deformities. As an external examiner, he has undertaken external consultancy work on curriculum design as well as staff development activities.

Contents

Preface

We are pleased to present *Spinal Deformities in Adolescents, Adults and Older Adults*, a unique book with a wide scope of coverage of the topic. It presents readers with under-reported topics and treatments in spinal deformity. It also includes a very interesting case study/autobiography in which one of the authors discusses his self-management approach to his own deformity. This volume is written by specialists worldwide, all of whom have experience working with patients with spinal deformities and/or conducting valued research in the field.

The chapters examine the evidence relating to spinal deformities together with assessment tools, treatment modalities, and the various types, benefits, and side effects of these diverse treatment approaches. The book also bravely provides a more balanced view of different treatment methods, including more subjective research on the experiences of patients in treatment, an aspect that is greatly needed in this area. It also provides recent reviews on the evidence base of well-researched areas such as adolescent idiopathic scoliosis treatment. Instead of focusing on conservative treatment only, the book also includes a chapter on improving surgical outcomes. It courageously embarks upon the wider functional and psychosocial exploration of the impacts of spinal deformities as a global disease. Furthermore, the book sets a much wider focus on the research area by demonstrating a more holistic person-centered approach and collaboration with patients in their treatments, while still focusing on the needs of the patient group.

We hope clinicians working with patients, researchers, and patients and their families will find this book useful. We also hope that it will inspire further research and new innovations and patient experiences in the field of spinal deformity.

Josette Bettany-Saltikov and Gokulakannan Kandasamy
School of Health and Life Sciences,
Allied Health Department Teesside University,
United Kingdom

Chapter 1

Bracing Adult Scoliosis: From Immobilization to Correction of Adult Scoliosis

Jean Claude de Mauroy, Fabio Gagliano, Rosario Gagliano and Piera Lusenti

Abstract

Unlike adolescent idiopathic scoliosis, bracing was used in adults less and was used more as a way of reducing pain. There is little publication of adult scoliosis series in the literature. The use of very high-rigidity and high-precision CAD/CAM technologies currently makes it possible to create corrective braces for the adult. The digital CAD/CAM cast in three blocks allows for precise correction at the pelvic, lumbar, and thoracic levels. This chapter presents the results of a series of 62 consecutive adult scoliotic patients treated with a corrective asymmetric detorsion brace of very high rigidity made in 2014–2016. Tolerance and angular correction results will be compared to those of 158 patients treated with the former bivalve polyethylene overlapping immobilization brace mainly used for lumbar scoliosis. The new Lyon adult ARTbrace is a detorsion brace adapted to all the curvatures which controls the sagittal plane. Despite a resistance four times greater than that of polyethylene of the same thickness, the tolerance of the Europlex'O is excellent as it is a "shock absorber," and the anterior opening facilitates the use for very old people. Consequently, the aim of this chapter is to consider if it is possible to envisage for some patients an alternative to surgery, thanks to the new technologies of bracing.

Keywords: adult scoliosis, bracing, de novo scoliosis, camptocormia, Lyon method, nonsurgical, PSSE, ARTbrace

1. Introduction

1.1 Adult scoliosis instability

1.1.1 Bracing history

Lyon has always had a great tradition of orthopedic, and Charles Gabriel Pravaz was not only the inventor of the syringe, but he also created in Lyon a great orthopedic institute to treat scoliosis 200 years ago. The first Lyon brace, which was made of leather and steel, was created by Stagnara 70 years ago. It undergone a first change with the replacement of leather by polymethacrylate. This brace was used in adults in addition to surgery while waiting for the graft fusion, at a time when osteosynthesis did not have the current quality. In 2013, the use of adult ARTbrace in Europlex'O in polyamide and asymmetry allowed to avoid the plaster cast which

IntechOpen

has always been the characteristic of the Lyon management. The use of polyamide and digital allows treatment of thoracic and double major curves.

1.1.2 Frequency of adult scoliosis

Vanderpool et al. [1] shows that the frequency of scoliosis in adults increases steadily with age, from 6% of scoliosis after the patient reaches 40 years until it reaches 10% of the population at age 65. The sex ratio was 2 females to 1 male. It is women who have the most painful instabilities and imbalances. Their bone mass is lower than that of men with a vertebral fracture threshold at age 65. Pregnancy and menopause could be also aggravating factors [2].

1.1.3 Adult patients are different

Akbarnia et al. [3] described the key features as curve stiffness, degeneration of the discs, osteoporosis, spinal imbalance both coronal and sagittal, rotary subluxation, spinal stenosis, and higher rate of complications (pulmonary, etc.). The esthetic aspect is not negligible, and even surgery performed during adolescence does not solve everything. Edgar and Mehta [4] has shown that self-image representation and social life is different after surgery in adolescence. 82% of adult scoliosis without surgery was married compared to 60% of scoliosis operated in adolescence. O'Brien [5] analyzes the consequences of scoliosis in adulthood. He noted that for adult scoliosis abnormal physical appearance and diminished self-esteem may always be present, but breathing limitations, inability to function, and other quality of life issues generally become the driving forces for clinical examination, diagnosis, and treatment.

1.1.4 Complications of surgical treatment vs. non-operative

The complications were analyzed by many authors. For Baron and Albert [6] the incidence of medical complications ranges between 40 and 86%. Local complications include infection, pseudarthrosis or failure of instrumentation, and neurological and adjacent-level degeneration or instability. Common medical complications include pneumonia, atelectasis, ileus, delirium, and cerebrovascular incidents. Smith et al. [7] studied the incidence of complications according to age. His conclusions were the following: the oldest age group (65–85 years) has nearly four times the number of minor complications and nearly five times the number of major complications when compared with the youngest age group (25–44 years). As invasive surgical therapy needs a perfect understanding of risk/benefit, Ogilvie [8] suggests that the decision to proceed with surgical treatment even if justified in many cases must be based on a thorough understanding of the anticipated benefits from surgical treatment and the risk of serious complications. These potential complications lead to multiple surgeries with results that can be less desirable than the original condition. The results of conservative orthopedic treatment are more difficult to assess. Kluba et al. [9] compares surgical and conservative treatment for degenerative lumbar scoliosis. He finds a significantly higher rate of spinal stenosis and degenerative spondylolisthesis in the group of patients with surgery. However no significant difference was evident between the two groups in terms of lumbar back pain after 4 years, respectively.

Everett and Patel [10] conducted a systematic review of non-operative treatment. There is indeterminate, level III/IV evidence on the effectiveness of any conservative option; level IV evidence on the role of physical therapy, chiropractic care, and bracing; and level III evidence for injections in the conservative treatment of adult deformity. The use of rigid or hard bracing in adult scoliosis is generally not recommended. This is due to the risk of muscle weakening effects from hard bracing and the fact that this could accelerate the degenerative process in some cases. Chuah et al. [11] notes that bracing may sometimes help the symptoms, but it has no effect on curve progression.

Pain is not synonymous with deformity progression. Some stable scoliosis patient report pain, and others evolve without pain. It will be necessary to try to make the difference between the "physical" pain and the "emotional" suffering when the patient does not support his deformation anymore.

1.2 Anatomo-pathological classification of painful instabilities

a. Thoracolumbar pain often corresponds to minor joint instability.

b. The pain of convexity is of muscular origin.

c. The pain of the concavity is posterior: facet syndrome.

d. The lumbosacral pain is of ligament origin.

These pains respond perfectly to physiotherapy.

When scoliosis progresses, it is either (1) the evolution in adulthood of an adolescent idiopathic scoliosis, (2) a de novo scoliosis usually of discal origin, or (3) a camptocormia of muscular origin. In all cases, there may be a disc disease with sometimes rotatory dislocation, postural impairment with imbalance, extrapyramidal muscle involvement, and bone involvement (osteoporosis). In these progressive cases of instability, bracing or surgery may be necessary.

1.3 Classification of painful instabilities according to age

a. From 20 to 30 years old, the main problem is the anatomical pain.

b. From 30 to 50 years old, the main problem is the discal decompensation.

c. After 50 years old, there are two main problems: degenerative scoliosis very rigid with arthrosis and camptocormia reducible with paravertebral muscular atrophy.

1.4 Natural history of idiopathic scoliosis from adolescent to adulthood

Early works on scoliosis progression in adulthood were pessimistic [12], but at this time, idiopathic scoliosis, especially rachitic infantile, is mixed with neurological poliomyelitis that no longer exists.

In 2003 Weinstein published the spontaneous evolution of 117 idiopathic scolioses over more than 50 years [13]. Thoracic curves of more than 50 degrees at skeletal maturity progressed with an average of 29.4 degrees. Thoracolumbar curves between 50 and 75 degrees increased with an average of 22.3 degrees. Lumbar curves had the most progression, especially when the L5 vertebra was not well seated and when the apical rotation was greater than 33%. He does not observe a functional respiratory or painful repercussion below 70°. This angulation could be currently the functional surgical Cobb limit. Pregnancy does not change the progression of scoliosis in adulthood, except in cases of twin pregnancy.

1.5 The two distinct entities

In 2007 Marty-Poumarat [14] describes two specific adult scoliosis entities: adolescent scoliosis in adult (ASA) and degenerative de novo scoliosis (DDS).

Group A (ASA) = adult progression of AIS > 40° with first dislocation at 45 years. The progression can be sometimes regular, sometimes chaotic.

Group B (DDS) = de novo scoliosis with low Cobb after 50°, first dislocation at 52 years after menopause. DDS is more progressive than AIS. Because DDS is a result of degenerative disc instability, it is almost always progressive. Lumbar and thoracolumbar are the most progressive degenerative curves. Duval-Beaupere and Dubousset [15] have first described the mechanism of rotatory subluxation. Following their work, many authors have insisted on the importance of the lumbo-pelvic parameters [16–18].

1.6 Risk factors for instability

The radiological risk factors for instability are (1) rotatory dislocation with lateral olisthesis (**Figure 1**), (2) L3–L4 inclination, (3) hypolordosis, and (4) increased thoracolumbar kyphosis [19–20].

1.7 Indications of bracing

The physical activity and fracture rate of adult scoliosis is identical to that of the general population, except for operated patients who have less physical activity [21]. Unlike adolescence, when bracing is systematic when scoliosis progresses, the corrective bracing indication in adults is less related to Cobb angulation but more to the instability which results in pain, abnormal angular evolution, or imbalances (**Figure 2**).

From a database started in 1998, we selected all adult scoliosis in which conservative orthopedic treatment has been proposed to, even if the treatment had not been achieved by the patient. Scoliosis treated during adolescence and monitored in adulthood were excluded [22]. In this case series study, we analyzed 779 patients referred for nonsurgical treatment, and we correlated three parameters: the etiology, age, and Cobb angulation (**Table 1**).

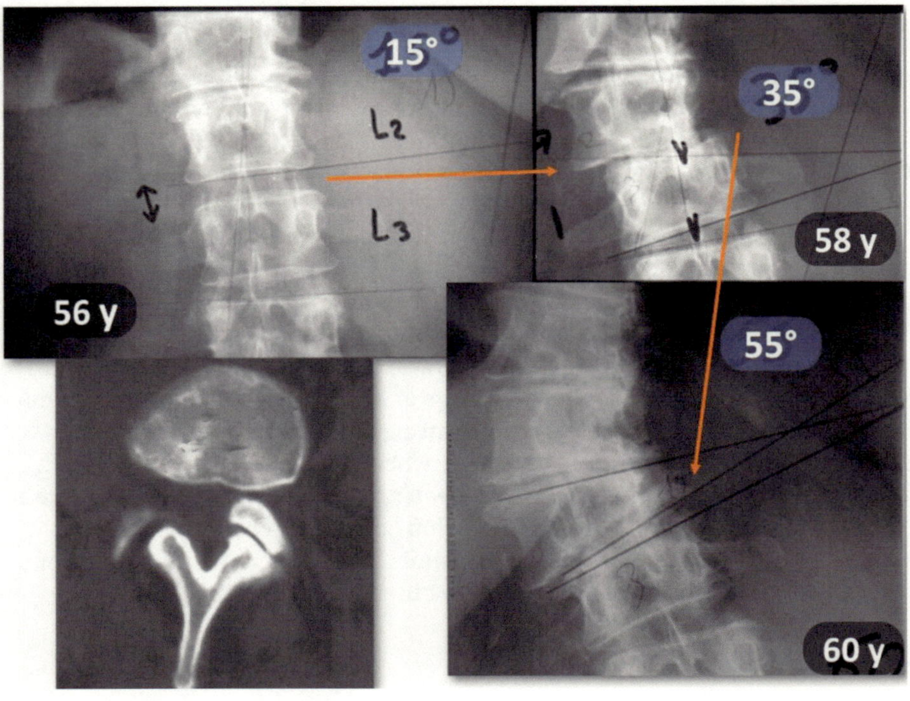

Figure 1.
De novo scoliosis with constitution of a rotatory dislocation in 2 years, then scoliosis worsening by osteoporotic cuneiformization.

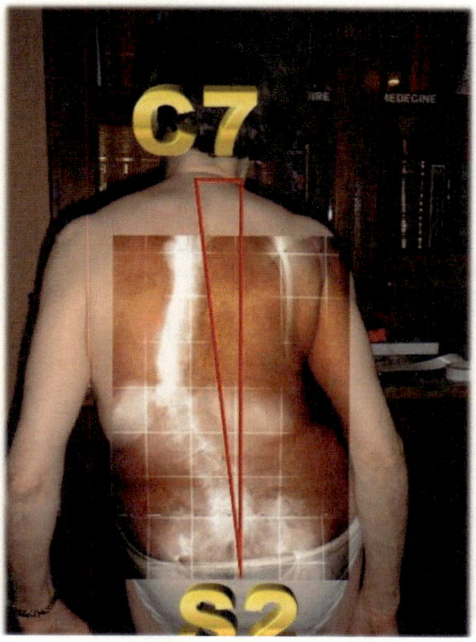

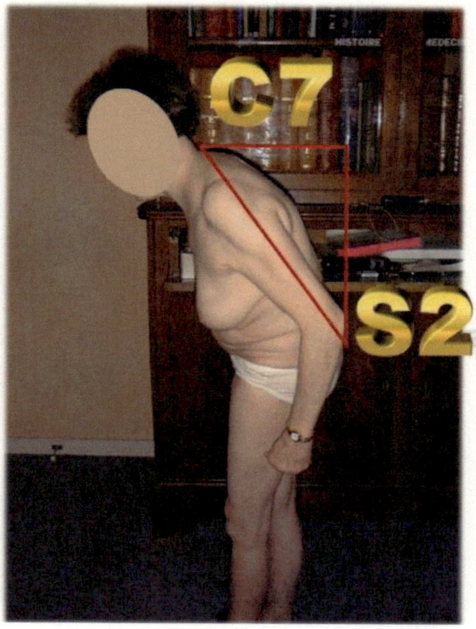

Figure 2.
Clinical imbalances in the frontal and the sagittal planes.

Indications ARTbrace adult (n = 779)	Rate %	Mean age	Mean angulation
Rotatory dislocation (n = 361)	46.5%	59.73 y ± 13.50	39.08° ± 16.56
Segmental instability (n = 150)	19%	46.03 y ± 15.49	25.29° ± 12.29
Instability post-surgery (n = 86)	11%	53.09 y ± 12.91	40.49° ± 15.38
Camptocormia (n = 68)	9%	69.78 y ± 12.19	38.09° ± 14.23
Kyphosis (thoracolumbar) (n = 62)	8%	60.73 y ± 15.51	43.34° ± 21.48
Disabling pain (n = 33)	4%	48.36 y ± 13.73	36.45° ± 21.48
Spondylolisthesis and spinal stenosis (n = 19)	2.5%		

Table 1.
Main indications for adult scoliosis bracing with frequency classification.

The rate of dropout patients not wearing the brace is 17% which is not excessive, especially since the plaster cast at that time was made before the brace discouraged patients.

A tentative classification according to etiology, age, and angulation is proposed (**Figure 3**).

More than half of the indications concern the rotational dislocation, which is the specific complication of adult scoliosis. The rotary dislocation is visible on the CT scan with subluxation and joint narrowing on the sliding side and widening of the articular space on the opposite side.

One-fourth of the indications concern disc instability, which can be considered as the early stage of rotational dislocation.

The other etiologies are less frequent: lumbar-pelvic-femoral kyphosis, secondary instability under arthrodesis, root pain, and rarely spinal stenosis which requires neurosurgery. Camptocormia is linked to weakness of the deep posterior musculature [23]. The patient increases kyphosis gradually to tighten his weak paravertebral muscles. There is often an extrapyramidal context of Parkinson's

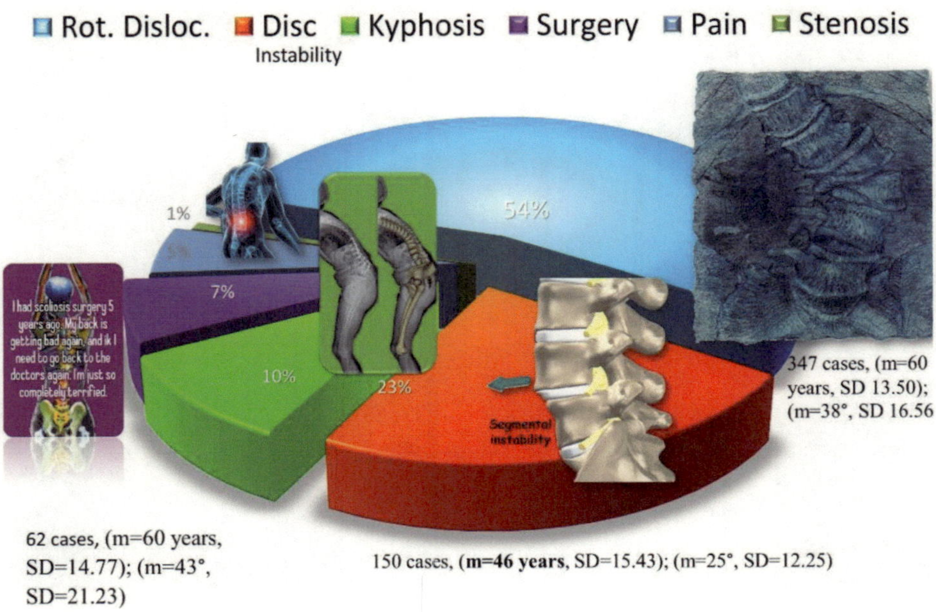

Figure 3.
Indications of nonsurgical treatment by etiology (n = 739).

disease [23]. MRI cross sections highlight the fatty degeneration. Some authors have mentioned paravertebral myopathy [24].

According to age, there is no Cobb angle difference between patients aged 39 and 80 years old, even if we notice a slight worsening between patients aged 80 and 90 years old. It can be concluded that after 40 years, for the same angulation, the risk of decompensation does not depend on age [22].

If we examine in more detail the distribution of patients according to Cobb angle, we find that Cobb angle is not a discriminating factor like aging.

1.8 Eligibility test

One of the bracing eligibility tests especially for camptocormia is self-correction by using the hands on the thighs, even if this self-correction does not last long in time. The second test of reducibility is carried out in supine position. The occipital patient must rely on the plane of the examination table. The placement of the ARTbrace is performed by the patient who stabilizes the brace at the pelvic level then unrolls the spine using the rigidity of the posterior bar and finally blocks the upper part. As for children, the "mayonnaise tube" effect of the two lateral hemi-valves completes the correction in the sagittal plane.

2. Methodology and results

2.1 Evolution of management

Adult scoliosis bracing is performed only in technically equipped medical clinics. Hospitalization is not essential because the use of the brace must be integrated into the patient's environment. On the other hand, physiotherapy scoliosis-specific exercises (PSSE) is mandatory.

The brace wearing time protocol is a total time of 24 hours a day during 3 weeks with a plaster cast (or digital cast) to adjust the length of the ligaments with plastic

Management	Wearing time	Particularity	Follow-up examination
First 3 weeks	Total time 24/24	Only 10′ for shower, no work interruption	At the end of total time without X-ray
First 6 months	4 hours/24	Systematically for 2 hours after physical activity	At 6 months with X-ray
6 m to 2 years	On demand and 2 hours after sport	In case of pain, in prevention before major efforts	At 2 years with X-ray
After 2 years	No specific indication	Brace is kept for safety	AT 5 years with X-ray, then every 5 years

Table 2.
Adult bracing management (Lyon ARTbrace).

deformation and, then, at least 4 hours per day for a minimum of 6 months, including systematically for 2 hours after the practice of sports activity (**Table 2**).

Wearing the brace for a "total time" allows the patient to relearn all the gestures of daily living in a good posture, for example, the sitting writing posture with feet behind the chair and buttocks in front of the seat. The lower part of the chest touches the anterior edge of the table, and the forearms rest on the desktop.

The digital cast is made in three blocks according to the deviations as in the teenager, but in deep inspiration. In many cases, only a scan in maximum corrective posture perfectly balanced is performed. The corrective posture is derived from Schroth. The sagittal plane and the frontal plane are simultaneously corrected, ensuring the overall balance of the spine. The spine is placed in maximum extension to promote lumbar lordosis and reduce thoracic hyperkyphosis. The convex hand is placed on the vertical support, the concave hand is placed on the head, and the operator supports the patient's elbow (**Figure 4**).

The thickness of Europlex'O used in adults is 3 mm. The digital cast is made in blocks according to the deviations as in the teenager, but in deep inspiration. The advantages are manifold: (1) The patient can maintain the maximum corrected position for a few seconds while standing; (2) breathing is controlled, and the patient can be asked to perform maximum inspiration; and (3) the accuracy of the eight structure sensors is less than 1 mm. The 3 mm Europlex'O with very high rigidity can be used instead of polyethylene. It is possible to work bare skin, but the thin optical vest in jersey allows the use of landmarks for the superposition of the

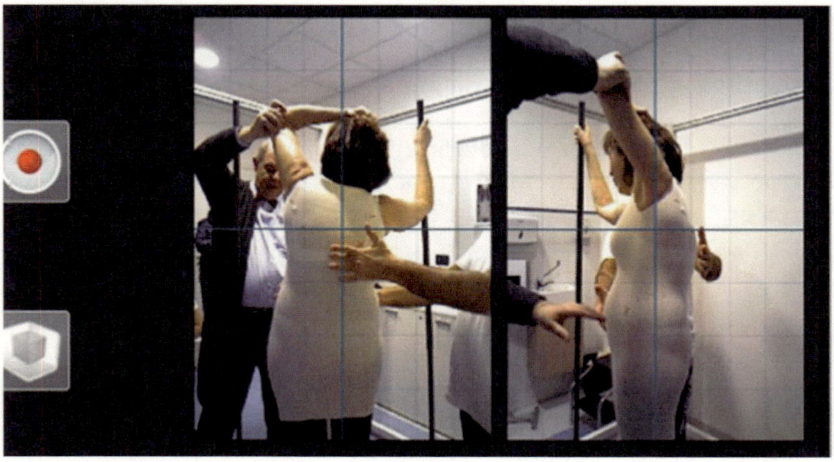

Figure 4.
Digital cast with simultaneous correction in the frontal and in the sagittal planes.

three blocks. The processing with a specific software allows the creation of a positive which will be milled by a digital milling machine. The CPO has all the tools to rework on the captured shapes. After a period of 3 weeks of "total time," the brace is worn for a minimum of 4 hours/24 for 6 months, then on demand.

2.2 Aims of rigid bracing

2.2.1 Instability pain management

Instability pain management is obtained by:

- A skin contact of the brace like a massage.
- A discharge of the lumbar discs and vertebral body by the "composite beam effect." The discharge of 30% is provided by the waist grip in the frontal plane, while the sagittal plane is free to prevent an excessive abdominal pressure.
- A rebalancing spine in the frontal and sagittal plane.
- A limitation of extreme postures.

2.2.2 Muscle strengthening

The rigid brace is an active brace. The patient spontaneously tends to contract the paravertebral musculature in the sense of self-active axial elongation. Associated physiotherapy is however essential.

2.2.3 Esthetics

The brace can reshape the waist. It can also symmetrize the body for the largest scoliotic curves by the adjunction of a foam cushion in the concavity.

2.2.4 Saving spine: development of compensations

The lock automatically performed by the brace facilitates motion and strengthens the musculature of the lower limbs. There is also a better mobility of shoulder girdle because of the stabilization of shoulder blades in a more physiological position.

2.3 Lyon method of physiotherapy for adult scoliosis

The wearing of a rigid brace is obligatorily supplemented by physiotherapy scoliosis-specific exercises. The ideal is to act when the spine begins to disrupt or becomes painful, indicating instability. The therapeutic progression is usual:

2.3.1 Aims

- Analgesia.
- Preventing muscle atrophy lumbo-abdominal strengthening in isometric and improving paravertebral deep muscles (**Figure 5**).
- Promoting more flexible self-active axial elongation (**Figure 6**).

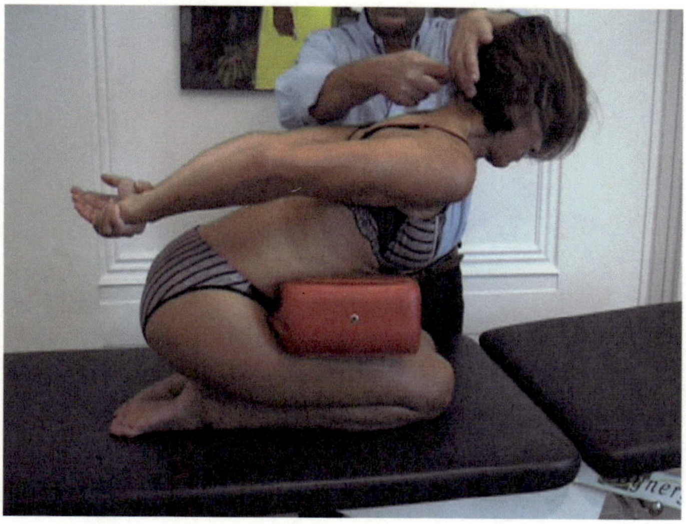

Figure 5.
Isometric strengthening of the deep front line with correction of thoracolumbar kyphosis.

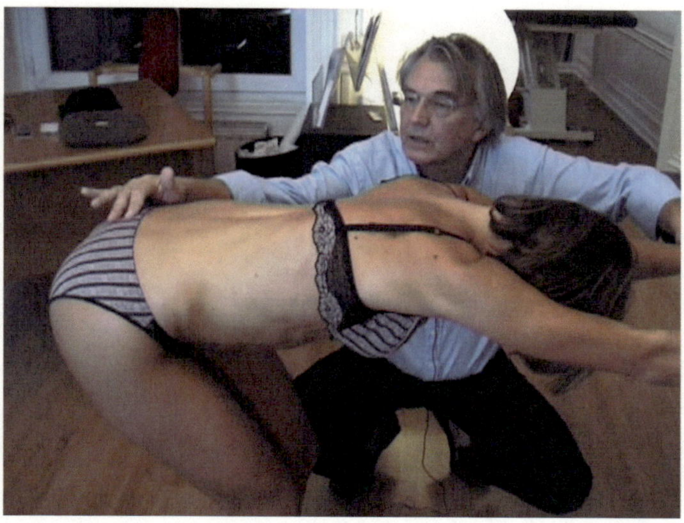

Figure 6.
Self-active axial elongation in closed kinetic chain (hands/espalier).

- Correcting 3D spine balance: in the frontal plane, rebalance of the occipital axis; in the sagittal plane, restoration of sagittal lumbar and pelvic curvatures (pelvic anteversion and lumbar lordosis (strengthening of the iliopsoas)); and in the horizontal plane, dissociation of pelvic and shoulder girdles.

- Developing compensation at the lower and upper limbs: relaxation under pelvic extension (hamstring stretching) (**Figure 7**).

- Stimulating the mechanisms of postural correction with reharmonization of the paravertebral tensions (muscular chains) (**Figure 8**).

The main differences between adolescent and adult scoliosis are demonstrated in **Table 3**.

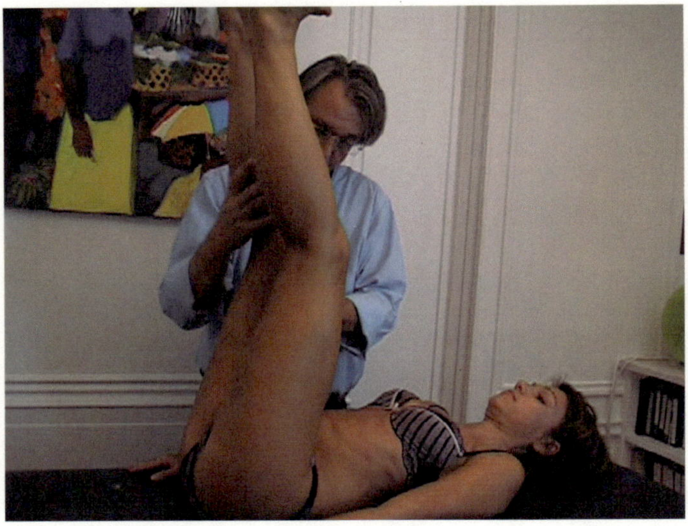

Figure 7.
Posture of stretching posterior chains of the lower limbs.

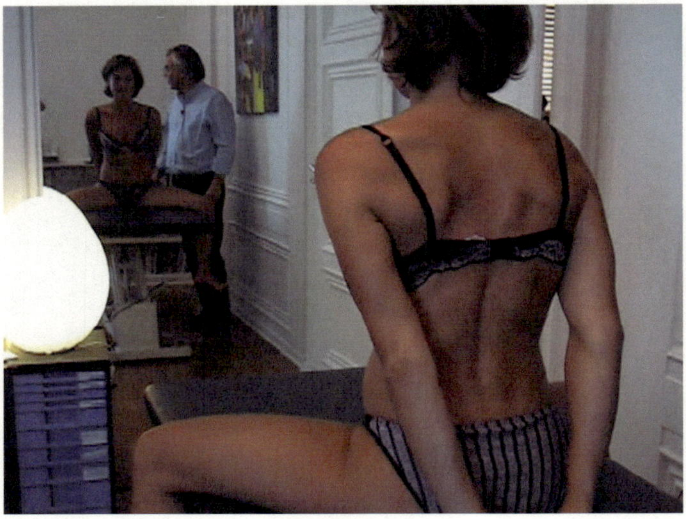

Figure 8.
Reharmonization of paravertebral tensions with mirror control.

2.3.2 Lyon method during the total time

First week. Physiotherapy is for analgesic purposes and is performed in the supine position by soft traction and a muscular work with irradiation of the short external rotators. Breathing is controlled because of the limitation of the abdominal expansion. The thoracic breathing is facilitated by the mobilization of the intercostal muscles.

Second week. The iliolumbar angle is mobilized to adjust tension at the iliolumbar level. The hump can be modeled with progressive closure of the ratcheting buckle. Physiotherapy is performed in sitting position.

Third week. Physiotherapy is more global, more general, more tonic, and stronger. The lever arm of shoulder and pelvic girdles is used. The sessions are made in standing position.

Physiology and biomechanics	Adolescent	Adult
No specific pain in adolescents. Painful instability in adults	No pain relief techniques	Pain relief techniques, massage, and others
Flat back in the teenager. Loss of lordosis and hyperkyphosis in adults	Restoration of physiological sagittal curves (arms projected forward)	Physiotherapy in lumbar lordosis (hands crossed in the back)
The brace aims to stiffen the spine (rust the spring). Spine mobilization in adults can lead to curve progression	Spine mobilization during cast and brace in all the amplitudes	No spine mobilization beyond the corrected posture
Strengthening muscle fibers (adult sarcopenia)	Reinforcement of the reticulospinal system (aerobic)	Reinforcement of voluntary musculature in anaerobic metabolism.
Translation along the vertical axis	Active axial self-elongation in standing position (grand porter) Open kinetic chain	Active axial self-elongation trunk bent at 90°, hands resting on the espalier. Closed kinetic chain
Lumbo-pelvic region	Opening the iliolumbar angle	Anterior lumbo-pelvic strengthening (iliopsoas, abdo, quad)
Lower limbs	No specific stretching. Global training without excessive resistance	Stretching of the posterior chain at the level of the lower limbs
One-third of the thorax volume develops after the end of the stature growth	Resistance breathing exercises (inflating a balloon)	Breathing exercises in forced expiration

Table 3.
Main differences between adolescent and adult scoliosis Lyon method physiotherapy.

2.3.3 Physiotherapy during partial time bracing

We first determine the sagittal direction of muscular work, usually lordosis for lumbar and thoracolumbar scoliosis. For each session there is a progression from supine to sitting and standing position.

2.3.3.1 Examples of basic exercises

Rib hump erasing. Having refocused the spine from the vertical in the sagittal plane and in the frontal plane, the patient is asked to lengthen from the brace at the rib hump level. The movement is controlled manually. The trapezius muscle is relaxed.

Sagittal tensioning girdles. The aim is to relax the posterior chain muscles while avoiding cervical lordosis. The exercise is made with control of inspiration breathing.

Self-axial lengthening. The patient straightens his head, his hands resting on the anterosuperior part of the brace. It can be done in a sitting position using a proprioceptive system. When the head is at the correct high position, a sound and a light stimulate the patient. If the spine is close to a wall, a cushion at the cervical level must be stabilized by the patient. This exercise can be completed with the upper limb extension.

Posture memorization. Exercise can be more complete with the work of the lower limbs. The starting position is knees bent for self-axial elongation of the spine; the upper limbs are fixed on the espalier. The patient is asked to stand up to a position of global extension. This exercise improves the quadricep muscle that will be key to saving the spine.

Strengthening of weak muscles: quadriceps and abdominals. The exercise will be started in a supine position. The pelvis is locked in the brace posture. This work is associated with an isometric tension of the posterior chain and expiration. This exercise is completed by a stabilization of the shoulder girdle with a stick and control of the rotation of the hip by a ball between the knees. The solicitation is obtained by an oblique manual push on the side of the patient. By gradually lowering the legs, it also seeks the rectus femoris. The anterior chain has been stretched, and it is in this posture of extension that strengthening is performed with isometric contract-relax muscular work.

Stretching strong muscles: hamstrings and short external rotators. It starts at the lumbosacral junction with pelvic-femoral, tricep, and hamstring stretch in lumbar lock controlled by the brace. It also stretches the psoas and rectus femoris. We can stimulate muscular work by manual push on the pelvis. The buttocks and the latissimus dorsi are solicited in the prone position, emphasizing the control of the cervical lordosis. When sitting, it stretches the anterior chain by adjusting the hip. Stretching can also be controlled at home on a stair. The exercise at the bar also allows global stretching.

Proprioceptive rehabilitation. On a Klein Vogelbach ball, it transfers the body weight in all plans, with emphasis on relaxation of tone and breathing control. The muscle tonicity is improved by changes in posture, standing, and lying and by the addition of loads. The global proprioceptive work prepares the patient for the definitive weaning of the brace.

2.3.4 Advice

In case of major disc degeneration, physiotherapy will be conducted in physiological lordosis, rather than in a standing position.

In case of major facet joint degeneration, physiotherapy will be conducted in physiological lordosis in prone position, legs bent or in a sitting position.

In case of leg length discrepancy, the feet imbalances adjustment with a shoe lift of 5 mm if it improves both pelvic and spine alignment.

In the sagittal plane, one can use small high heel stubs from 3 to 5 cm to reduce a lumbar kyphosis.

The food control helps to reduce overweight.

The postural control concerns mainly the workstation.

The regular practice of physical activity outside is essential. It is necessary to insist on the strict brace wearing during 2 hours after the sports activity.

2.3.5 Difficulties

Excessive mobilization of passive structures may lead to a progression of scoliosis, so the hyper flexibility is avoided and a position closest to that of the brace is better.

High thoracic breathing is less efficient than the usual abdominal breathing, and we must insist on improving the vital capacity for thoracic or double major curves. If lumbar scoliosis is treated, the risk of an increase of scoliosis during inspiration is low; however, breathlessness is to be avoided.

As the brace can be asymmetrical in the direction of the rebalancing of the spine, it will, however, always ensure the balance of the shoulder girdle.

2.3.6 Practice of sport

When the body is fully developed, we advise high-impact sports such as running and dance, to favor the fixation of the calcium on the bone and the constitution of an important bony mass.

In a specific way when ribs are asymmetric, we recommend avoiding deep and quick inhalation which favors the vertebral rotation and therefore the breathlessness during the practice of sports.

For lumbar curves, we advise, as well, against the quick flexions of the trunk forward or the position extending with an anterior flexion of the trunk.

During the period of maximal tensegrity up to 40 years, all sports can be performed at a high level as long as the spine is straight.

After 40 years, decreased intervertebral disc height and sarcopenia reduce the body's performance.

After 65 years, osteoarthritis is predominant. Swimming avoids overloading the lower limbs and helps maintain lumbar lordosis (**Table 4**).

2.4 Results

2.4.1 Bivalve polyethylene short brace with lateral overlap for lumbar scoliosis

Immobilization braces made of polyethylene have been used for more than 50 years in case of mechanical pain. They complement classical physiotherapy by reducing load by 30% at the lumbar spine. We specifically studied the 158 patients with 5-year follow-up from our prospective database [25].

The principle of bracing is completely different from that of adolescent scoliosis. Indeed, we try to:

1. Decompress the discs with the "sandglass effect" lifting the trunk under the ribs and transferring the load on the pelvis.

2. Rebalance the spine in both the frontal plane and in the sagittal planes, mostly by recreating lumbar lordosis.

3. Relieve pain by the analgesic effect of rigid low back brace.

A specific frame is used to stabilize the patient in the most corrective posture in the frontal and the sagittal plane.

For those patients who had a progressive scoliosis, Cobb angle is stabilized or improved by more than 5° in 80% of cases, and only 20% of scoliosis remain candidates for surgery [25].

The frontal and horizontal clinical parameters are improved, but not the sagittal parameters with the forward trunk projection (**Figure 9**).

The sternoclavicular support is poorly tolerated, and due to reduced dexterity in the older person, lateral closure is a handicap for elderly patients, even if adaptations are possible, that is why we currently use the 3 mm Europlex'O.

Age (girls)	Physiology	Activity (example)
15–21 years	Before complete bone mass	Jogging and running Axial impact and spiral chains
21–40 years	Before sarcopenia and osteopenia (tensegrity)	Fitness, sports reinforcing spiral chains
40 to retirement	Before extrapyramidal weakness (postural system)	Nordic walking, cycling
Retirement	Osteoarthritis, Pisa syndrome	Swimming

Table 4.
Sports activity according to the age.

2.4.2 Nonsurgical orthopedic treatment of 62 adult vertebral deviations treated with adult ARTbrace

Instability in adulthood is frequent, and surgery is the most frequently offered solution despite the high rate of complications, as there was no alternative to date for thoracic and thoracolumbar curves. Only overlapped bivalve polyethylene braces were used for lumbar scoliosis with good frontal stabilization but no control in the sagittal plane (**Figure 9**). The ARTbrace in Europlex'O which allows an average reduction of 70% for the children has been used since 2015 in the adult for all the deviations.

The results of a consecutive series of 62 patients (6.2% of all ARTbrace patients) were treated between 2015 and 2016, as an alternative to surgery.

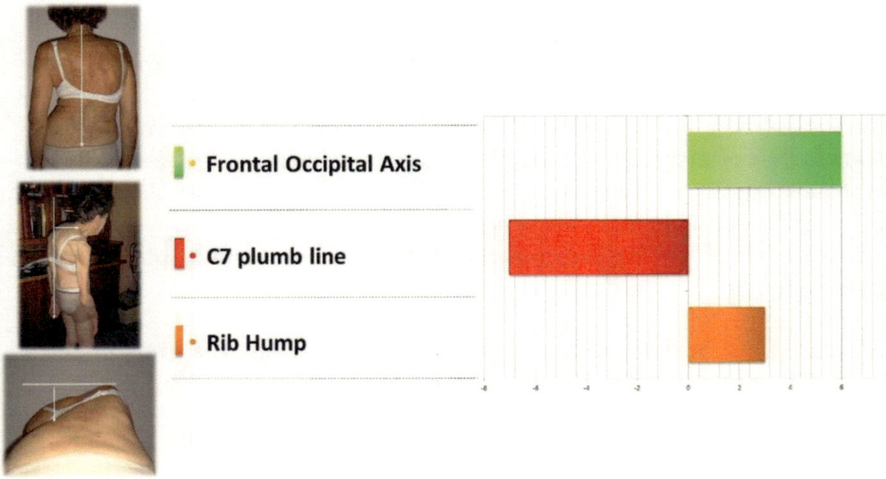

Figure 9.
Insufficient correction in the sagittal plane.

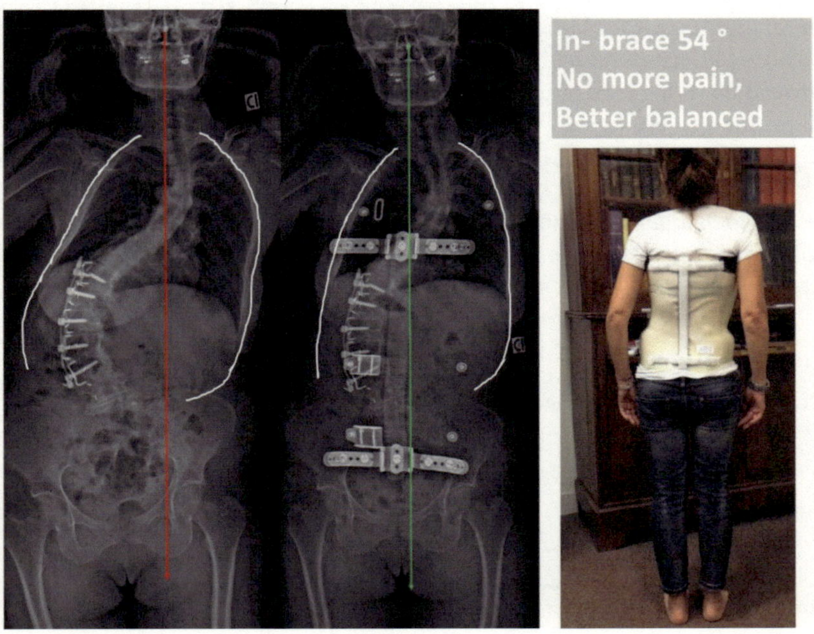

Figure 10.
Reduction in the frontal plane after decompensation upon arthrodesis.

Nine patients (15%) which constitute the dropout were not seen at 6 months, which is very little considering the general condition and age of patients. The percentage of dropouts is identical to the previous series of lumbar curves treatments.

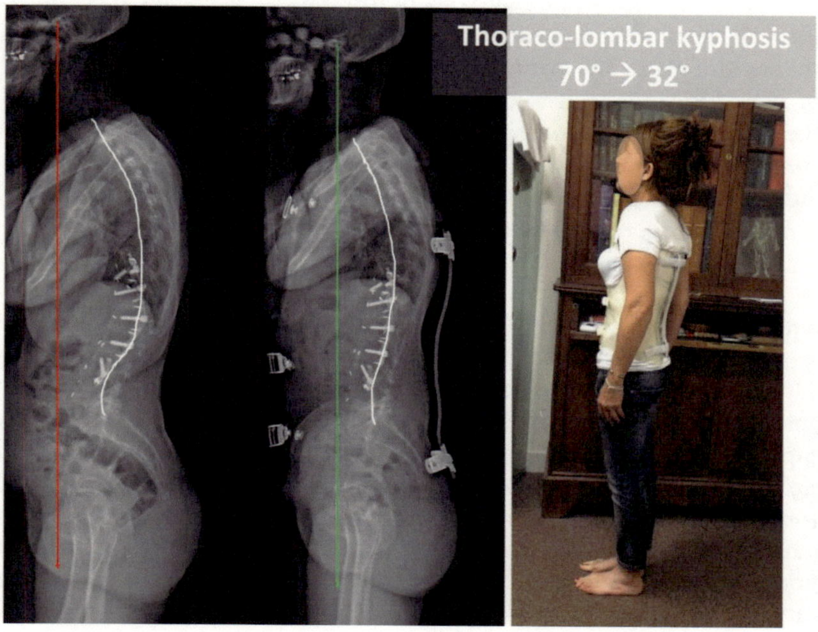

Figure 11.
Correction of kyphosis in the sagittal plane.

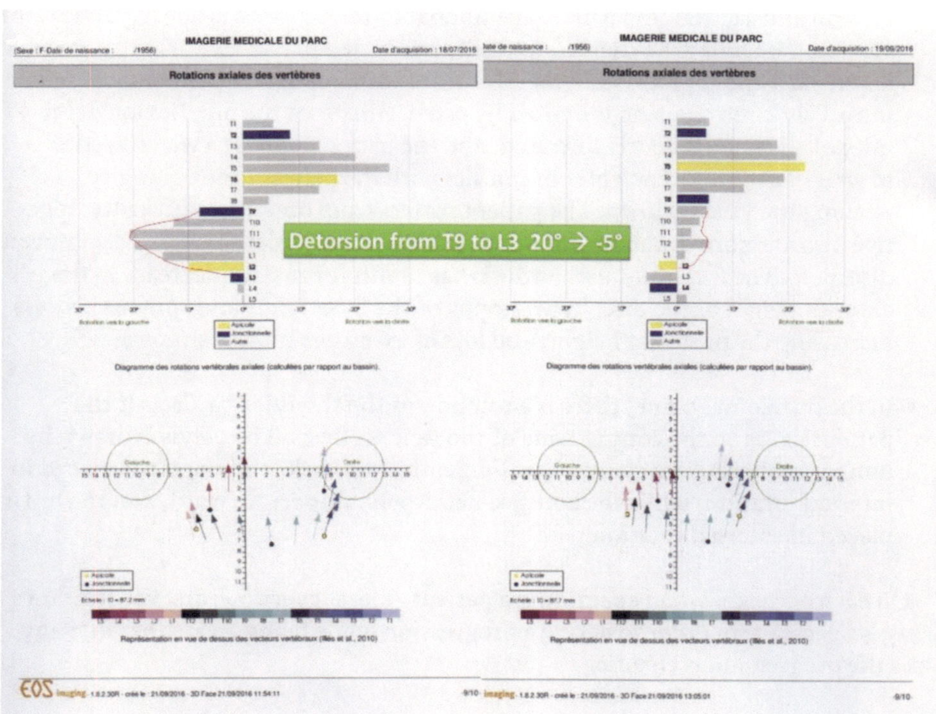

Figure 12.
EOS 3D confirms thoracolumbar spine detorsion in ARTbrace.

Despite the very high rigidity, Europlex'O which needs a precision of 1 mm is therefore as well tolerated as polyethylene.

In the frontal plane, the average in-brace reduction is 27%, slightly higher for lumbar and thoracolumbar curvatures. The reduction to 2 years without brace is 15%, and especially the symptomatology of instability disappears. It is now possible to stabilize all thoracolumbar, thoracic, and double major scoliosis (**Figure 10**).

In the sagittal plane, the average in-brace reduction is 32% and at 2 years without brace of 25% (**Figure 11**).

In the horizontal plane, some characteristic case study with EOS 3D confirms that adult ARTbrace is indeed, as in the child, a detorsion brace. Adult ARTbrace is the only brace to correct kyphosis and thus compensate for the insufficiency of polyethylene whose sternoclavicular support was not tolerated (**Figure 12**).

3. Discussion

Adult deformity is a major demographic health issue in the geriatric population. Surgeons are often very conservative in the treatment of adult scoliosis because of the complication rates associated with the surgeries and the marginal bone quality endemic to this population. Medical complications are a major concern in adult spinal deformity surgery [26]. The incidence ranges between 40% and 86%, but there is indeterminate level III/IV evidence on the effectiveness of any usual conservative care option. There is currently a lack of consensus on the most efficacious conservative treatments for adult deformity.

Very few results have been published concerning scoliosis adult bracing. Most of them only concern low back pain [27, 28]. Pain is the usual reason of medical consultation. Pain means instability when combined with the following clinical signs:

- Frontal and sagittal Imbalance. The lumbar kyphoscoliosis is due to pelvic retroversion. The hips are extended under a retroverted pelvis, femurs were oriented downward and forward, and knees and ankles compensate with flexion deformity. Pelvic retroversion is limited by osteoarthritis of the hip, flexion deformity of the knee is poorly tolerated, and the patient will use a walking stick to walk. The thorax can enter in conflict with the pelvis at the concavity level pushing the viscera down. The patient suffers from breathing difficulty; digestive disorders are common and promote abdominal hypertension and sphincter disorders. The loss of lumbar lordosis has multiple causes: a decrease in the anterior height of the disc, hypertrophy of the facet joints and spinous process increasing the posterior height, and loss of extensors muscle strength [29].

- In the horizontal plane, there is a rotation of the shoulder girdle as if the patient looks on the concave side of thoracic scoliosis. The pelvis is drawn by lumbar scoliosis. The convex hemi-pelvis moves back, and the hip is placed in internal rotation, while the concave hemi-pelvis moves forward, and the hip is placed in external rotation.

On each occasion when examining a patient at least every 5 years, verification X-ray is necessary in order to define a progression while being aware that in many cases the progression is chaotic.

- The most characteristic sign of decompensating is the disc height loss that can sometimes exceed 10 mm. The disc corruption results in loss of physiological lordosis and ligament instability by hypermobility.

- The losses of the gluteal muscles are very distinct when we make the plaster cast. It explains in part the pelvic retroversion; the spine tends to relocate along the line of gravity.

Muscular atrophy is a common criticism for rigid braces. In fact, the conservative orthopedic treatment does not suffer approximation. Its teamwork incorporates a specific physical therapy, the continuation of normal activity, and the practice of regular physical activity. No patient is wearing the brace for pleasure. The risk of overtreatment is zero.

Usually the total time bracing relieves pain, and the partial time bracing extends the improvement obtained. When the patient is not relieved, we can discuss the surgery with better arguments. The nonsurgical treatment treats the cause of lumbar instability mainly by discharging the pressure in the disc and stabilizing the lumbar area in lordosis to restore the tensegrity of the spine.

The esthetic improvement of the rib hump and asymmetrical waist is logical; the orthopedic brace is the best way to remodel a trunk. The cosmetic result continues 5 years after starting the treatment, with improvement of the rib hump measured with the plumb line and the Bunnel angle of trunk rotation (**Figure 9**).

The nonsurgical treatment can fit into a therapeutic progression. The indications may be progressive: observation, physiotherapy, medicine, conservative orthopedic Treatment, and surgery.

The good surgical indications concern the degenerative scoliosis not relieved by bracing, or relieved by total time, but insufficiently by partial time and especially if there is a spinal stenosis. It can also be used to complete surgery if remaining instability.

The Greek study [30] associating Schroth and Chêneau brace shows that patients have great difficulty to follow the protocol. For the quarter of patients following the protocol, the results are correct on pain and posture, but in 39% of patients, Cobb angle continues to increase.

Josette Bettany [31] confirms that for adult scoliosis, there are only a few studies on the effectiveness of PSSEs and a conclusion cannot yet be drawn. Recently a RCT proves the effectiveness of a motor and cognitive rehabilitation [32].

3.1 Differences between adult and non-adult bracing

The motivation of the patient is fundamental. The brace should be designed as a tool to facilitate physiotherapy.

The use of an instantaneous and accurate CAD/CAM is better because the adult patient can only maintain the corrected position for a few seconds.

The scan is made in deep inspiration to not limit the vital capacity.

The management is 4 hours a day including systematically for 2 hours after any physical activity. Physiotherapy is even more important than during adolescence [33].

4. Conclusion

The frequency of adult scoliosis makes it a public health problem. The new digital technologies have changed the adult scoliosis bracing, and conservative care in general may be a helpful option for adult deformity, but evidence for this decision was lacking. Lyon nonsurgical treatment is effective and offers new perspectives to adult scoliosis bracing. Not only does the brace relieve pain and support the spine, but for the first time, it corrects deviations in the frontal, sagittal, and horizontal planes. Immobilization braces in polyethylene allow a treatment of the cause of pain without side effects. Worn a few hours in the day, they complement physiotherapy. The first results confirm the excellent tolerance of Europlex'O adult ARTbrace with its ease of implementation and corrections unmatched to date in adults. These corrections make it possible to restore stability of the deviations without surgery. Adult scoliosis bracing as an alternative to surgery could be possible. Initially reserved for the most severe cases, this management deserves to be more widely used for adult scoliosis. The increasing number of CPO using the most modern CAD/CAM technologies should facilitate research in the field of very high rigidity.

Acknowledgements

Thanks to my daughter Agnès Thornton de Mauroy, for proofreading in English.

Acronyms and abbreviations

ARTbrace	asymmetrical rigid torsion brace
ASA	adolescent scoliosis in adult
CAD/CAM	computer-aided design/computer-aided manufacturing
CPO	certified prosthetist/orthotist
CT scan	computed tomography scan
DDS	degenerative de novo scoliosis
EOS	low-dose X-ray imaging
MRI	magnetic resonance imaging
PSSE	physiotherapy scoliosis-specific exercises
RCT	randomized controlled trial

Author details

Jean Claude de Mauroy[1*], Fabio Gagliano[1], Rosario Gagliano[2] and Piera Lusenti[3]

1 Clinique du Parc, Lyon, France

2 ROGA, Enna, Italy

3 Poliambulatorio Baia del Re, Piacenza, Italy

*Address all correspondence to: demauroy@aol.com

References

[1] Vanderpool DW, James JI, Wynne-Davies R. Scoliosis in the elderly. Journal of Bone and Joint Surgery. 1969;**51**:446-455

[2] Schroeder JE, Dettori JR, Ecker E, Kaplan L. Does pregnancy increase curve progression in women with scoliosis treated without surgery? Evidence-Based Spine-Care Journal. 2011;**2**(3):43-50

[3] Akbarnia BA, Ogilvie JW, Hammerberg KW. Debate: Degenerative scoliosis: To operate or not to operate. Spine. 2006;**31**:S195-S201

[4] Edgar MA, Mehta MH. Long term follow-up of fused and unfused idiopathic scoliosis. Journal of Bone and Joint Surgery. 1988;**70-B**:712-716

[5] O'Brien J. Living with scoliosis: An adult perspective. Scoliosis. 2010;**5**:O43

[6] Baron EM, Albert TJ. Medical complications of surgical treatment of adult spinal deformity and how to avoid them. Spine. 2006;**31**:S106-S118

[7] Smith JS, Shaffrey CI, Glassman SD, Berven SH, Schwab FJ, Hamill CL, et al. Risk-benefit assessment of surgery for adult scoliosis. An analysis based on patient age. Spine. 2010;**36**:817-824

[8] Ogilvie JW. Adult scoliosis: Evaluation and nonsurgical treatment. Instructional Course Lectures. 1992;**41**:251-255

[9] Kluba T, Dikmenli G, Dietz K, Giehl JP, Niemeyer T. Comparison of surgical and conservative treatment for degenerative lumbar scoliosis. Archives of Orthopaedic and Trauma Surgery. 2009;**129**(1):1-5

[10] Everett CR, Patel RK. A systematic literature review of nonsurgical treatment in adult scoliosis. Spine. 2007;**32**:S130-S134

[11] Chuah SL, Kareem BA, Selvakumar K, Borhan TA, Harwant S. The natural history of scoliosis: Curve progression of untreated curves of different etiology, with early (mean 2 year) follow-up in surgically treated curves. The Medical Journal of Malaysia. 2001;**56**(suppl C):37-40

[12] Weinstein SL, Zavala DC, Ponsetti I. Idiopathic scoliosis; long-term follow-up and prognosis in untreated patients. Journal of Bone and Joint Surgery. 1983;**63A**:702-712

[13] Weinstein SL, Dolan LA, Spratt KF, Peterson KK, Spoonamore MJ, Ponseti IV. Health and function of patients with untreated idiopathic scoliosis: A 50-year natural history study. Journal of the American Medical Association. 2003;**289**(5):559-567

[14] Marty-Poumarat C, Scattin L, Marpeau M, Garreau de Loubresse C, Aegerter P. Natural history of progressive adult scoliosis. Spine (Phila Pa 1976). 2007;**32**(11):1227-1234. discussion 1235

[15] Duval-Beaupere G, Dubousset J. La dislocation rotatoire progressive du rachis. Processus mécanique commun aux cypho-scolioses évolutives génératrices de troubles neurologiques. A propos de 16 observations. Revue de Chirurgie Orthopédique. 1972;**58**:323-334

[16] Hong JY, Suh SW, Modi HN, Hur CY, Yang JH, Song HR. Correlation of pelvic orientation with adult scoliosis. Journal of Spinal Disorders & Techniques. Oct 2010;**23**(7):461-466

[17] Murata Y, Takahashi K, Hanaoka E, Utsumi T, Yamagata M, Moriya H. Changes in scoliotic curvature and lordotic angle during the early phase of degenerative lumbar scoliosis. Spine. 2002;**27**(20):2268-2273

[18] Ploumis A, Liu H, Mehbod AA, Transfeldt EE, Winter RB. A correlation of radiographic and functional measurements in adult degenerative scoliosis. Spine. 2009;**34**(15):1581-1584

[19] Schwab FJ, Smith VA, Biserni M, Gamez L, Farcy JP, Pagala M. Adult scoliosis: A quantitative radiographic and clinical analysis. Spine (Phila Pa 1976). 2002;**27**(4):387-392

[20] Naresh-Babu J, Viswanadha AK, Ito M, Park JB. What should an ideal adult spinal deformity classification system consist of?: Review of the factors affecting outcomes of adult spinal deformity management. Asian Spine Journal. 2019;**13**(4):694-703

[21] Diarbakerli E, Grauers A, Danielsson A, Gerdhem P. Adults with idiopathic scoliosis diagnosed at youth experience similar physical activity and fracture rate as controls. Spine (Phila Pa 1976). 1 Apr 2017;**42**(7):E404-E410

[22] de Mauroy JC, Lecante C, Barral F, Pourret S. Bracing in adult with scoliosis: Experience in diagnosis and classification from a 15-year prospective study of 739 patients. Scoliosis and Spinal Disorders. 2016;**11**(Suppl 2):29

[23] Schulz-Schaeffer WJ. Camptocormia in Parkinson's disease: A muscle disease due to dysregulated proprioceptive polysynaptic reflex arch. Frontiers in Aging Neuroscience. 2016;**8**:128

[24] Lenoir T, Guedj N, Boulu P, Guigui P, Benoist M. Camptocormia: The bent spine syndrome, an update. European Spine Journal. 2010;**19**(8):1229-1237. DOI: 10.1007/s00586-010-1370-5

[25] de Mauroy JC, Lecante C, Barral F, Pourret S. Prospective study of 158 adult scoliosis treated by a bivalve polyethylene overlapping brace and reviewed at least 5 years after brace fitting. Scoliosis and Spinal Disorders. 2016;**11**(Suppl 2):28

[26] Smith JS, Shaffrey CI, Glassman SD, Berven SH, Schwab FJ, Hamill CL, et al. Spinal deformity study group. Risk-benefit assessment of surgery for adult scoliosis: An analysis based on patient age. Spine (Phila Pa 1976). 2011;**36**(10):817-824

[27] Weiss HR, Dallmayer R, Stephan C. First results of pain treatment in scoliosis patients using a sagittal realignment brace. Studies in Health Technology and Informatics. 2006;**123**:582-585

[28] Gallo D. Case reports: Orthotic treatment of adult scoliosis patients with chronic back pain. Scoliosis. 2014;**9**:18. DOI: 10.1186/1748-7161-9-18

[29] York PJ, Kim HJ. Degenerative Scoliosis. Current Reviews in Musculoskeletal Medicine. 2017;**10**(4):547-558

[30] Papadopoulos D. Adult scoliosis treatment combining brace and exercises. Scoliosis. 2013;**8**(Suppl 2):O8. DOI: 10.1186/1748-7161-8-S2-O8

[31] Bettany-Saltikov J, Turnbull D, Ng SY, Webb R. Management of spinal deformities and evidence of treatment effectiveness. The Open Orthopaedics Journal. 2017;**11**(Suppl-9, M6):1521-1547

[32] Monticone M, Ambrosini E, Cazzaniga D, Rocca B, Motta L, Cerri C, et al. Adults with idiopathic scoliosis improve disability after motor and cognitive rehabilitation: Results of a randomised controlled trial. European Spine Journal. Oct 2016;**25**(10):3120-3129. Epub 2016 Mar 25

[33] de Mauroy JC, Vallèse P, Lalain JJ. Lyon conservative treatment of adult scoliosis. Minerva Ortopedica e Traumatologica. 2011;**62**(5):385-396

Chapter 2

Posture and Back Shape Measurement Tools: A Narrative Literature Review

Gok Kandasamy, Josette Bettany-Saltikov and Paul van Schaik

Abstract

The clinical assessment of spinal deformities often involves the assessment of posture and back shape together with the associated mobility of the spine, pelvis and rib cage. Currently, there is a wide range of posture and back shape assessment tools available for clinical use. The choice varies from conventional approach to advanced structured light methods. The advanced methods like ultrasound, 3D radiography and inertial sensors are not easily accessible to most clinicians, as they are either expensive, require specialist training or are complex and/or difficult to use. Thus, simple conventional methods like eyeballing, photography and the plumb line are still used within clinical practice today. The primary aim of this article is to give an overview of different tactile and non-tactile measurement systems that have been developed for the measurement of posture and whole-body analysis.

Keywords: posture, back shape, tactile, non-tactile, objective, whole body

1. Background

The term 'spinal deformity' indicates the abnormal alignment or shape of the vertebral column and rib cage. Schwab et al. identifies the most common spinal deformities found in the population are scoliosis, lumbar lordoscoliosis, pelvic obliquity and either increased or decreased lumbar lordosis, with a high prevalence rate of 68% [1]. These spinal deformities are often linked to a range of different types of pain, physical dysfunction and psychosocial wellbeing [2–5]. The clinical assessment of these spinal deformities often involves the assessment of posture and back shape together with the associated mobility of the spine, pelvis and rib-cage. Currently, there are a wide range of posture and back shape assessment tools available for clinical use. The choice varies from conventional approaches to advanced structured light methods. The advanced methods like ultrasound [6], 3D radiography [7] and inertial sensors [8] are not easily accessible for most clinicians, as they were either expensive, require specialist training or are complex or difficult to use. Thus, simple conventional methods like "eyeballing" photography [9] and the plumb line [10] are still used within clinical practice.

A comprehensive literature review was undertaken firstly to search and retrieve research papers related to the tools and scientific methods for assessing posture and back shape and secondly to critique which methods were best for assessing posture and back shape with regard to their cost, safety, reliability, validity, ease of use and duration. The primary research question for the current narrative review was 'what are the different types of tactile and non-tactile measurement systems, for the measurement of posture and whole-body analysis in adults with spinal disorders?'. And the secondary research question is related to the critical evaluation of assessment methods in terms of cost, safety, reliability and validity of the tools.

2. Methods

2.1 Search strategy

A comprehensive literature search was performed in the following databases, PubMed, EMBASE, Scopus, CINAHL, Medline and Science Direct, for articles on posture and back shape from 1980 to 2017. The search keywords were 'posture', 'back shape', 'spinal mobility', 'postural assessment', 'back surface measurement', 'postural alignment', 'posture' and 'reproducibility', 'posture' and 'reliability', 'posture' and 'accuracy', 'posture' and 'validity', 'posture' and 'spinal pain' and 'posture' and 'low back pain'. The author also combined each human body segment with 'posture' as keywords, 'head posture', 'neck posture', 'cervical posture', 'thoracic posture', 'trunk posture', 'lumbar posture', 'shoulder posture', 'arm posture', 'upper limb posture' and 'lower limb posture'. In addition, the author searched for related articles from references cited in the articles identified from the original search. The search was limited to articles only written in English. No wildcards were used in this study.

2.2 Criteria for inclusion and exclusion

All articles that assessed posture and back shape were considered in order to identify all possible methods for the evaluation of posture. Reviews of postural assessment and articles that discussed posture in some manner that could help the discussion were also included. Letters to the editor and conference proceedings were excluded.

3. Data collection and analysis

The titles, keywords and abstracts of all research articles identified during the search were read to confirm whether they satisfied the inclusion criteria. Full text copies of all articles that met the inclusion criteria were obtained for analysis and data extraction. Preference was given to recent reviews on posture and back shape assessment and research papers on new or unusual forms of postural evaluation. Older articles with the same information contained in newer ones were excluded.

4. Results and discussion

The author identified 66 articles representing 15 principal instruments that are currently used to assess posture and back shape (please refer to the PRISMA diagram in **Figure 1**). These included tactile, non-tactile, two-dimensional as well as three-dimensional (3D) methods. Tactile measurement methods are defined as methods used to measure posture or back shape through contact, for example, the flexiruler and goniometry, whereas non-tactile measurement methods measure

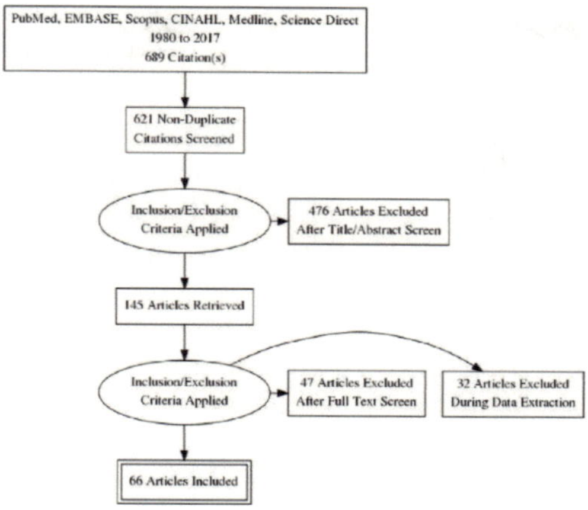

Figure 1.
PRISMA flow diagram of literature search and selection process.

posture and back shape without any direct contact to the skin by the operator. These included, for example, X-rays and photogrammetric methods. The literature primarily documented the reliability and validity of each postural measurement tool in normal individuals including a few patients with spinal deformities. Each method is described and critiqued below.

4.1 Two-dimensional analysis of posture and back shape

4.1.1 Tactile methods of measurement

4.1.1.1 Flexiruler

The flexiruler for the evaluation of posture is common for clinical and research purposes [11, 12]. This objective method of postural measurement requires the manual placement of the flexiruler onto the contours or curvatures of the spine followed by the tracing and calculation of these angles onto paper (see **Figure 2A** and **B**).

Greenfield et al. [13] used a flexiruler to measure the mid-thoracic curvature, while Rheault et al. [14] observed the inter-rater reliability of the flexiruler for measuring cervical lordosis in two different positions (neutral and fully flexed) in 20

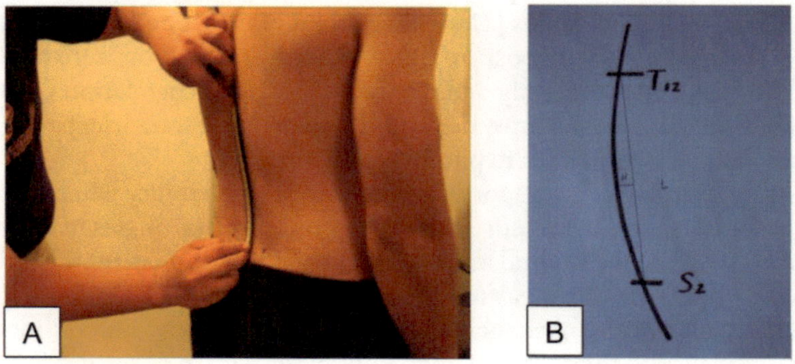

Figure 2.
An example of the flexiruler method (A) data collection and (B) measurement of lumbar lordosis based on the captured data [15].

healthy subjects [13, 14]. In both studies, the flexiruler was placed on the curvature of the spine, with its tip at the most proximal part of the curvature and the other end at the distal end of the spine.

Following the measurement of the spine, the flexiruler was placed on a paper, to trace its curve. Greenfield et al. [13] reported good to moderate Pearson correlation for intrarater (r = 0.90) and interrater reliability (r = 0.70). Furthermore Rheault et al. [14] reported no significant difference between raters (t = 1.24; p>0.05) at the two different positions of the cervical spine. The results of both Greenfield et al. and Rehault et al. studies suggest that the flexible ruler is a reliable measuring tool between raters for measuring sagittal plane curvature.

Concerning validity, many researchers have demonstrated a high correlation between radiographic and surface measurements for measuring the lumbar spine curvature [16, 17]. For example, Hart and Rose [18] compared the angles of the curve taken with a flexible ruler to the angle obtained by the standard roentgenographic technique and found good validity with the Pearson product moment correlation of +0.87. Burton further substantiated the result by reporting a correlation of +0.87 for the validity of the flexible ruler in comparison to the radiographic method for measuring lumbar lordosis [16]. Even though the above studies demonstrated good validity, the main limitation was that the results were based on a very low sample size (n = 8). In addition, the measurement of postural variables through a flexiruler is always two-dimensional. The presentation of spinal curvature is not necessary always two-dimensional. There is a possibility of the deviation of curvature being in more than one plane. In this scenario, the obtained spinal curvature angle might not represent the real degree.

It is important to note that most of the above studies reported their results based on the data collected from young normal healthy participants. Although the use of the flexible ruler is important for this population, there is a possibility that the flexible ruler may be more difficult to use for patients with pain, disease, or postural deformity. Other limitations of this method of postural assessment are the following. Firstly, it is difficult for patients to maintain one position during data collection. Secondly, the literature reports only one measurement plane (sagittal). It is difficult to measure both the frontal and the transverse plane posture variables. Third, this method of postural assessment has a high possibility of manual error during data collection and angle measurement [19].

4.1.1.2 Goniometry

In clinical practice, goniometers are commonly used to measure joint range of motion (ROM) [20]. Icn et al. reported the use of a goniometer for the assessment of a number of posture variables [21]. This method of direct body measurement used a goniometer to quantify posture variables with a value from zero to 360 degrees. The results of their study demonstrated moderate correlation (r = 0.47) to measure the tibiotarsal angle, knee flexion/extension angle, quadriceps angle as well as the sub-talar angle in relation to photogrammetry.

Conversely, Harrison et al. reported poor interrater reliability when using manual goniometry for the measurement of sagittal postural angles in the neck inclination angle (craniovertebral angle) and cranial rotation (sagittal head tilt) (see **Figure 3**) [22]. The ICC measures were found to be r = 0.68 and r = 0.34 for the cervical rotation angle and neck inclination angle, respectively. The authors attributed the poor results to the difficulty in maintaining the arm of the goniometer parallel with the horizontal axis.

Fortin et al. ([9], pp. 381-382) suggest that the main limitation for this type of individual measurement of postural variables is the lengthy evaluation process

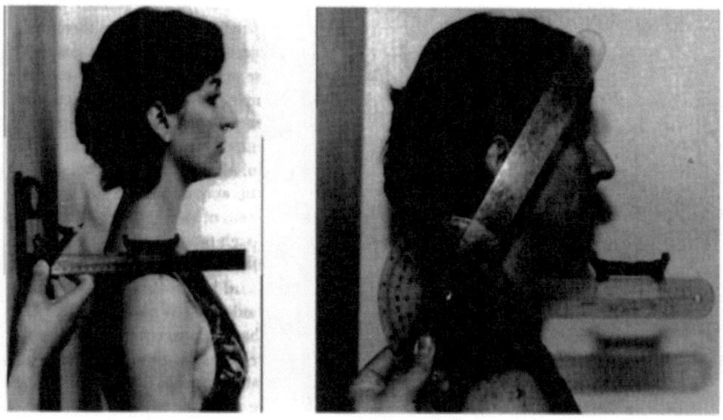

Figure 3.
Measurement of shoulder and neck inclination angle using goniometer (reproduced from Harrison et al. [22]).

involved for both the therapist and the patient. The author states that 'this approach may be appropriate for the assessment of one body segment or a variable, but not for the whole body or posture'.

4.1.2 Non-tactile methods of measurement

4.1.2.1 Plumb line method

The two-dimensional evaluation of posture, using a plumb line, is very common, due to its low-cost and simplicity [23]. Kendall et al. postulated guidelines to evaluate posture in accordance with the alignment of the ideal plumb line for the measurement of the sagittal and frontal planes [24]. Kendall et al. state that the ideal alignment of sagittal plane posture is when the plumb line intersects the ear lobe, through the shoulder joint; then through the greater trochanter of the hip, just in front of the knee joint; and finally slightly in front of the lateral malleolus of the ankle before it reaches the floor. Williams and McClay reported that the plumb line method had a good intra-rater reliability for measuring postural variables with an average ICC of 0.80 in both 10 and 90% of body weight bearing scenarios in standing [10]. The standard error of the mean (SEM) reported was between 2 and 5 mm for the lower limb indices and from 5 to 10 mm for patients with a trunk list or lateral shift. List is defined as 'the lateral displacement, in millimetres, of a surface marking of the spinous processes of T12 from that of S1' (McKenzie and May [25], p. 214). Furthermore, Hickey et al. evaluated the reliability of using the plumb line to measure resting head posture in a large sample size of 122 healthy volunteers (80 women and 42 men, ages 18–60 years) [26]. In this study, all participants were screened for cranial, cervical and/or upper thoracic dysfunction. The results of this study demonstrated the plumb line method to have high intra-rater reliability with ICCs ranging from 0.83 to 0.84 for the measurement of resting head posture. Although the plumb line method has been reported to have good intra-rater reliability and is a useful and easy to use instrument for measuring posture, its limitations include the difficulty of minimising movement error or postural sway [9, 27]. Additionally, this plumb line method only measures one plane.

4.1.2.2 Radiography

Schwab et al. considers the radiographic method of spinal screening to be the traditional and "gold standard" method for the assessment and screening of patients with spinal deformities [28]. Furthermore, Schwab et al. suggests that radiography is an essential tool for the accurate diagnoses of spinal abnormalities/deformities and accurately reveals the degree and severity of the problem [29].

In this method, an X-ray image is captured when a beam of X-ray light is passed through the spine and the amount of radiation emerging on the other side is recorded. Since the bones of the spine absorb the radiation and soft tissues allow it to pass through, a clear image of the spine is captured. McVey et al. suggests that the captured radiographic image provides essential information on spinal bone structure, which can be used to analyse individual vertebrae and the overall contour of the spine [30].

In addition to the assessment of spinal curvature, X-rays are also used to record and monitor the progression of spinal deformities and dysfunction [31, 32]. Therefore, in adolescent patients it is performed every few months in order to detect any changes in the progression of the spinal deformity.

The main drawback of the radiographic method of spinal assessment is associated with the increased radiation that has been found to increase the incidence of cancer in later years [33, 34]. Doody et al. in their retrospective cohort study estimated the carcinogenic risk and the patterns in breast cancer mortality among female patients with scoliosis [35]. This study included a large sample size (5,573 female patients with scoliosis, or abnormal curves). The results suggested that due to the high exposure to cumulative x-ray radiation of 10.8 cGy (from childhood to adolescence), breast cancer risk increased by 70%. Similarly, Beir in his review, reported that the exposure to radiation during periods of rapid growth, potentially amplified the deleterious biological effects [36].

Due to its high cost and risk of exposure towards harmful radiation, studies by van Niekerk et al. and Kilinç et al., recommended using alternative non-invasive methods for the assessment and screening of postural variables [37, 38]. In the next section, photogrammetry tools, together with methods to analyse postural variables are discussed. As stated by Furlanetto et al., the simplicity and convenience, has made the photogrammetry method very popular among clinical practitioners [39].

4.1.2.3 Photogrammetric method

In the last two decades, the photogrammetric method of postural evaluation and its applicability has been widely reported in the literature [9, 39]. Low-cost, quantitative evaluation together with its use in reducing the exposure to radiation, makes this method much more feasible for healthcare practitioners to use within their clinical practice. The following research studies have assessed the reliability, and validity of photogrammetry together and its application in different scenarios. Souza et al. and Fortin et al. have proposed a number of diverse photographic methods for evaluating postural variables and conducting postural diagnosis [9, 40]. Several authors [41, 42] have reported the use of photographic methods for the quantification together with the reliability of measuring postural variables. Santos et al. (2009) reported good to excellent inter-rater reliability (interclass correlation coefficient [ICC] values were between 0.84 and 0.99) for the photographic measurement of 33 postural variables in standing in 122 normal healthy children aged 7–10 years [41].

However, Souza et al. in their study on measuring 20 postural variables found mixed results. The ICC values for inter and intra-rater reliabilities for trunk and hip angle were found out to be 0.62 (*p* value was 0.12) and 0.56 (*p* value was 0.43) respectively. The level of reliability of these two angles was thus classified as not acceptable. The ICC values for lower leg postural variables (bilateral hind foot angle) ranged from 0.74 to 0.86 ($p < 0.05$). This level of reliability was classified as good and acceptable. The interrater reliability for the remaining sixteen posture angles reported excellent ICC values (greater than 0.90). Except for the trunk and hip angles, the rest of the sixteen variables yielded non-repeatable intra-rater values. The authors of this study concluded that frontal-view postural variables, such as the alignment of the head, trunk and lower limbs, measured using the photography method were reliable for measuring various postural asymmetries.

Although numerous studies [9, 43, 44] have reported the photogrammetric method of posture analysis, the most common limitation is the inconsistency used in the data collection procedure. For example, the distance between the subject and the placement of the camera varied between studies. The body segment length increases or decreases depending on how close the camera is to the surface of the human body. Additionally, from 2D photographic methods, it is very difficult to study deformities which have a rotational component in the transverse plane [9, 45]. Similarly, in the sagittal plane, there is a possibility that the muscle mass of the erector spinae can obscures the median furrow of the back surface; thereby it is very difficult to study the true spinal curvature [46].

In summary, two-dimensional spinal assessment tools do not provide a complete description of the three-dimensional nature of the back and other spinal deformities. To obtain the detailed three-dimensional description of spinal deformities together with the information of the 3D back surface, various three-dimensional surface and posture measurements tools have been reported in recent years. In the following section, three-dimensional measurement systems (both tactile and non-tactile methods) have been used to assess posture and back shape variables. These are reviewed below.

4.2 Three-dimensional analysis of posture and back shape

In the last decade, three-dimensional analysis of posture and back shape has not only developed significantly, but its use in both the spinal research and clinical environment has also been extended to include both tactile and non-tactile instruments, which will be discussed below.

4.2.1 Tactile tools of measurement of spinal curvature

4.2.1.1 Posturometer-S

The Posturometer-S is a specially designed, electronic, objective, non-invasive body posture measuring device [47] (see **Figure 4**). This tool consists of three coupled systems: 'P' which is a pointer to indicate the position of a measured point (mechanical), an element to compute the position of the pointer in a three-dimensional space (electronic) and an 'informatique' which is used to analyse the results obtained. This system not only enables a practitioner to visualise the curvature of the spine in all three planes but also provides a quantitative description of the postural parameters.

Previous research [47, 48] has demonstrated not only the reliability of the posturometer but also its applicability in the assessment of posture in different age groups. Lichota et al. using the Posturometer-S examined the postures of 46 athletes who were aged between 20 and 24 years [49]. A total of four sports groups were examined, namely, handball (n = 16), athletics (n = 9), taekwondo (n = 5) and

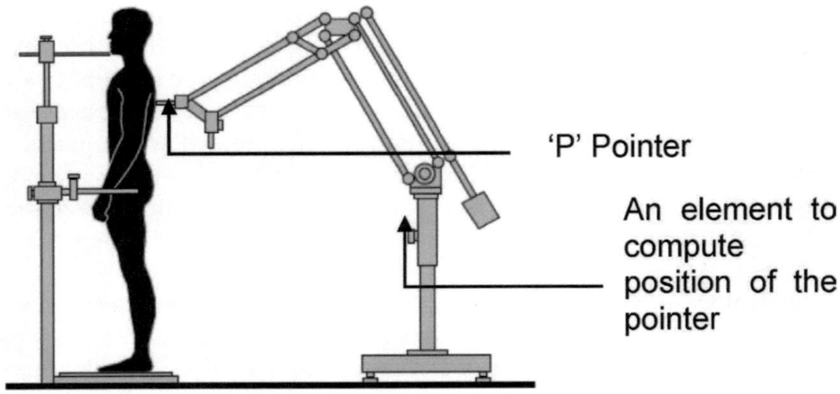

Figure 4.
Schema of Posturometer-S device (source: Stachoń et al. [47]).

volleyball (n = 13). In this study, the 'Posturometer-S' was used to describe various angles of the spine, for example, lumbar lordosis, thoracic kyphosis, upper thoracic segment (α angle), the thoracolumbar segment (β angle) and the lumbosacral segment (γ angle). The highest values for α angle, β angle and γ angle were reported in volleyball (15.2°), athletics (12.6°) and taekwondo (14.0°) groups, respectively. The lowest values for the α angle, β angle and γ angle were observed in athletics (12.4°), handball (8.8°) and handball (8.0°) groups, respectively. The authors contended that posture was affected by the specific type of sports training and that the type of sport influenced the type of posture. The main limitation the authors reported in the study was that the Posturometer-S was not user-friendly, consumes more space in the room and requires a thorough understanding of the equipment together with training before it can be used.

4.2.1.2 Ultrasound

Cheung et al. demonstrated the use of a radiation-free three-dimensional ultrasound system for the assessment of spinal curvature in 29 scoliosis patients [6]. Similarly, Kowalski et al. used an ultrasound-based volume projection imaging method to compare the lumbar lordosis and thoracic kyphosis angle in patients with scoliosis as well as normal subjects or other people with spinal disorders [50]. In this volume projection imaging method, the 3D representation of the spinal anatomy was generated using the ultrasound images together with the corresponding 3D spatial information (see **Figure 5**). The structure of the spine anatomy was reconstructed from image data ranging from 16 to 96 MB in size [6]. The results of this feasibility study showed good intra- and interrater reliability with ICCs larger than 0.92 ($p < 0.001$). The results also showed that the spinal curvature obtained by the new method had a good linear correlation with the X-ray Cobb method ($r^2 = 0.8$; $p < 0.001$).

Although these results suggest that the ultrasound volume projection imaging method can be a promising approach for the assessment of spinal deformity, there were still a number of factors that contributed to errors. For example, the ultrasound system and its data were susceptible to the distortion of the electromagnetic field, leading to a system offset/counteract or transient jitter in the spatial and orientation data. Therefore, precaution must be taken especially if the supporting frame is made of metal. The additional limitations of using the ultrasound volume projection imaging method were as follows: (a) heavy to carry around,

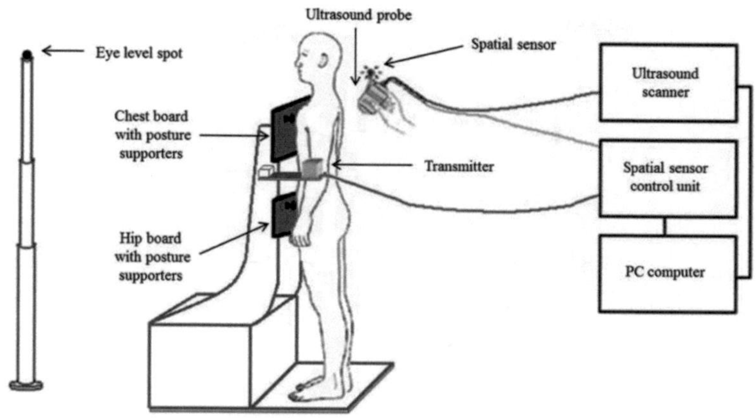

Figure 5.
Illustration of 3-D ultrasound system for the measurement of spinal deformity [6].

(b) expensive, (c) relatively dependent on the skilled operator [51, 52], (d) only measures the spinal curvature and not the whole back and (d) time-consuming for the assessment of the whole spine. Therefore, this suggests that it is not an appropriate tool for clinical practice.

In summary, the main disadvantage of all tactile posture measurement systems is the error produced due to electromagnetic and patient interference during data acquisition process. This is because it is difficult for patients to maintain a static standing position for a long time.

4.2.2 Non-tactile tools of measurement of spinal curvature

In the following section, non-surface measuring systems, such as 3D radiographic imaging systems and inertial measuring units, will be discussed. This is followed by various surface measurement tools, such as Moiré topography, integrated shape imaging system, laser triangulator system and the Kinect sensor system.

4.2.2.1 Non-surface measuring systems

4.2.2.1.1 3D radiographic imaging

Cheriet et al. demonstrated the use of biplanar X-ray images for the reconstruction of the three-dimensional spine and rib cage [7]. These images are useful in evaluating patients with spinal deformities like scoliosis. In this method, the reconstruction of images is based on a direct linear transformation technique (DLT), which requires the explicit calibration of an object with known 3D coordinates (see **Figure 6**). This method produced accurate 3D reconstruction of six manually identified anatomical landmarks per vertebra (centres of superior and inferior vertebral endplates and the tips of both pedicles). Similarly, the absolute differences between the Cobb angle obtained with the standard DLT and the explicit calibration methods were as low as 0.3 ± 0.42°. The absolute differences of the frontal and sagittal balance were 0.15 ± 0.15°and 0.37 ± 0.25°, respectively.

Using 3D X-rays for clinical or research purposes has the same motion and radiation issues as the use of 2D X-rays. Additionally, most of these tools are complex to set up, are heavy and only can be applied in laboratory environments.

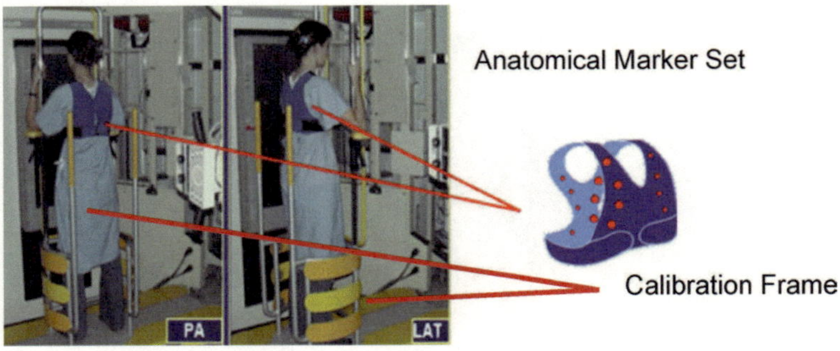

Figure 6.
Biplanar X-ray (posterior anterior (PA) and lateral view) acquisition system with calibration apparatus (Cheriet et al. [7]).

4.2.2.2 Inertial sensors

The recent advancement and application of electronic systems and sensors, namely, accelerometers, gyroscopes, flexible angular sensors, electromagnetic tracking systems and sensing fabrics, have enhanced the quality of clinical practice. Godfrey [53] and Fathi [8] all reported the use of sensors in the evaluation of human posture. The following section reviews their clinical applications, together with their problems and limitations.

An inertial measurement unit (IMU) is an electronic device that primarily contains accelerometers, gyroscope and magnetometer sensors. All these sensors are based on measuring and converting the global position of human body segment, momentum/inertia or changes of path length. An accelerometer is a sensor which measures a specific force and acceleration. In this context, an accelerometer is used to determine the orientation of the spinal segment in relation to the Earth's gravitational field. A gyroscope sensor measures the rate of change of angles. Using these sensors, a three-dimensional (3-D) position together with displacement data is calculated by combining inertial sensors orientation data, together with its known distance between the sensors [54, 55].

Kent et al., in their randomised controlled study, used dorsaVi's hardware (which contains two IMU movement sensors) (see **Figure 7**) to measure posture and movement in subacute and chronic low back pain patients (n = 58) [56]. The results not only demonstrated that the procedure was suitable for posture measurement but also demonstrated its applicability in providing postural biofeedback. Similarly, Fathi and Curran demonstrated the effective application of wireless IMU sensors to detect the curvature of the spine with 85–95% accuracy in ankylosing spondylitis patients [8].

Other portable, non-invasive sensors used in the assessment of posture are e-textiles. Many studies [57, 58] have reported the use of textile sensors to detect the curvature of the spine. The specially designed fabric contains an inductive sensor, a circuit board and a piezoelectric actuator (a component of a machine responsible for moving and controlling the piezoelectric system) (see **Figure 8**). Any change in posture and spinal movement is calculated by a change in the length or position of the sensors together with the percentage of change in electrical resistance.

Sardini et al. compared the e-textile output data with an optical motion system (Vicon) [58]. The trials performed on four subjects obtained on different days demonstrated that the wireless wearable sensor described in this paper is capable of producing reliable data compared with the data obtained with the optical system.

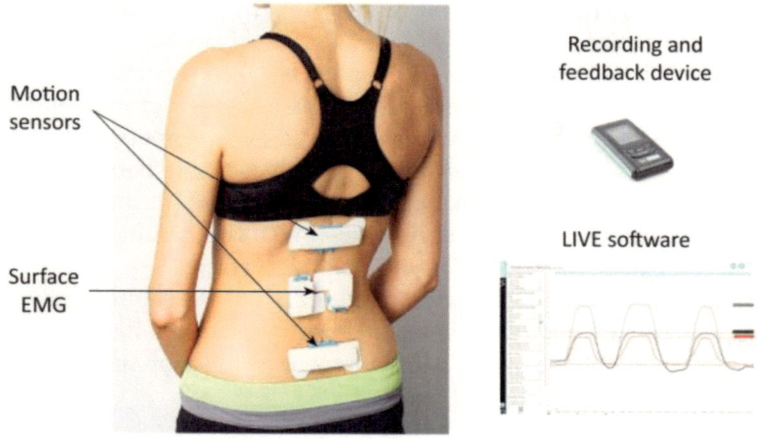

Figure 7.
ViMove wearable motion-sensor system with IMU sensors and surface EMG electrodes (Kent et al. [56]).

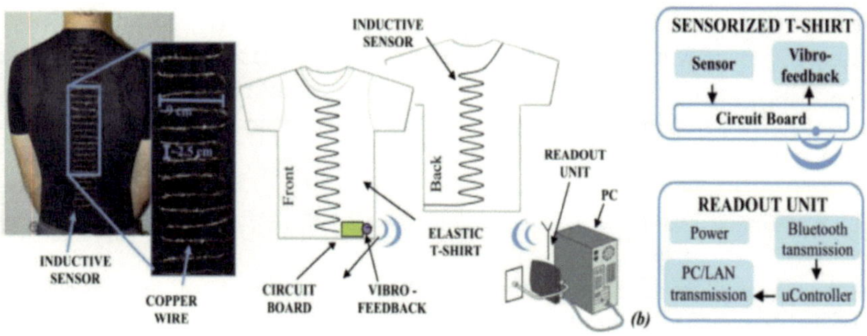

Figure 8.
E-textile with inductive sensors [58].

As the above IMU and e-textile tools were low-cost, portable and easy to use, it might be appropriate to use these for monitoring movement. The reliability of the above tools for measuring spinal curvatures or other back parameters has not yet been reported. The potential limitation of the IMU and e-textile tools is that their interaction with metal in the environment could affect the sensor data extraction due to its capacity to distort electromagnetic waves. In addition, these tools do not provide back surface and whole-body data.

4.2.2.3 Surface measuring systems

Berryman et al. detail that back surface observation and measurement methods have been widely used by both clinicians and researchers for the evaluation of posture and spinal curvature in patients with spinal disorders [59]. The following section aims to review both the qualitative and quantitative studies that describe skin surface measurement tools.

4.2.2.3.1 Moiré topographic methods

Moiré topography and rastereo photography systems are the most valuable and widely used non-radiographic tools in the measurement of posture/back surface. Additionally, these instruments are also used for screening three-dimensional spinal deformities and furthermore for quantifying the progression of the 3D spinal curvature.

The above topographical systems work on the basis of projecting a structured light onto the back surface. Based on the reflection of the structured light from the subject, Moiré topography images are produced (see **Figure 9**). The contour map image helps to visualise back asymmetry and record the spatial information of the subject's three-dimensional back shape and posture. The quantification of Moiré fringes typically involves the derivation of quantitative angular and/or linear measures by comparing the left and right side back surfaces.

Numerous authors [60, 61] have described the use of the Moiré topography method to evaluate back shape and spinal deformity. The main limitation of the Moiré topography method is that the measurement depends on the absolute order of Moiré fringes.

A Moiré pattern is a low-frequency line image produced from two high-frequency line images or grids. For example, by projecting a high-frequency grid onto an object and viewing the reflection of this projected pattern through another high-frequency grid is called Moiré fringes [62]. The formation of the Moiré fringes depends on a patient's position. A slight change in the patient's position or movement can produce considerable changes in the Moiré topogram. Thus, a direct inspection of Moiré fringes may be misleading. Further Stokes and Moreland states that the data analysis is a complex procedure, requiring much expertise [63]. Additionally, Nissinen et al. also reported that the correlation of Moiré topographs with X-rays is poor and ranges from r = 0.24–0.45 [64].

4.2.2.3.2 The integrated shape imaging system 1 and 2 (ISIS1 and 2)

The Integrated Shape Imaging System (ISIS) is a widely used optical scanning system for the measurement of human back shape and posture within a clinical environment [65, 66]. The ISIS system consists of an optical scanner (A), which projects a horizontal beam of structured white light onto the patient's back (B). The camera (C), mounted below the projector, captures the position of the light blade on the back from different perspectives (see **Figure 10**). Based on the geometry of the illumination/camera system together with the coordinates of the blade of light, the three-dimensional shape information is derived.

The validation of this system was carried out in the late 1980s and early 1990s [67, 68]. Although the reliability and validity of this tool was good to excellent for clinical use, the original ISIS system was getting old and data acquisition was slow which led to potential movement errors. The system was modified and redesigned

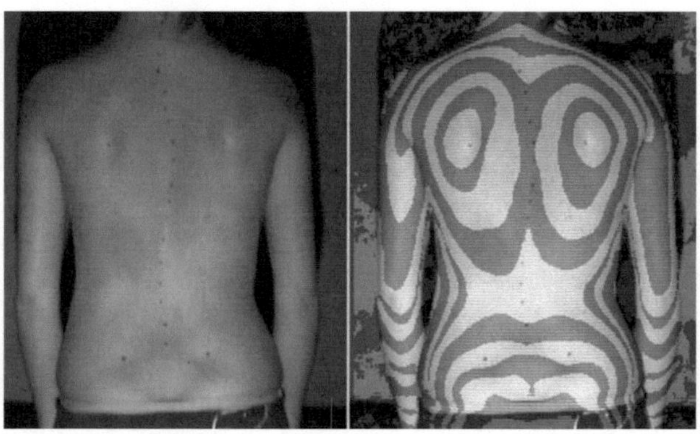

Figure 9.
Example of Moiré topographic images of a subject with scoliosis (reproduced from Kotwicki et al. [60]).

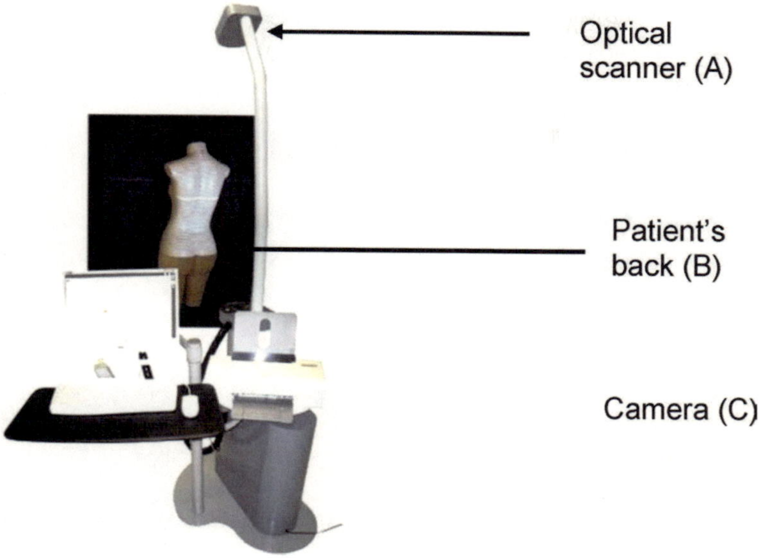

Figure 10.
Integrated shape imaging system (ISIS2) (reproduced from Porto et al. [73]).

by Berryman et al. with the new addition of a clinical parameters and renamed ISIS2 [59]. This automated non-invasive surface topography system measures three-dimensional shape of the back with improved speed, accuracy, reliability and ease of use [69].

Berryman et al. [59] described the data collection procedure, involving palpation and marking bony landmarks on the subject's back with small coloured stickers. A digital camera is then used to take a photo. The projector then projects a grid of horizontal black lines onto the patient's back. The pixel size is approximately 0.5 mm with fringe frequency of approximately 0.16 fringes/mm. Fourier transform profilometry is used to convert the distortion of the reference grid lines into a three-dimensional surface map of the back.

The data processing with ISIS2 takes only 40 s, compared to 10 min in ISIS. Knott et al. [70] suggest that by reducing the duration of data collection, the error due to natural postural sway of the body decreases, thereby increasing the accuracy (±1 mm). The results are stored in a database so that the data of the particular patient can be recalled at any given point of time. ISIS2 helps in the screening and monitoring of the development of spinal deformity over time [71, 72].

Zubović et al. [69] carried out a study to validate the ISIS2 system against X-rays. They reviewed 520 ISIS2 scans on 242 scoliosis patients not only for quantifying postural variables but also to assess their validity. The average number of scans per patient was 2.01 with a range of 1–10 scans. The median values and 95% CI were reported for the linear, angular and volumetric asymmetry of scoliosis patients. The results of this study showed no statistically significant differences in their investigations between ISIS measurements and X-ray images.

Similarly, Berryman et al. [59], in their study on measuring three-dimensional back shape in scoliosis patients, also found good correlations (r = 0.84) between the Cobb angle and the lateral asymmetry of the ISIS scans.

As seen in **Figure 11**, the ISIS2 system provides additional data to simple radiographic examination, describing the three-dimensional characteristics of the back surface [59, 74]. Previous studies [71, 72] have demonstrated that the ISIS2 produces reliable, valid and accurate data that can monitor the progression of spinal deformities. Berryman et al. [59], Frerich et al. [75], Sadani et al. [76], Brewer et al. [77]

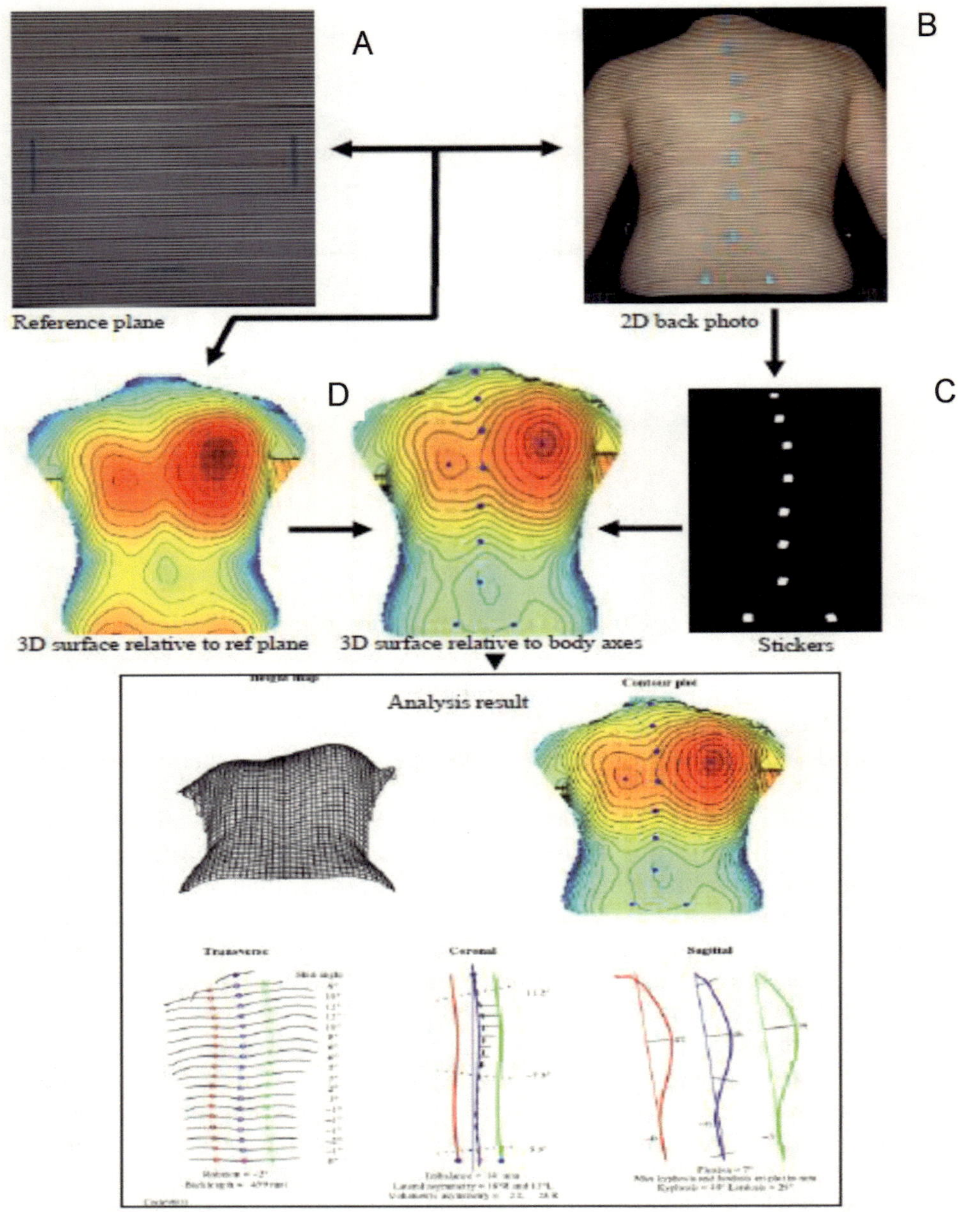

Figure 11.
Illustration of data processing and a sample report of ISIS2 method [74]. (A) the reference frame with calibration markers; (B) example of patient image with fringes projected onto the back; (C) representation of symmetry line analysis in frontal and sagittal planes to obtain lateral deviation, kyphosis and lordosis angles; (D) back height map with rib hump, contour plot (representing the shape using contour lines and colour; blue lowest to red highest); and (E) example of ISIS2 report with representation of contour plot and quantification of curve in all planes.

and Knott et al. [33] suggest that the additional advantage of ISIS2 is to reduce the exposure to radiation.

However, Fortin et al. [9] and Bettany-Saltikov et al. [46] identify the ISIS2 system as being very heavy, is not easily moved and requires skilled clinicians to operate it. In addition, Berryman et al. [59] suggests that identifying the bony landmarks for marking spinous process is more difficult for patients who are extremely obese or have heavy musculature. Similarly, the above authors also found it difficult to mark bony landmarks in patients with congenital curves that had little rotation.

The main limitation of the ISIS2 system is that it can only measure back shape and not the whole body. Non-contact optical imaging techniques for the assessment of back shape and posture has also been achieved by using the laser triangulators method.

4.2.2.3.3 Laser triangulators

Čelan et al. [78] and Poredoš et al. [79] used the laser triangulation method to evaluate the three-dimensional human spine curvature. The main purpose of these studies was to estimate the spatial bend of the thoracic and lumbar spine curvatures in all three planes. The laser triangulation imaging system used in Poredoš et al.'s study consisted of two basic elements: a greyscale camera (A) and a laser line projector (B) (see **Figure 12**). The spinal path or region of interest (ROI) of the human model is manually marked by the palpation of the subject's bony landmarks. The laser projector illuminates the light onto the subject's back, and the intersection of the laser line with the spinal path or ROI provides the intersection curve, which is then measured using a greyscale camera. The distance between the laser projector and the camera is known. The intersection angle in 3D space is calculated using the triangular method [80].

The laser scanning triangulation method was assessed for both validity and repeatability. Using a point-to-point analysis, the average error (±1 mm S.D) (distance between markers) for a regular shape (cylinder) was as low as 4.99 ± 1.56 mm, versus 6.91 ± 2.29 mm for an irregular shape (mannequin) [81]. Research by Majid et al. [82] demonstrated the performance of the 3D laser scanning system. In this laboratory-based study, craniofacial measurements of mannequins demonstrated that the photogrammetric/3D laser scanning system had an accuracy of ±0.7 mm (1 standard deviation [SD]).

The same measurement in human models demonstrated an accuracy of ±1.2 mm. This decrease in accuracy was due to facial movement during data acquisition.

However, this method also has limitations. The manual spinal path determination is also likely to cause palpation errors. This limits the usage of the system to only experienced healthcare practitioners who have good palpation skills.

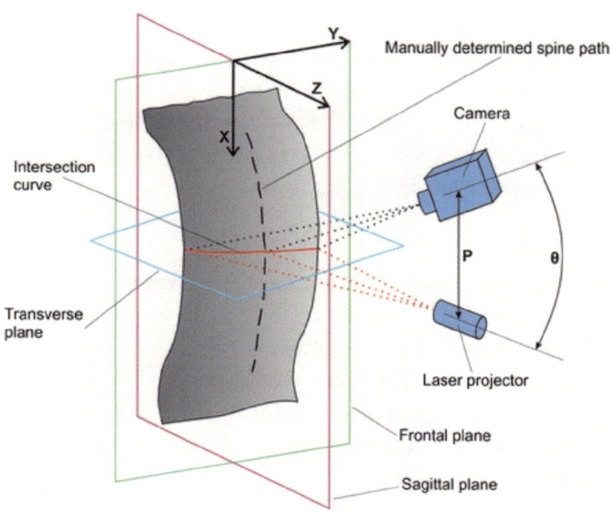

Figure 12.
Illustration of one-laser-plane triangulation method in all planes (reproduced from Poredoš et al. [79]).

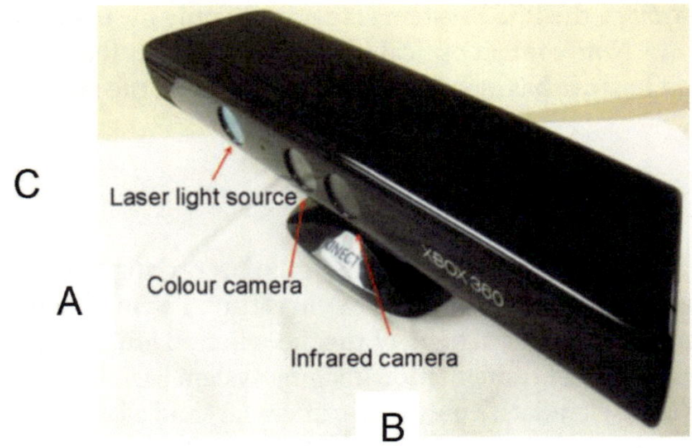

Figure 13.
Microsoft Kinect sensor.

Additionally, this tool is capable of only measuring the shape of the human spine and not the complete back or human body.

4.2.2.3.4 Kinect sensors

Microsoft kinetic sensors are currently being used in a range of disciplines from biomechanics to clinical applications [83, 84]. Castro et al. [85] described the use of the Microsoft's Kinect™ to measure back surface and posture. The Kinect sensor consists of two cameras, a colour camera (RGB camera) (A) and a depth (infrared IR) camera (B), and a projector (C) (please see **Figure 13**). These cameras do not require passive markers to determine anatomical landmarks. By measuring the deformations of the projected speckle pattern, a 3D map of the dorsal skin surface is created by using the appropriate software.

The results from previous studies have demonstrated that the depth sensor is valid in measuring 3D back surface in patients with scoliosis and in healthy volunteers [85, 86]. The Microsoft Kinect™ system had comparable intertrial reliability (ICC difference = 0.06 ± 0.05; range, 0.00–0.16) and excellent concurrent validity against a benchmark reference, a multiple-camera 3D motional analysis system, with Pearson's r-values >0.90 for the majority of measurements (r = 0.96 ± 0.04; range, 0.84–0.99).

Whilst the Microsoft Kinect™ is inexpensive, portable and offers good repeatable of the 3D map of the back surface, it also has a few limitations. The measurements are limited only to the back surface and not the whole body. Additionally, the Kinect system software is mainly restricted to the Microsoft operating system and is not applicable to any other mobile applications.

5. Conclusion and requirements for a novel system

A number of different techniques for the assessment of posture and back shape within clinical practice and research have been described above. Most are expensive, are difficult to use, need specialised training, are heavy to move or cannot be used for regular clinical use (Fortin et al. [9]). When considering a new system, the following requirements are necessary:

1. A novel tool needs to be simple, portable, low-cost, easy to use and less time-consuming for the purpose of using within clinical practice. This can be

achieved by innovatively using a mobile low-cost scanner, such as the Structure Sensor™ together with freeware software. This has previously been used in the construction and fashion industry [87, 88].

2. The most conventional photographic systems, used in clinical practice at present, do not provide the three-dimensional information of patients' posture and back shape. A novel portable system providing three-dimensional information of patient's posture and back shape would help to better understand the three-dimensional nature of spinal deformities.

3. Most existing systems described in this review provide information on either back shape or spinal posture and not the whole body. A system providing information on the whole body and its relation to spinal posture would yield more information on the relationship between the orientations of the extremities to the trunk.

4. Technological advances in imaging and computerised image-processing led to the development of new 3D image acquisition techniques. There is a demand for bridging the gap between technological advancement and medical practice for the assessment and treatment of spinal disorders [89, 90]. The continuous increase in 3D imaging technology provides opportunities for the development of a novel system that provides reliable and valid results for assessment of whole-body posture and back shape.

Author details

Gok Kandasamy[1*], Josette Bettany-Saltikov[1] and Paul van Schaik[2]

1 School of Health and Life Sciences, Teesside University, United Kingdom

2 School of Social Sciences Humanities and Law, Teesside University, United Kingdom

*Address all correspondence to: g.kandasamy@tees.ac.uk

References

[1] Schwab F, Dubey A, Gamez L, et al. Adult scoliosis: Prevalence, SF-36, and nutritional parameters in an elderly volunteer population. Spine (Phila Pa 1976). 2005;**30**:1082-1085

[2] Fällström K, Cochran T, Nachemson A. Long-term effects on personality development in patients with adolescent idiopathic scoliosis. Influence of type of treatment. Spine (Phila Pa 1976). 1986;**11**:756-758

[3] Burt S, Punnett L. Evaluation of interrater reliability for posture observations in a field study. Applied Ergonomics. 1999;**30**:121-135

[4] Danielsson AJ, Wiklund I, Pehrsson K, et al. Health-related quality of life in patients with adolescent idiopathic scoliosis: A matched follow-up at least 20 years after treatment with brace or surgery. European Spine Journal. 2001;**10**:278-288

[5] Tyson SF, DeSouza LH. A clinical model for the assessment of posture and balance in people with stroke. Disability and Rehabilitation. 2003;**25**:120-126

[6] Cheung C-WJ, Zhou G-Q, Law S-Y, et al. Ultrasound volume projection imaging for assessment of scoliosis. IEEE Transactions on Medical Imaging. 2015;**34**:1760-1768

[7] Cheriet F, Laporte C, Kadoury S, et al. A novel system for the 3-D reconstruction of the human spine and rib cage from biplanar X-ray images. IEEE Transactions on Biomedical Engineering. 2007;**54**:1356-1358

[8] Fathi A, Curran K. Detection of spine curvature using wireless sensors. Journal of King Saud University. 2017;**29**:553-560

[9] Fortin C, Ehrmann Feldman D, Cheriet F, et al. Clinical methods for quantifying body segment posture: A literature review. Disability and Rehabilitation. 2011;**33**:367-383

[10] Williams DS, McClay IS. Measurements used to characterize the foot and the medial longitudinal arch: Reliability and validity. Physical Therapy. 2000;**80**:864-871

[11] Elabd A, Ibrahim A, Elhafez H. Kinesio taping versus postural correction exercises on mechanically triggered neck dysfunction. International Journal of Therapy and Rehabilitation. 2017;**24**:155-162

[12] Raupp EG, Candotti CT, Marchetti BV, et al. The validity and reproducibility of the Flexicurve in the evaluation of cervical spine Lordosis. Journal of Manipulative and Physiological Therapeutics. 2017;**40**:501-510

[13] Greenfield B, Catlin PA, Coats PW, et al. Posture in patients with shoulder overuse injuries and healthy individuals. The Journal of Orthopaedic and Sports Physical Therapy. 1995;**21**:287-295

[14] Rheault W, Ferris S, Foley JA, et al. Intertester reliability of the flexible ruler for the cervical spine. The Journal of Orthopaedic and Sports Physical Therapy. 1989;**10**:254-256

[15] Hecimovich MD, Stomski NJ. Lumbar sagittal plane spinal curvature and junior-level cricket players. International Journal of Athletic Therapy and Training. 2016;**21**:47-52

[16] Burton AK. Suggestion from the field: Measurement of "regional" lumbar sagittal mobility. The Journal of Orthopaedic and Sports Physical Therapy. 1987;**9**:166-169

[17] Bryan JM, Mosner E, Shippee R, et al. Investigation of the validity of postural evaluation skills in assessing

lumbar lordosis using photographs of clothed subjects. The Journal of Orthopaedic and Sports Physical Therapy. 1990;**12**:24-29

[18] Hart DL, Rose SJ. Reliability of a noninvasive method for measuring the lumbar curve. The Journal of Orthopaedic and Sports Physical Therapy. 1986;**8**:180-184

[19] Wu W, Liang J, Du Y, et al. Reliability and reproducibility analysis of the cobb angle and assessing sagittal plane by computer-assisted and manual measurement tools. BMC Musculoskeletal Disorders. 2014;**15**:33

[20] Hogeweg JA, Langereis MJ, Bernards ATM, et al. Goniometry-variability in the clinical practice of a conventional goniometer in healthy subjects. European Journal of Physical and Rehabilitation Medicine. 1994;**4**:2-7

[21] ICN S, BWC Q, et al. Reliability of photogrammetry in relation to goniometry for postural lower limb assessment. Revista Brasileira de Fisioterapia. 2007;**11**:411-417

[22] Harrison DD, Janik TJ, Troyanovich SJ, et al. Comparisons of lordotic cervical spine curvatures to a theoretical ideal model of the static sagittal cervical spine. Spine (Phila Pa 1976). 1996;**21**:667-675

[23] Perry J, Klopfer E, Norton M, et al. AR gone wild: Two approaches to using augmented reality learning games in zoos. In: Proceedings of the 8th International Conference on International Conference for the Learning Sciences-Vol. 3. 2008. pp. 322-329

[24] Kendall FP, McCreary EK, Provance PG, et al. Muscles; Testing and Function with Posture and Pain. Williams and Wilkins. Seoul 2005; 52, 61, 159

[25] McKenzie R, May S. The Lumbar Spine: Mechanical Diagnosis and Therapy. New Zealand: Orthopedic Physical Therapy, Spinal Publications; 2003

[26] Hickey ER, Rondeau MJ, Corrente JR, et al. Reliability of the cervical range of motion (CROM) device and plumb-line techniques in measuring resting head posture (RHP). Journal of Manual and Manipulative Therapy. 2000;**8**:10-17

[27] Perry M, Smith A, Straker L, et al. Reliability of sagittal photographic spinal posture assessment in adolescents. Advances in Physiotherapy. 2008;**10**:66-75

[28] Schwab FJ, Patel A, Ungar B, et al. Adult spinal deformity — Postoperative standing imbalance assessing alignment and planning corrective surgery. Spine (Phila Pa 1976). 2010;**35**:2224-2231

[29] Schwab FJ, Smith VA, Biserni M, et al. Adult scoliosis: A quantitative radiographic and clinical analysis. Spine (Phila Pa 1976). 2002;**27**:387-392

[30] McVey G, Sandborg M, Dance DR, et al. A study and optimization of lumbar spine X-ray imaging systems. The British Journal of Radiology. 2003;**76**:177-188

[31] O'neill TW, Felsenberg D, Varlow J, et al. The prevalence of vertebral deformity in European men and women: The European vertebral osteoporosis study. Journal of Bone and Mineral Research. 1996;**11**:1010-1018

[32] Rea JA, Steiger P, Blake GM, et al. Morphometric X-ray absorptiometry: Reference data for vertebral dimensions. Journal of Bone and Mineral Research. 1998;**13**:464-474

[33] Knott P, Pappo E, Cameron M, et al. SOSORT 2012 consensus paper: Reducing x-ray exposure in pediatric patients with scoliosis. Scoliosis. 2014;**9**:1-9

[34] Zhang Y, Chen Y, Huang H, et al. Diagnostic x-ray exposure increases the risk of thyroid microcarcinoma: A population-based case-control study. European Journal of Cancer Prevention. 2015;**24**:439

[35] Doody MM, Lonstein JE, Stovall M, et al. Breast cancer mortality after diagnostic radiography: Findings from the US scoliosis cohort study. Spine (Phila Pa 1976). 2000;**25**:2052-2063

[36] Council NR, others. Committee on the biological effects of ionizing radiation. In: Heal Eff Expo to Low Levels Ioniz Radiat (BEIR V). National Academics; 1990

[37] van Niekerk S-M, Louw Q, Vaughan C, et al. Photographic measurement of upper-body sitting posture of high school students: A reliability and validity study. BMC Musculoskeletal Disorders. 2008;**9**:113

[38] Kilinç F, Yaman H, Atay E. Investigation of the effects of intensive one-sided and double-sided training drills on the postures of basketball playing children. Journal of Physical Therapy Science. 2009;**21**:23-28

[39] Furlanetto TS, Sedrez JA, Candotti CT, et al. Photogrammetry as a tool for the postural evaluation of the spine: A systematic review. World Journal of Orthopedics. 2016;**7**:136

[40] Souza JA, Pasinato F, Basso D, et al. Biophotogrammetry: Reliability of measurements obtained with a posture assessment software (SAPO). Revista Brasileira de Cineantropometria & Desempenho Humano. 2011;**13**:299-305

[41] Santos MM, Silva MPC, Sanada LS, et al. Photogrammetric postural analysis on healthy seven to ten-year-old children: Interrater reliability. Brazilian Journal of Physical Therapy. 2009;**13**:350-355

[42] Thigpen CA, Padua DA, Michener LA, et al. Head and shoulder posture affect scapular mechanics and muscle activity in overhead tasks. Journal of Electromyography and Kinesiology. 2010;**20**:701-709

[43] JLP R. Biomechanical assessment of human posture: A literature review. Journal of Bodywork and Movement Therapies. 2014;**18**:368-373

[44] Ruivo RM, Pezarat-Correia P, Carita AI. Cervical and shoulder postural assessment of adolescents between 15 and 17 years old and association with upper quadrant pain. Brazilian Journal of Physical Therapy. 2014;**18**:364-371

[45] Viazzi S, Bahr C, Van Hertem T, et al. Comparison of a three-dimensional and two-dimensional camera system for automated measurement of back posture in dairy cows. Computers and Electronics in Agriculture. 2014;**100**:139-147

[46] Bettany-Saltikov J, Martin D, Wellburn S, et al. Information provided to patients with adolescent idiopathic scoliosis (AIS) at the first point of diagnosis in the hospital clinic: A survey of UK NHS scoliosis consultants. Scoliosis. 2012;**7**:O36

[47] Stachoń A, Burdukiewicz A, Andrzejewska J, et al. The imaging and evaluation of body posture defects in hearing impaired children. Bio-Algorithms and Med-Systems. 2012;**8**:221-236

[48] Mroczkowski A. The effect of aikido exercises on shaping spinal curvatures in the sagittal plane. Journal of Combat Sports and Martial Arts. 2013;**2**(2):173-177

[49] Lichota M, Plandowska M, Mil P. The shape of anterior-posterior curvatures of the spine in athletes practising selected sports. Polish Journal of Sport and Tourism. 2011;**18**:112-116

[50] Kowalski IM, Kotwicki T, Siwik P. Analysis of diagnostic methods in trunk

deformities in the developmental age. Polish Annals of Medicine. 2013;**20**:43-50

[51] Scholten-Peeters GGM, Franken N, Beumer A, et al. The opinion and experiences of Dutch orthopedic surgeons and radiologists about diagnostic musculoskeletal ultrasound imaging in primary care: A survey. Manual Therapy. 2014;**19**:109-113

[52] Thoomes-de Graaf M, Scholten-Peeters GGM, Duijn E, et al. Inter-professional agreement of ultrasound-based diagnoses in patients with shoulder pain between physical therapists and radiologists in the Netherlands. Manual Therapy. 2014;**19**:478-483

[53] Godfrey A, Conway R, Meagher D, et al. Direct measurement of human movement by accelerometry. Medical Engineering & Physics. 2008;**30**:1364-1386

[54] Wong WY, Wong MS. Trunk posture monitoring with inertial sensors. European Spine Journal. 2008;**17**:743-753

[55] Voinea G-D, Butnariu S, Mogan G. Measurement and geometric modelling of human spine posture for medical rehabilitation purposes using a wearable monitoring system based on inertial sensors. Sensors. 2016;**17**:3

[56] Kent P, Laird R, Haines T. The effect of changing movement and posture using motion-sensor biofeedback, versus guidelines-based care, on the clinical outcomes of people with sub-acute or chronic low back pain-a multicentre, cluster-randomised, placebo-controlled, pilot trial. BMC Musculoskeletal Disorders. 2015;**16**:131

[57] Rajdi NNZM, Bakira AA, Saleh SM, et al. Textile-based micro electro mechanical system (MEMS) accelerometer for pelvic tilt mesurement. Procedia Engineering. 2012;**41**:532-537

[58] Sardini E, Serpelloni M, Pasqui V. Wireless wearable T-shirt for posture monitoring during rehabilitation exercises. IEEE Transactions on Instrumentation and Measurement. 2015;**64**:439-448

[59] Berryman F, Pynsent P, Fairbank J, et al. A new system for measuring three-dimensional back shape in scoliosis. European Spine Journal. 2008;**17**:663-672

[60] Kotwicki T, Kinel E, Stryla W, et al. Discrepancy in clinical versus radiological parameters describing deformity due to brace treatment for moderate idiopathic scoliosis. Scoliosis. 2007;**2**:18

[61] Rankine L, Liu XC, Tassone C, et al. Reproducibility of newly developed spinal topography measurements for scoliosis. The Open Orthopaedics Journal. 2012;**6**:226

[62] Chiang C. Moiré topography. Applied Optics. 1975;**14**:177-179

[63] Stokes IAF, Pekalsky JR, Moreland MS. Surface topography and spinal deformity. In: Proceedings of the 4-th International Symposium. New York: Gustaw Verlag; 1987

[64] Nissinen M, Heliövaara M, Tallroth K, et al. Trunk asymmetry and scoliosis anthropometric measurements in Prepuberal school children. Acta Paediatrica. 1989;**78**:747-753

[65] Turner-Smith AR, Harris JD, Abery JM, et al. Back shape measurement. Oxford Orthopaedic Engineering Centre. 1981;**8**:41-49

[66] Turner-Smith AR, Harris JD, Houghton GR, et al. A method for analysis of back shape in scoliosis. Journal of Biomechanics. 1988;**21**:497-509

[67] Legaye J, Lokietek W, Orban C, et al. The ISIS optic scanner: Its use in the evaluation and control of spinal deviations. Acta Orthopaedica Belgica. 1992;**58**:66-72

[68] Berdishevsky H, Lebel VA, Bettany-Saltikov J, et al. Physiotherapy scoliosis-specific exercises - a comprehensive review of seven major schools. Scoliosis and Spinal Disorders. 2016;**11**:20

[69] Zubović A, Davies N, Berryman F, et al. New method of scoliosis deformity assessment: ISIS2 system. Studies in Health Technology and Informatics. 2008;**140**:157-160

[70] Knott P, Smith K, Mack L, et al. A comparison of static vs dynamic surface topography measurements in the evaluation of scoliosis. Scoliosis. 2012;**7**:P12

[71] Talasila SSA, Gorantla M, Thomas V. A study on screening for scoliosis among school children in the age group of 10-14 using a cost effective and an innovative technique. The International Journal of Community Medicine and Public Health. 2017;**4**:2118-2123

[72] Pino-Almero L, M'inguez-Rey MF, Rodr'iguez-Mart'inez D, et al. Clinical application of back surface topography by means of structured light in the screening of idiopathic scoliosis. Journal of Pediatric Orthopaedics. Part B. 2017;**26**:64-72

[73] Porto F, Gurgel JL, Russomano T, et al. Moiré topography: Characteristics and clinical application. Gait & Posture. 2010;**32**:422-424

[74] Anwary AR. Statistical Shape Analysis for the Human Back Statistical Shape Analysis for the Human Back. Openrepository.com, University of Wolverhampton; 2012

[75] Frerich JM, Hertzler K, Knott P, et al. Comparison of radiographic and surface topography measurements in adolescents with idiopathic scoliosis. The Open Orthopaedics Journal. 2012;**6**:261-265

[76] Sadani S, Jones C, Seal A, et al. A pilot study of scoliosis assessment using radiation free surface topography in children with GMFCS IV and V cerebral palsy. Child: Care, Health and Development. 2012;**38**:854-862

[77] Brewer P, Berryman F, Baker D, et al. Influence of cobb angle and ISIS2 surface topography volumetric asymmetry on Scoliosis Research Society-22 outcome scores in scoliosis. Spinal Deformities. 2013;**1**:452-457

[78] Čelan D, Papež BJ, Poredoš P, et al. Laser triangulation measurements of scoliotic spine curvatures. Scoliosis. 2015;**10**:25

[79] Poredoš P, Čelan D, Možina J, et al. Determination of the human spine curve based on laser triangulation. BMC Medical Imaging. 2015;**15**:2

[80] Amann M-C, Bosch TM, Lescure M, et al. Laser ranging: A critical review of unusual techniques for distance measurement. Optical Engineering. 2001;**40**:10-20

[81] Chang Y-C, Detchev I, Habib A. A photogrammetric system for 3D reconstruction of a Scoliotic torso [A Master Thesis]. University of Calgary; 2008; 1: 126-137

[82] Majid Z, Chong AK, Ahmad A, et al. Photogrammetry and 3D laser scanning as spatial data capture techniques for a national craniofacial database. The Photogrammetric Record. 2005;**20**:48-68

[83] Bonanno DR, Zhang CY, Farrugia RC, et al. The effect of different depths of medial heel skive on plantar pressures. Journal of Foot and Ankle Research. 2012;**5**:20

[84] Nguyen CV, Izadi S, Lovell D. Modeling kinect sensor noise for improved 3d reconstruction and tracking. In: Second International Conference on 3D Imaging, Modeling, Processing, Visualization and Transmission (3DIMPVT). 2012. pp. 524-530

[85] Castro APG, Pacheco JD, Lourenço C, et al. Evaluation of spinal posture using Microsoft Kinect™: A preliminary case-study with 98 volunteers. Porto Biomedical Journal. 2017;**2**:18-22

[86] Lachat E, Macher H, Mittet MA, et al. First experiences with kinect V2 sensor for close range 3D modelling. International Archives of the Photogrammetry, Remote Sensing and Spatial Information Sciences - ISPRS Archives. 2015;**40**:93-100

[87] D'Apuzzo N. 3D body scanning technology for fashion and apparel industry. In: Electronic Imaging. International Society for Optics and Photonics; 2007. pp. 64910O-64910O

[88] Yap YL, Yeong WY. Additive manufacture of fashion and jewellery products: A mini review: This paper provides an insight into the future of 3D printing industries for fashion and jewellery products. Virtual and Physical Prototyping. 2014;**9**:195-201

[89] Eysenbach G, Köhler C. How do consumers search for and appraise health information on the world wide web? Qualitative study using focus groups, usability tests, and in-depth interviews. The BMJ. 2002;**324**:573-577

[90] Gammon D, Årsand E, Walseth OA, et al. Parent-child interaction using a mobile and wireless system for blood glucose monitoring. Journal of Medical Internet Research. 2005;**7**(5):e57

Chapter 3

An Anatomical and Pathological Classification of Thoracolumbar Adjacent Segment Disease

David Christopher Kieser and Niels Hammer

Abstract

Structural failure of the spine adjacent to the level of a previous spinal fusion is commonly observed. It may be defined by the radiologic degree of adjacent deformity, often termed junctional level kyphosis, proximal junctional kyphosis or junctional level failure, or the symptomatic failure of the spine above the level of an operation, termed adjacent segment disease (ASD). ASD can be further specified according to its anatomical location of failure, which provides insight into the specific pathological cause of failure and the optimal subsequent management. This chapter describes the anatomical and pathological classification of ASD in order to help clinicians understand the cause of failure and thereby reduce its rate and offer a treatment algorithm if it occurs.

Keywords: adjacent segment disease, thoraco-lumbar fusion, pathological cause, junctional level kyphosis

1. Introduction

Adjacent segment disease (ASD) is the symptomatic structural failure of the spine or sacrum adjacent to an area of previous operative intervention, most notably fusion [1]. Internationally, the numbers of spinal fusions being performed is increasing. Within the USA approximately 457,500 adult spinal fusions and 38,000 paediatric spinal deformity corrections are performed annually, with similar rates per capita reported worldwide [2]. Of concern is that more than 20% of patients undergoing lumbar deformity surgery will develop ASD within 8 years, most of which occurs early with 40% requiring revision within 6 months [3–9]. This has a significant clinical effect on patient outcomes, with pain, neurological, emotional, social and occupational concerns, but also carries a large financial burden, with an estimated cost in the USA for revision being $77,432 USD per patient [10, 11]. This would suggest that over 500 million USD is spent annually on the surgical treatment of ASD. Yet, a complete understanding of the aetiology of this problem has not been compiled.

It is believed that the cause of ASD is multifactorial [12]. These causes can be separated into non-modifiable, potentially modifiable and modifiable risk factors.

Non-modifiable risk factors include patient age and expected baseline motion segment degeneration that cannot be modified with current known treatments [13, 14]. These factors are particularly pertinent in the adult population where their index procedure is often related to degeneration which itself renders patients at higher risk of degeneration at other levels.

Potentially modifiable risk factors include bone density, which may be amenable to medical treatment [15]. Others include fusion without instrumentation and limiting the fusion length, however the pathology often dictates the length of fusion and implant requirement [13, 16].

Modifiable risk factors include intraoperative surgical techniques, notably motion preservation to reduce the adjacent segment load, avoiding circumferential fusion of the most cranial segment that increases the stresses on the adjacent level, ensuring spinal balance, avoiding extensor musculature and ligamentous damage, protecting the adjacent facets, endplates and intervertebral disc (IVD) [13, 14].

While multiple classification systems and definitions have been proposed, none have attempted to group these into anatomical or pathological considerations. Our classification broadly categorises ASD into five groups according to the anatomical region of failure which can then determine the likely pathological cause and offer treatment direction.

2. The Kieser and Hammer classification system

2.1 Type 1: global failure (implant pull-out)

This form of ASD is seen when metalware pulls out of the vertebrae (**Figure 1**). This failure is not seen in anterior interbody constructs, unless supplementary posterior or lateral instrumentation is utilised. This is because it is recognised as persistent spinal malalignment, which requires interconnected rigid implants to remain in one position and the spine to displace from the rigid instrumentation. However, with lateral implants (plates, stapes, etc.) and a failure to restore coronal balance or posterior implants and a failure to restore sagittal balance, the metalware can pull out of the bone producing a type 1 failure.

This failure is therefore almost always due to malalignment, but can be sub-classified into:

1a. Bone failure: osteoporosis.
1b. Implant failure: insufficient fixation.
1c. Combination.

In type 1a, the bone quality is insufficient to hold the implanted device in a given configuration, with the effect that the metalware pulls out. Similarly, in type 1b the implant configuration is insufficient to stabilise and anchor in the bone and

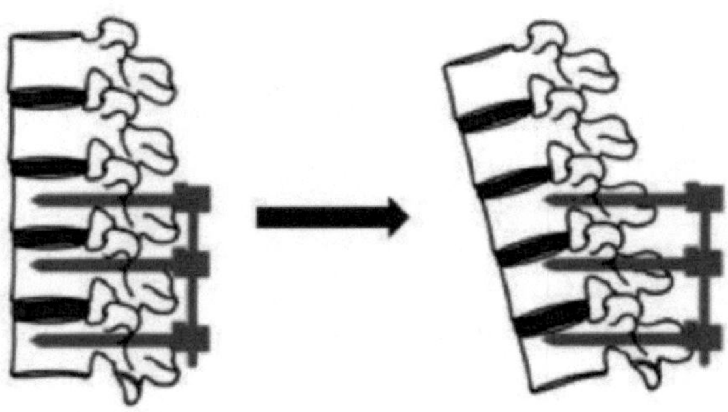

Figure 1.
Type 1 (global failure).

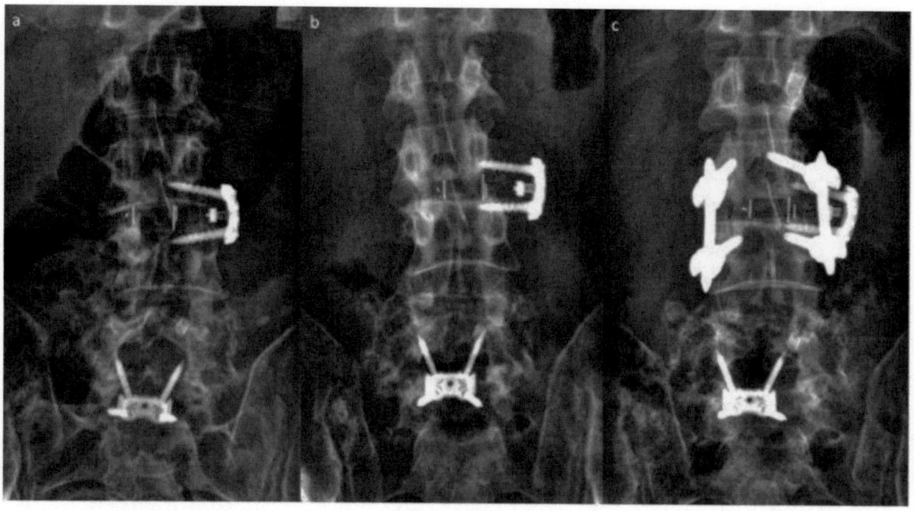

Figure 2.
Antero-posterior X-rays of a patient with a previous L4-S1 fusion who developed type 4d ASD of L3/4 causing foraminal stenosis and therefore underwent a lateral interbody fixation and plate (a. immediate postoperative) but with failure to completely restore coronal balance and insufficient fixation resulting in implant pull-out and progressive coronal imbalance with recurrence of symptomatic foraminal stenosis (b. 6 weeks postoperative). Therefore supplementary percutaneous pedicle screw insertion to augment fixation and bracing was undertaken, which resulted in sufficient fixation to permit definitive fusion (c. 6 months postoperative).

therefore it pulls out (**Figure 2**). In most cases it is a combination of both poor bone stock and insufficient implant fixation.

In an asymptomatic patient without skin compromise, the practitioner or surgeon advises bracing to prevent further progression until the fusion has developed. In contrast, in symptomatic patients or those with progressive failure amendable to operative intervention, the treatment of type 1 failure is revision surgery with restoration of spinal alignment and supplementary bracing until fusion has developed. In addition, for each sub-classification we advocate.

1a. Bone supplementation with medical management of osteoporosis (e.g. calcium, vitamin D, bisphosphonates, etc.) and increased fixation (e.g. cemented screws, HA coated screws, sublaminar bands, etc.).
1b. Increase fixation of the operative levels. May require extension of fusion if adequate fixation of the operative levels is not possible.
1c. Both.

It should be recognised that bone supplementation takes a prolonged period of time to achieve clinical benefit and most of these patients require semi-urgent surgical intervention. Thus, in symptomatic patients with deficient bone quality, increased fixation should be provided in addition to the medical management of osteoporosis. Furthermore, bracing should be considered to supplement the spinal stability provided by the surgery until fusion has occurred.

2.2 Type 2: adjacent bone failure (failure of the cranial or caudal uninstrumented vertebrae)

This form of ASD occurs when an adjacent, uninstrumented vertebrae fails, typically with a compression type fracture (**Figures 3** and **4**). This is most commonly caused by poor bone quality and/or malalignment and is therefore subclassified as:

2a. Poor bone stock.
2b. Malalignment.
2c. Combination.

Most patients have a combination of malalignment and osteoporosis but are predominantly affected by their poor bone quality. Unlike type 1 failures, these patients are rarely in need of an urgent surgical intervention. Therefore, a conservative approach can be initially trialled. Bracing as well as vertebroplasty or kyphoplasty should be considered to avoid progressive collapse and deformity. However, the clinician should recognise that vertebral body cementation may affect subsequent extension of fusion if necessitated, particularly if pedicle screws are considered necessary. Therefore, surgeons treating these patients should consider alternative fixation techniques, such as cortical trajectory screws, in the cemented vertebrae if extension is subsequently required. In those that become asymptomatic these fractures should be treated as osteoporotic compression fractures. In those that remain symptomatic and are amenable to operative intervention, the treatment should be:

2a. Bone supplementation ± bracing until fracture union is achieved. In a globally aligned spine with union of the fracture, no operative intervention is required.
2b. Deformity correction with extension of fusion and increased fixation. Increased fixation is necessary because the bone has shown evidence of weakness, even in the absence of global osteoporosis, and therefore increased fixation is necessitated.
2c. a ± b: Bone supplementation and bracing if the global malalignment is acceptable OR bone supplementation and deformity correction with extension of fusion, increased fixation and bracing if the malalignment is unacceptable.

2.3 Type 3: endplate failure

This is one of the most common forms of ASD and it occurs when the most cranial instrumented vertebral body collapses (**Figures 5** and **6**). It can occur with posterior or anterior/lateral implants and its causes can be classified as:

3a. Poor bone stock.
3b. Devascularisation of the endplate.
3c. Excessive endplate load.
3d. Combination.

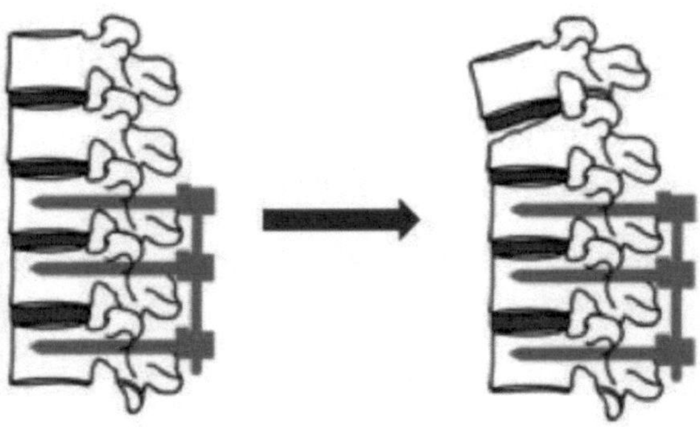

Figure 3.
Type 2 (adjacent bone failure).

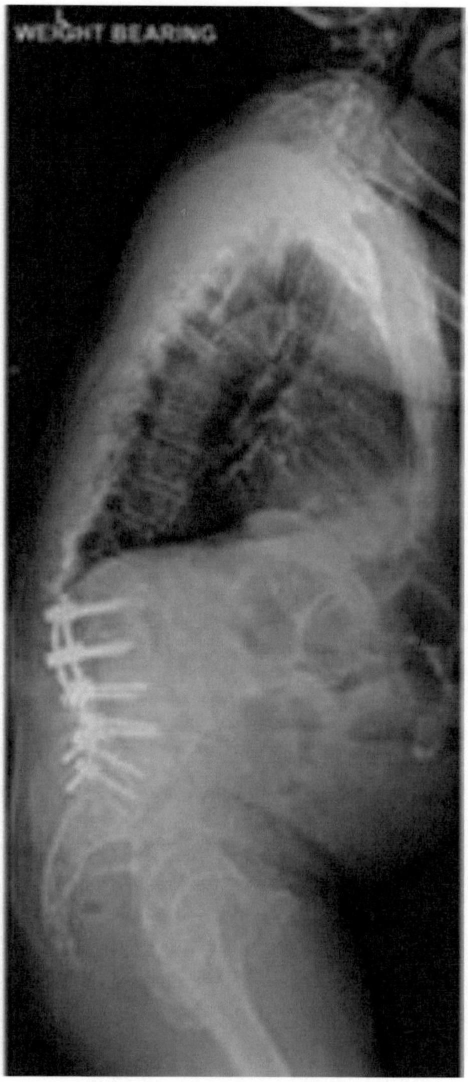

Figure 4.
A lateral standing full spine x-ray of a patient who had undergone an L2-S1 fusion with a failure to correct sagittal balance who developed an adjacent compression fracture of L1 that accentuated the spinal imbalance and over a 6-year period, despite attempted compensation with pelvic retrolisthesis and thoracic hypokyphosis, they developed a progressive anterolisthesis of T11/12 causing thoracic myelopathy.

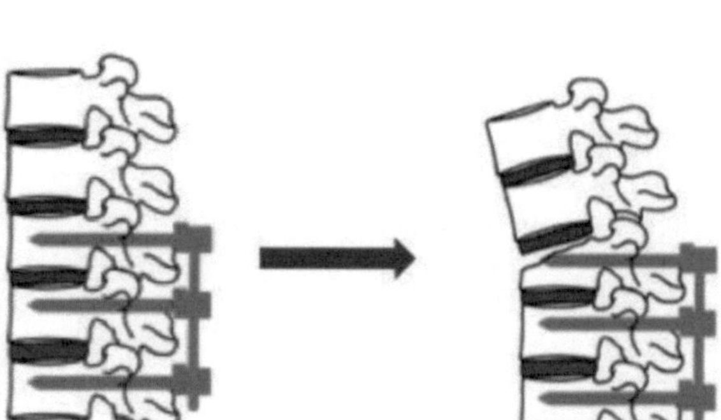

Figure 5.
Type 3 failure (endplate failure).

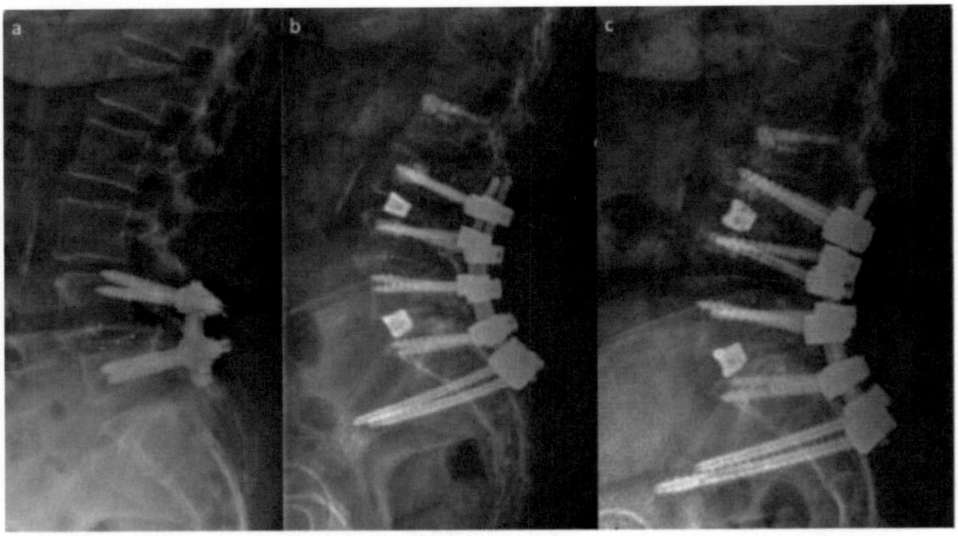

Figure 6.
Lateral standing X-rays of an obese osteoporotic patient who had previously undergone an L4/5 circumferential fusion complicated by global sagittal imbalance, pedicle screw malposition causing right L5 radiculopathy and dysfunction as well as progressive type 4d ASD of L3/4 causing critical central stenosis (a). They underwent revision of their instrumentation with L3-S2 fusion and correction of their sagittal balance, supplemented with cranial vertebroplasty (b). However, the patient developed type 3d ASD (c).

Most are thought to occur because of poor bone stock and therefore mimic osteoporotic compression fractures. However, end-plate devascularisation, either from a direct injury to the end arteries of the endplate by subcortical screws or by damage of the nutrient vessels to the endplate by anterior dissection can occur [17]. Similarly, with interbody devices the excessive load induced by rigid constructs can surpass the endplates' biomechanical tolerance and induce fracture.

Treatment depends on the severity of symptoms and the degree of compression of the vertebrae. In asymptomatic patients bracing to prevent further compression and bone supplementation may need to be considered if there is poor bone stock. In symptomatic patients amendable to operative intervention, treatment should consist of:

3a. Treat as osteoporotic compression fractures. Bone supplementation ± bracing. If metalware protrudes into the adjacent IVD consider deformity correction with increased fixation.
3b. Bracing. If metalware protrudes into adjacent IVD consider deformity correction. While the cause is endplate vascular compromise, there is to date no evidence that changing the surgical technique for the extension of fusion will reduce the risk, however surgeons should consider avoidance of cranial endplate compromise if possible (e.g. cortical trajectory screws, sublaminar bands or hooks).
3c. Deformity correction with extension of fusion and avoidance of a rigid interbody device at the most cranial fusion level.
3d. Treat as osteoporotic compression fractures. Bone supplementation ± bracing. If metalware protrudes into adjacent IVD consider deformity correction with extension of fusion and avoidance of both cranial endplate compromise and a rigid interbody device at the most cranial fusion level.

2.4 Type 4: IVD failure

This is a common form of ASD and is most commonly seen as a late complication of fusion (**Figure 7**). It may be related to inherent disc degeneration that would have occurred whether fusion was performed or not. However, it may also be caused by:

4a. Acute hyper-load which presents as an acute IVD prolapse.
4b. Diffusion insufficiency and/or chronic excessive loading which presents with progressive IVD desiccation.

Hyperload is caused by the rigidity imparted by the fusion. Typically, with circumferential fusions at the most cranial level this causes acute hyperload and acute disc prolapse. In contrast, isolated posterior or isolated interbody devices cause chronic overload as the fusion develops and micromotion of the fusion construct reduces. This causes progressive disc failure of the adjacent level (**Figure 8**). Similarly, implants that induce rigidity of the end-plates, such as subchondral pedicle screws limit the usual motion of the endplate. This motion, which mimics that of a trampoline, aids diffusion of nutrients into, and waste products out of the IVD. Thus, limiting its motion affects disc health by affecting its nutrient supply.

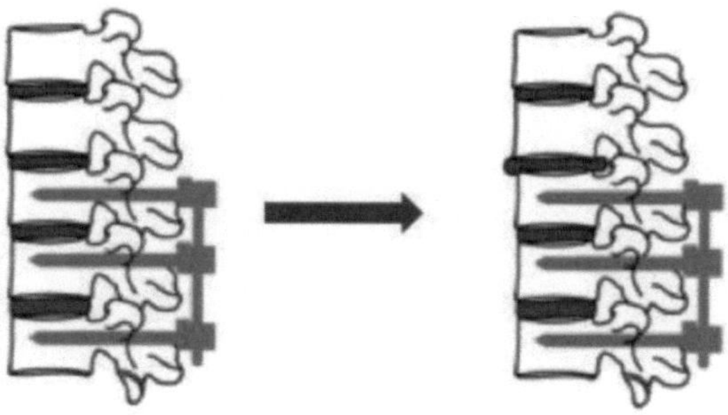

Figure 7.
Type 4 failure (IVD failure).

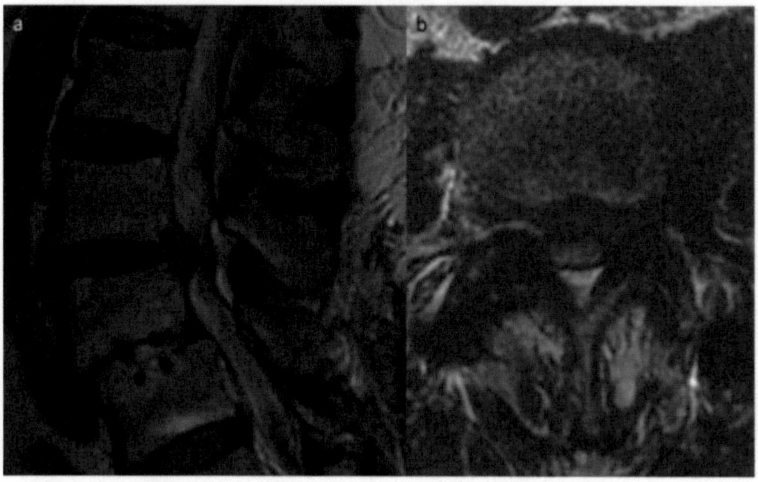

Figure 8.
Sagittal (a) and axial (b) MRI sequences of a type 4b failure above a L4/5 circumferential fusion. The IVD prolapse caused central stenosis and neurogenic claudication.

The treatment of this form of ASD depends on the symptoms and is the same for both 4a and 4b:

a. If neural compromise without instability: decompression alone.

b. If neural compromise with instability: decompression and single level fusion.

c. If discogenic pain or instability: single level fusion.

In patients with malalignment, deformity correction should be considered.

2.5 Type 5: facet failure

This form of ASD occurs when the facets joints fail, usually through hypermobility in the early stages and degeneration in the later stages (**Figures 9** and **10**). Hypermobility may occur in anterior procedures due to excessive stretch from oversized interbody devices, but this affects the motion segment that is fused and is therefore rarely a symptomatic problem once fusion occurs, but may cause long-term symptoms in disc arthroplasty.

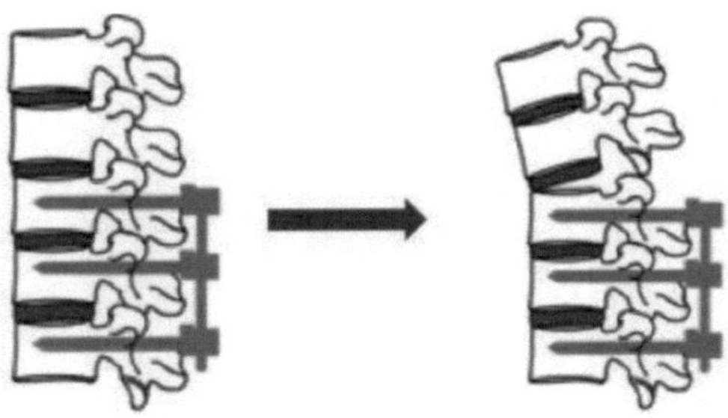

Figure 9.
Type 5 failure (facet failure).

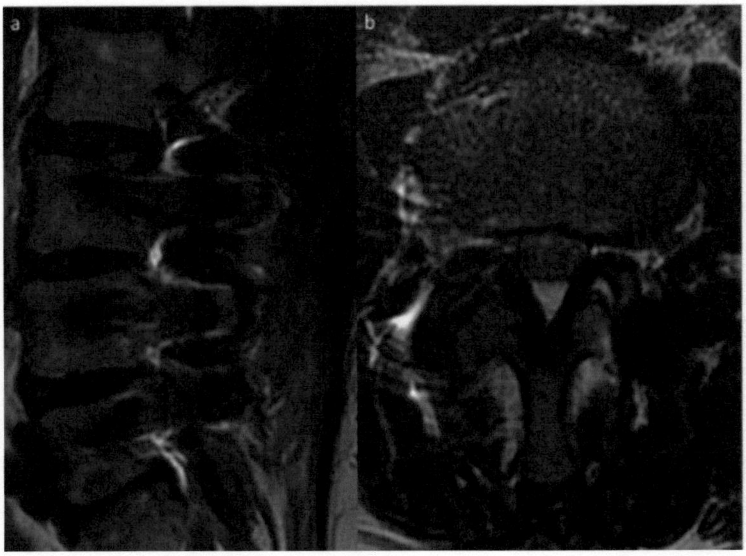

Figure 10.
Sagittal (a) and axial (b) MRI of a patient with a previous L3–5 postero-lateral fusion with left facet dysfunction causing a dynamic rotational deformity and unilateral retrolisthesis of L2/3 causing foraminal stenosis.

Type 5 failure is therefore predominantly seen with posterior instrumentation. The cause of type 5 failure is usually multifactorial and is classified as follows:

5a. Extensor mechanism dysfunction.
5b. Malalignment.
5c. Devascularisation and denervation of the adjacent facet joint.
5d. Metalware impingement on the adjacent facet joint.
5e. Combination.

To understand type 5 failure, one needs to appreciate the anatomy of the posterior spine. The extensor musculature acts to lordose the spine and is a dynamic control of spinal posture. It is innervated by posterior branches of the dorsal ramus, which run with the posterior vascular supply of these muscles, adjacent to the pars and is therefore at risk with the lateral dissection necessary for posterolateral fusion and standard pedicle screw insertion.

The extensor ligaments, namely the interspinous and supraspinous ligaments, and ligamentum flavum act as static restraints to kyphosis. In contrast, the intertransverse ligaments predominantly restrain lateral flexion. The facet capsule restrains excessive motion of the facet joint, particularly kyphosis. The facet joint itself is innervated and supplied by nerves and vessels that run with the dorsal muscular supply and are therefore at risk during posterolateral fusion and the dissection necessary for the insertion of standard pedicle screws.

We believe extensor mechanism dysfunction is caused by dysfunction of the dynamic or static restraints to segmental kyphosis. Dynamic restraint damage is caused by direct posterior musculature trauma and/or denervation and devascularisation of the paraspinal musculature most commonly induced by multi segment posterior dissection. This causes extension weakness, which results in adjacent segment kyphosis with load. Static restraint dysfunction is caused by transection of the cranial inter- and supraspinous ligaments or most cranial spinous process during the index procedure. The adjacent segment then relies on the ligamentum flavum and facet joint capsules as static restraints. Thus, adjacent flavectomy or direct capsular injury further disables the static restraints. Damage to the adjacent intertransverse ligaments is rarer, because the ligaments at risk are usually incorporated into the fusion, and the lateral IVD capsule offers significant restraint to lateral flexion. However, if a cranial transverse process fracture occurs the adjacent intertransverse ligament is affected and that increases the load on the lateral IVD capsule and may predispose to coronal failure.

Malalignment, particularly sagittal imbalance, puts excessive strain on both the dynamic and static restrains. This is particularly important if there is already dysfunction of the extensor mechanism, as the additional load induced by malalignment needs to be compensated for by the extensor mechanism.

The facet joints themselves are also commonly injured with posterior instrumentation. This is caused by the dissection necessary to insert posterior instrumentation, particularly standard pedicle screws through a midline approach, which involves far lateral dissection with stripping of the soft tissue from the posterior facet capsule and exposure of the pedicle entry point, which damages the neurovascular supply of the facet joints and extensor musculature.

Percutaneous insertion of the most cranial posterior implants is therefore preferable if possible, because this limits the degree of dissection necessary for insertion of the metalware, reducing the risk of neurovascular injury to the extensor mechanism and facet joints.

Metalware impingement on the adjacent facets is also common with pedicle screws, with estimates of up to 60% of pedicle screws breaching the facet [18–20].

Furthermore, even without facet joint breach, impingement can occur of the adjacent inferior articular process on the pedicle screw or rod with spinal extension, driving the adjacent level into kyphosis.

The treatment of asymptomatic patients or those not amenable to operative intervention remains non-operative. However, the treatment of symptomatic patients amendable to operative intervention is as follows:

5a. Single level extension of fusion, with protection of the extensor mechanism. This may involve the use of interbody fusion from anterior or lateral approaches, or a posterior approach with cortical trajectory screws or percutaneous insertion of cranial pedicle screws, with protection of the ligamentous restraints to kyphosis.
5b. Deformity correction and extension of fusion.
5c. Single level extension of fusion, with protection of the adjacent facet, often with anterior or lateral approaches, or a posterior approach with cortical trajectory screws or percutaneous insertion of pedicle screws.
5d. Dependent on facet function

- Facet non-functional: single level adjacent fusion.

- Facet functional: remove or reposition metalware depending on fusion of instrumented levels.

5e. Deformity correction with extension of fusion and avoidance of extensor mechanism and adjacent facet injury.

This classification broadly classifies ASD into anatomical and pathological groups, in order to further our understanding of its aetiology and treatment. However, as with any classification, it has limitations. Some patients with ASD fit more than one category and others fail in an atypical way. In such cases, the causes may be multifactorial and therefore the treatment may differ from those proposed in this classification system. Clinicians should be aware of these nuances and treat patients accordingly.

Understanding this anatomical and pathological based classification system allows treating clinicians to limit the modifiable risk factors for ASD after thoracolumbar fusion. By optimising bone quality preoperatively, the surgeon reduces the risk of bone failure, such as type 1a, 1c, 2a, 2c, 3a and 3d. In addition, ensuring spinal alignment and balance, reduces the risks of all failure mechanisms. Furthermore, ensuring adequate fixation at the time of operative intervention surgeons will reduce the risk of type 1b and 1c failure. However, this must be achieved without complete rigidity, which imparts excessive load through the cranial endplate and adjacent IVD motion to type 3c and type 4 failure. In addition, posterior dissection should be limited to avoid type 5a, 5c and 5e failure and the most cranial implants should avoid damage of the cranial endplate causing type 3b failure and the adjacent facet causing type 5d failure. Abiding by these principals reduces the risk of ASD, but does not prevent ASD because there remain non-modifiable risk factors for the condition.

Similarly, if ASD does develop, the clinician should critically appraise the causes of the failure, to ensure that optimal treatment is provided. In the setting of bone failure, bone supplementation should be provided, however, these alone fail to resolve the problem and therefore bracing or further surgical intervention is necessary. In all revision procedures, spinal alignment and balance should be considered. Abiding by the same principals as discussed above, clinicians will reduce the risk of recurrence.

Lastly, this classification is the first to describe the pathophysiology of ASD and therefore provides a framework on which further work can expand the prevention and treatment of this increasingly common condition.

In conclusion, this anatomical and pathological based classification system allows treating clinicians to limit the modifiable risk factors for ASD, understand the causes of ASD and offer a treatment algorithm for ASD. Furthermore, understanding this classification and the causes of failure allows clinicians to not only diagnose and treat ASD, but also offers a clearer understanding of what modifiable factors should be addressed during the index procedure. In addition, it illustrates that new technologies to eliminate modifiable risk factors are necessary, which should stimulate research and industry to find solutions to this common problem.

Acknowledgements

The authors are grateful to Glynny Kieser for her editorial input, and Amelie Poilliot for her illustrative input.

Author details

David Christopher Kieser[1*] and Niels Hammer[2]

1 Department of Orthopaedics and Musculoskeletal Medicine, University of Otago, Christchurch, New Zealand

2 Department of Orthopaedic and Trauma Surgery, University of Leipzig, Leipzig, Germany

*Address all correspondence to: kieserdavid@gmail.com

References

[1] Zhang C, Berven SH, Fortin M, et al. Adjacent segment degeneration versus disease after lumbar spine fusion for degenerative pathology: A systematic review with meta-analysis of the literature. Clinical Spine Surgery. 2016;**29**:21-29

[2] Anderson G. The Burden of Musculoskeletal Disease in the United States. 3rd ed. USA: Bone and Joint Initiative; 2014

[3] Glattes RC, Bridwell KH, Lenke LG, Kim YJ, Rinella A, Edwards C. Proximal junctional kyphosis in adult spinal deformity following long instrumented posterior spinal fusion: Incidence, outcomes, and risk factor analysis. Spine. 2005;**30**(14): 1643-1649

[4] Kim YJ, Bridwell KH, Lenke LG, Glattes CR, Rhim S, Cheh G. Proximal junctional kyphosis in adult spinal deformity after segmental posterior spinal instrumentation and fusion: Minimum five-year follow-up. Spine. 2008;**33**(20):2179-2184

[5] Hyun SJ, Rhim SC. Clinical outcomes and complications after pedicle subtraction osteotomy for fixed sagittal imbalance patients: A long-term follow-up data. Journal of Korean Neurosurgical Association. 2010;**47**(2):95-101

[6] Kim HJ, Lenke LG, Shaffrey CI, Van Alstyne EM, Skelly AC. Proximal junctional kyphosis as a distinct form of adjacent segment pathology after spinal deformity surgery: A systematic review. Spine. 2012;**37**(22):S144-S164

[7] Mendoza-Lattes S, Ries Z, Gao Y, Weinstein SL. Proximal junctional kyphosis in adult reconstructive spine surgery results from incomplete restoration of the lumbar lordosis relative to the magnitude of the thoracic kyphosis. The Iowa Orthopaedic Journal. 2011;**31**:199-206

[8] Yagi M, Akilah KB, Boachie-Adjei O. Incidence, risk factors and classification of proximal junctional kyphosis: Surgical outcomes review of adult idiopathic scoliosis. Spine. 2011;**36**(1):E60-E68

[9] Hart R, McCarthy I, O'Brien M, Bess S, Line B, Adjei OB, et al. Identification of decision criteria for revision surgery among patients with proximal junctional failure after surgical treatment of spinal deformity. Spine. 2013;**38**(19):E1223-E1227

[10] Hart RA, Prendergast MA, Roberts WG, Nesbit GM, Barnwell SL. Proximal junctional acute collapse cranial to multi-level lumbar fusion: A cost analysis of prophylactic vertebral augmentation. Spine. 2008;**8**(6):875-881

[11] Theologis AA, Miller L, Callahan M, Lau D, Zygourakis C, Scheer JK, et al. Economic impact of revision surgery for proximal junctional failure after adult spinal deformity surgery. Spine. 2016;**41**(16):964-972

[12] Helgeson MD, Bevevino AJ, Hilibrand AS. Update on the evidence for adjacent segment degeneration and disease. Spine. 2013;**13**(3):342-351

[13] Cheh G, Bridwell KH, Lenke LG, Buchowski JM, Daubs MD, Kim Y, et al. Adjacent segment disease following lumber/thoracolumbar fusion with pedicle screw instrumentation: A minimum 5 year follow-up. Spine. 2007;**32**(20):2253-2257

[14] Lee JC, Kim Y, Soh JW, Shin BJ. Risk factors of adjacent segment disease requiring surgery after lumbar spinal fusion: Comparison of posterior lumbar interbody fusion and posterolateral fusion. Spine. 2014;**39**(5):E339-E345

[15] Toyone T, Ozawa T, Kamikawa K, Watanabe A, Matsuki K, Yamashita T, et al. Subsequent vertebral fractures following spinal fusion surgery for degenerative lumbar disease: A mean ten-year follow-up. Spine. 2010;**35**(21):1915-1918

[16] Park P, Garton HJ, Gala VC, Hoff JT, McGillicuddy JE. Adjacent segment disease after lumbar of lumbosacral fusion: Review of the literature. Spine. 2004;**29**(17):1938-1944

[17] Dunbar L, Vidakovich H, Loffler S, Hammer N, Gille O, Boissiere L, et al. Anterior cervical blood supply—A cadaveric study. Surgical and Radiologic Anatomy. 2019;**41**(6):607-611

[18] Chung KJ, Suh SW, Swapnil K, Yang JH, Song HR. Facet joint violation during pedicle screw insertion: A cadaveric study of the adult lumbosacral spine comparing the two pedicle screw insertion techniques. International Orthopaedics. 2007;**31**(5):653-656

[19] Patel RD, Graziano GP, Vanderhave KL, Patel AA, Gerling MC. Facet violation with the placement of percutaneous pedicle screws. Spine. 2011;**15, 36**(26):1749-1752

[20] Babu R, Park JG, Mehta AL, Shan T, Grossi PM, Brown CR, et al. Comparison of superior level facet joint violations during open and percutaneous pedicle screw placement. Neurosurgery. 2012;**71**:962-970

Chapter 4

The Use of a Dynamic Elastomeric Fabric Orthotic Intervention in Adolescents and Adults with Scoliosis

Martin Matthews and James Wynne

Abstract

The use of dynamic elastomeric fabric orthoses in the non-surgical management of scoliosis has been growing over the last 20 years in the paediatric populations and has now started to be used in adolescent and adult patients as well. The concepts of treatment concentrate on the use of movement and changes in the neurological pattern generation, to reduce scoliosis curve Cobb angles and pain that is sometimes experienced due to an altered positional sense. This chapter introduces research, including recent computer modeling, to demonstrate the effects of the combination of two different layered textiles which enable improved comfort, aesthetics as well as scoliosis clinical management. The textile combination enables a total body suit to use 3D scoliosis brace knowledge to assist in developing new orthotic interventions for adolescents and adults with both neurological and idiopathic onset scoliosis, for several different presentations.

Keywords: dynamic elastomeric fabric orthoses, spinal decompression, spinal translation, spinal tone management, pain relief, proprioception, exoskeleton

1. Introduction

There are different presentations of scoliosis, including genetic spinal deformities, neuropathic and idiopathic onset scoliosis, that develop in two to three percent of the population (depending on the research report) during skeletal development. Sometime this can cause complex management issues which can present at any age and continue well into adulthood and throughout the geriatric years. These presentations at times require differing orthopaedic, physical therapy and orthotic interventions to improve symmetry and pain management.

Rigid and semi-rigid bracing has been in existence for thousands of years. One of the earliest examples being an orthopaedic corset of a tree bark that was discovered painted in cliff dwellings of pre- Columbian Indians circa 900 AD (**Figure 1**) [1].

Furthermore, a number of interesting historical, almost medieval (by today's standards) devices have been designed to counter the deformities utilising complex metal designs to force the spine into a required position. A number of researchers have incorporated thigh fixation as described by German orthopaedists in the 19th and early 20th centuries (**Figure 2**) [1].

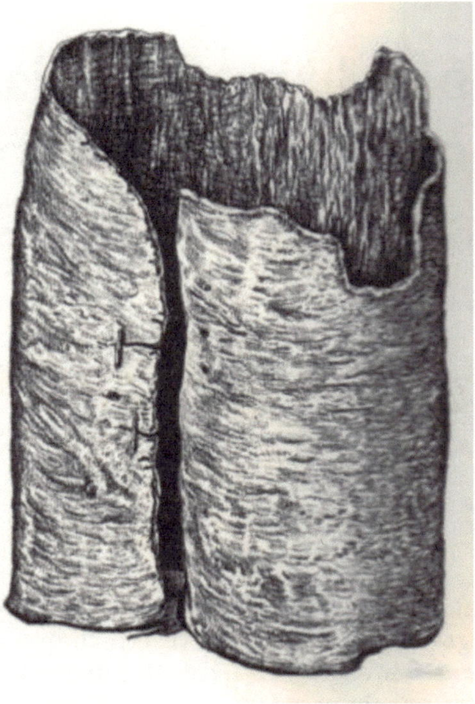

Figure 1.
Drawing of an orthopaedic corset of tree bark from the pre-Columbian Indians cliff dwellings Circa 900 AD. Colorado State Historical Museum (Denver).

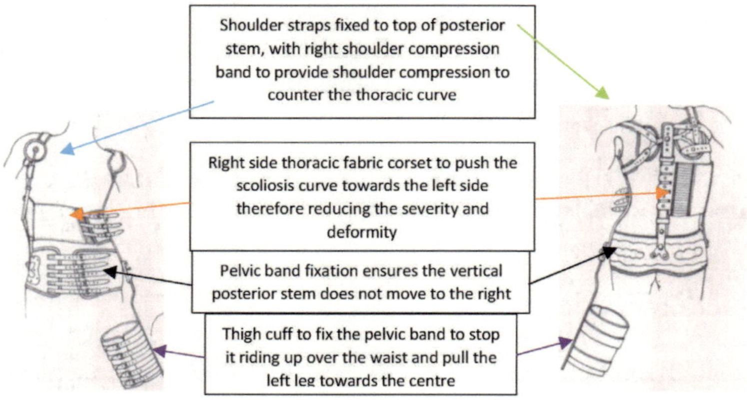

Figure 2.
Scoliosis brace with thigh attachment (Redrawn from an early print).

In 1971, the Boston modular rigid (**Figure 3**) and semi-rigid plastic spinal brace system was developed and has been used (and evolved) for over 40 years [2], becoming the stalwart of scoliosis management of both neurological onset and idiopathic scoliosis around the world.

Rigid bracing has been proven to be effective in preventing curves from progressing to the point of needing surgery and in some cases, have helped to reduce the curve magnitude [3]. The "Dose", the amount of time the patient wears the brace, has proven to be vital to bracing success. An international, partially randomized control trial (BRaist study) showed that if patients wore their full time brace an average of 12.9 hours per day or more, they had a 90–93% chance of not having

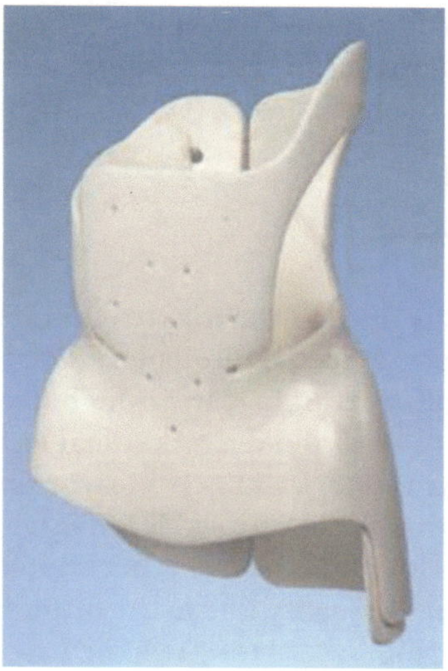

Figure 3.
Original Boston Brace made with 15 degrees of lumbar lordosis, fitted with compression pads and cut out to provide spinal asymmetry.

their curve progress to the point of requiring surgical intervention [4]. Wearing the brace for less than 6 hours per day, equated to a 42% chance of surgery requirement.

The opposite is true for neurological onset scoliosis, where a child with cerebral palsy (for instance), would wear similar corrective cast bracing. Spinal bracing would require "anniversary" casting (annual corrective brace casting) to ensure the brace was fit for purpose. The curve, however in neurological cases generally continues to worsen until the child reaches maturity in late adolescence and requires surgery to correct the spine. This happens even, with self-reported compliance. When compared to the natural history of neuromuscular scoliosis, bracing does not prevent the rate of curve progression [5], however there are reports that bracing improves seating [6], standing and walking postures as well as other benefits for people with neurological disorders.

Both idiopathic and neuropathic onset scoliosis presentations use the basic brace concept of marking up an x-ray to show the left/right lean and rotation of the vertebra at each level to inform the positioning of pads or pressure required to provide

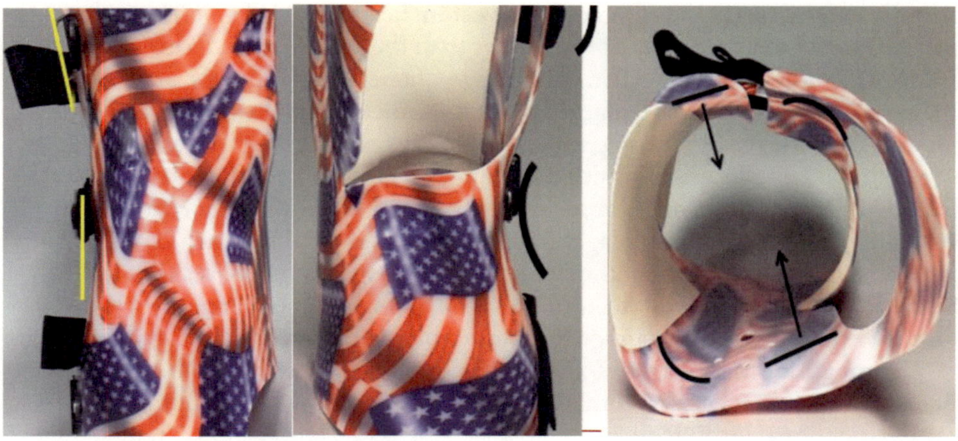

Figure 4.
Bston Brace 3D-custom fabricated from scan, built in asymmetry.

the corrective force on the body, known as "blue printing". Blue printing also informs the position of the cutaway areas of the brace. **Figure 4** illustrates the result, using computer aided design and manufacturing (CADCAM) to carry out this role.

2. Scoliosis presentations

Scoliosis presentations are due to numerous causes and include genetic changes and omissions to the bony structures; neurological dysfunction to the muscles that support and stabilize the spinal structure; hypo-mobility disorders (Ehler Danlos Syndrome); degenerative scoliosis and dysfunctional learnt patterns of movement. All learnt functions like sitting and walking is a learned pattern of movement, which rely on movement through error based learning to recalibrate a particular movement and altered position awareness [7]. In children, with cerebral palsy (CP) their image of self is different to reality due to the difference in their internal model of self [8]. This shows in sitting, where they feel they are sitting straight, however in reality they are sitting to one side. This loads one side of the spine and sets up a dysfunctional pattern, which they learn and understand as normal. This results in the complex scoliosis cases we see in adolescents and adults- particularly when requiring wheelchairs. Most of these issues are generally identified during childhood, however, they can affect adolescents and adults of all ages with scoliosis, whether idiopathic or neuropathic in origin. Bracing is therefore a major intervention in adolescents and adults who cannot or do not want to follow the surgical route. Although there are several different scoliosis causes, this section will concentrate on the two main causes of scoliosis in adolescents and adults, which require bracing: idiopathic onset scoliosis (IOS) and neuropathic onset scoliosis (NOS).

Idiopathic onset scoliosis is defined as a lateral curvature of the spine, that is greater than or equal to 10 degrees with no known cause. It is further defined by the age of initial presentation, infantile (zero to 3 years), juvenile (3–9 years of age) and, adolescent (10–17 years of age). Progression is related to growth, so patients are most vulnerable to curve progression during periods of rapid growth as occurs during the adolescent years. The Boston Brace, which introduced the concept of using a symmetrical form to fabricate the original modules which then, depending on the patient's x-ray analysis (blueprint) and physical presentation, is trimmed and had strategically placed pads added to make it asymmetrical. Numerous studies have shown this method to be effective [3, 9]. Recently, through the advent of scanning and CADCAM technologies, a custom fabricated asymmetric model of the patient is used to fabricate the brace rather than the symmetrical form. The Boston Brace 3D (**Figure 4**), the ARTbrace and Rigo Cheneau - type braces, are examples that utilise three point triangular sideways movement (known as translation) viewed from the posterior using x-rays of the back, re-aligning a small number of vertebra causing a localised positional change {segmental moulding [10]}. They included the combination of forces for regional and local de-rotation to achieve corrective balance and physiological alignment in the sagittal plane [11] **Figure 5**.

These coupled with physiotherapeutic scoliosis specific exercises (PSSE) like Schroth physiotherapy work to keep the spine mobile [12], but are also held physically by a brace, which encourage the re-alignment of the spine during wear.

Neuropathic onset scoliosis (NOS) typically appears in early childhood, particularly in children with cerebral palsy (CP), and continues into adulthood due to the dysfunctional loading on the spine which causes vertebral and rib remodeling. Twenty five percent of people with CP will develop scoliosis curves and range from 5% incidence for bilateral spastic to 74% in people with quadrilateral- spastic presentations due to the imbalance of muscle pull, and brain damage [13]. Most curves

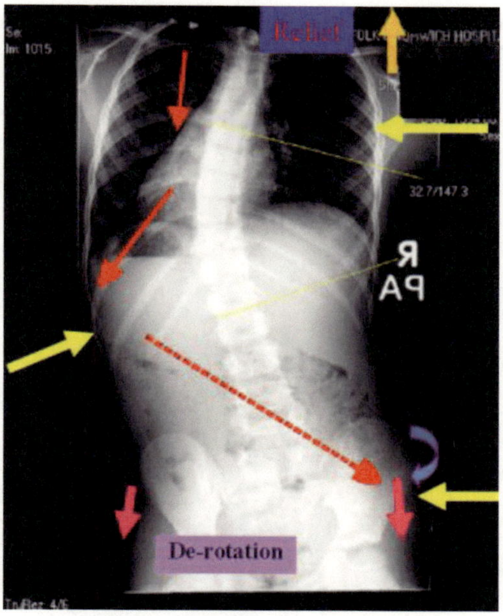

Figure 5.
Diagrammatic representation of X-ray blueprinting for dynamic elastomeric fabric scoliosis suit- identifying the three points of pressure (yellow arrows), distraction (orange arrow), downward compressive force (pink arrow) and de-rotational shoulder compression force (Red thin arrows).

present as a single thoracolumbar or lumbar "C" shaped curve associated with pelvic obliquity and hip dislocations, often seen in gross motor function classification scale (GMFCS) [14] Level 4/5 presentations.

The gross motor functional scale is a way of identifying what level of function a child with cerebral palsy can achieve and is divided into 5 levels.

Level 1 identifies children who can walk at home, school and in the community including outdoors with limited coordination, speed and balance when running and jumping.

Level 2 identifies children who can climb stairs holding on to a support rail, however they can experience difficulties in balancing and walking when on slopes and rough ground particularly when in crowded or confined areas.

Level 3 identifies children who need hand-held walking and mobility aids in doors and need supervision when climbing stairs. They will also tend to use self-propelled or powered wheelchairs for longer distances.

Level 4 identifies children with require physical assistance or powered mobility in most settings If physically assisted they can walk short distances around their homes and will often require powered wheelchairs and body weight support walkers. A self-propelled wheelchair or powered chair will be used whilst at school, outdoors and in the community.

Level 5 identifies children who are transported in manual wheelchairs in all areas. The children have a limited ability in maintaining head control and trunk posture [15]. They also have trouble with arm and leg control A classification at the age of 6 is unlikely to change level during adolescence into adulthood.

Therefore level 4 and 5 indicates that the child/young adults will be requiring wheel chair support, with basic or complex design dependent on severity [14]. A classification at the age of 6 is unlikely to change level during adolescence into adulthood. Twenty percent of scoliosis curves develop as a "S" shaped curve with balanced, symmetrical thoracic kyphotic and lumbar lordotic curves [13], normally associated with idiopathic scoliosis see **Figure 6a**, **b**.

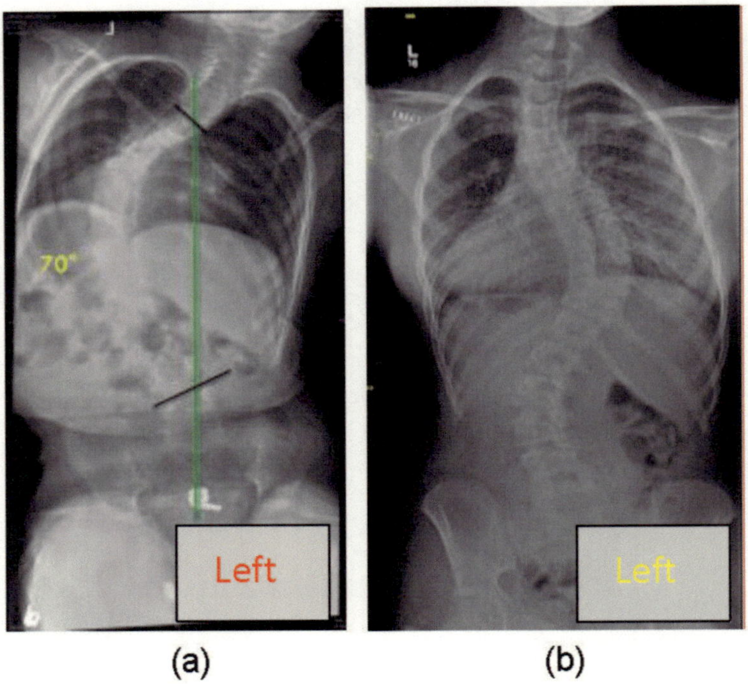

Figure 6.
(a) A typical "C" shaped curve to the left. (b) A typical "S" shaped curve with a left lumbar and right thoracic curve.

Adolescents with GMFCS Level 4/5 are dependent on wheelchairs for mobility, which due to a neuropathic or neuromuscular disease, have a 90% increased risk of progressive spinal deformities due to the impairments in postural balance and motor control [16]. There is also an increased risk of flexed sitting patterns due to hip flexion contractures, encouraging spinal deformity due to the loss of the protective lordosis and atypical loading patterns. These can lead to pain and discomfort leading to increased decline in the patients quality of life (QOL) [17].

Ehlers Danlos Syndrome is a group of disorders that affect the connective tissue that supports the tissues and human body organs, blood vessels, bones and skin [18]. The signs include extremely loose joints, which can sublux completely, coupled with extreme pain. In recent years, this connective tissue disease has been linked with young women presenting with scoliosis [19]. The women are often in their mid-thirties, following pregnancy and present with extreme pain, often due to nerve compression.

3. Elastic scoliosis bracing

Rigid and semi- rigid (foam based) spinal orthoses have been the common bracing option for adults, however the developments in dynamic elastomeric fabric orthoses (DEFO) using form fitting elasticated orthoses, have shown promise in the clinics based on the authors' clinical use. The use of "elastic" orthoses has become an additional bracing option, alongside rigid and semi-rigid scoliosis braces.

There are two variants of DEFOs that have evidence for use in scoliosis management, namely SpineCor® and Dynamic Movement Orthoses (DMO®). There are other Lycra suits, but they are mainly used in juvenile (less than 9 years of age) patients. As this chapter is concerned with adolescents (10–17 years of age) and adults (18 years of age and older) with scoliosis, they will not be discussed.

SpineCor® has a resemblance to an early somewhat simple, but controversial idea of using "Oblique and Spiral bandage" utilized by Richard Barwell of London in 1868 that purported to assist in scoliosis management (**Figure 7**).

An eminent surgeon of his time, Henry Bigg in 1877 [1], questioned the validity of this bandage. However, in recent years the use of diagonally activating compressive force correction now supports the early thinking behind the bandage type orthoses.

The SpineCor® brace has had some success in younger patients with idiopathic scoliosis, utilizing the compressive and de-rotative effects of strong elastic bands fixed to a bolero shaped vest and either a plastic anterior and posterior shell held in place by webbing straps, or shorts which enable fixation of the corrective straps. The original prospective observational study on the effectiveness of the SpineCor brace, used a standardised criteria proposed by the Scoliosis Research Society (SRS). The study included 170 patients (158 girls and 12 boys). Thirty-nine participants required spinal surgery, 12 withdrew and 14 participants were weaned out of the treatment as curve progression was deemed to be stable. Of the 105 remaining participants, 47 completed the 2-year brace follow up [20].

A more recent retrospective study evaluating the effects of the SpineCor brace that also followed the Scoliosis Research Society criteria for brace management of adolescent idiopathic scoliosis reported that the SpineCor® brace treatment could increase the risk of curve progression, when compared to the Boston Brace. Scoliosis curve progression occurs in the spine due to changes occurring naturally in the vertebra and intervertebral discs. If left without treatment the curve will increase exponentially [21]. The use of correctly fitted and function spinal brace will reduce the rate of curve progression and in most cases reducing the Cobb angle indicating curve regression. In the SpineCor brace study, a total of 243 patients were treated with either the Boston brace (146) or the SpineCor brace (97) with scoliosis

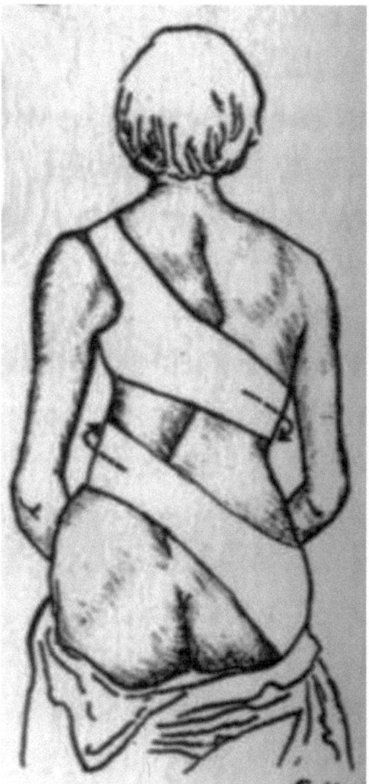

Figure 7.
Oblique and Spiral bandage utilised by Richard Barwell of London in 1868. (Page 182 Orthopaedic Appliances Atlas, Vol.1 1952).

curve progression recorded across the group. The average curve progression for the SpineCor cohort was 14.7° ±11.9°, compared to 9.6° ± 13.7°. The proportion of patients reaching 45° was 51% (SpineCor) and 37% (Boston Brace), however the proportion of patients referred for surgery was 39% (SpineCor) and 30% (Boston Brace). The paper concluded that the odds of reaching a ≥ 45 was 2.07 times greater when using a SpineCor brace [22].

Further comparison studies showed that the SPoRT (Symmetric, Patient oriented, Rigid, Three-dimensional, active braces) was more effective than SpineCor® [23, 24]. The SPoRT concept provides evidence of effect and is shared in three types of rigid braces. The Sforzesco brace joins two previous brace designs (Sibilla & Lapadula), to provide a new spinal concept which avoided the need for casting the worst scoliosis presentations. Brace compliance was a key driver for the new treatment journey and included mechanical efficacy, the active brace principle, versatility, and adaptability coupled with teamwork and patient compliance. Scoliosis correction is provided through the shape of the adjustable rigid body envelope, mechanical" pushes" encouraged the spine to move into a predetermined void, that adapted and remodeled body shape to unwind the scoliosis curve presentation (**Figure 8**).

A randomised controlled trial compared the SPoRT rigid concept with the SpineCor dynamic brace to identify the treatment effect over time. Using a retrospective controlled study, two groups were reviewed using clinical and X-ray evaluations. Data was recorded at the beginning and end of the study to record the scoliosis curve angles for SPoRT braces (20 patients) and SpineCor braces (41 patients). Both brace interventions proved to be effective in improving the aesthetics of the deformities, however the SPoRT brace was found to be more effective than SpineCor in avoiding scoliosis curve progression [23].

There is evidence that the SpineCor® brace relieves pain by improving posture following the reduction of mechanical strain on the neuromuscular system in adults. The brace enables spinal joint off-loading by reducing the misalignment of the spinal segments. Pain perception data from Marcotte [25] which reviewed the effect of SpineCor spinal braces used for between 18–28 months from 30 adults (26 females/4 males), which showed 77% overall improvement in pain recorded. Half of the patients reported total pain relief, although there was no significant reduction in spinal curvature in adults. This outcome may have been similar to the reasoning in the original designs in the 18th century.

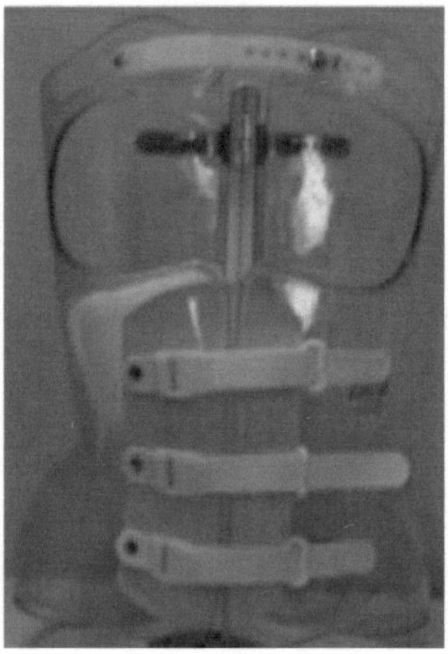

Figure 8.
The Sforzesco brace- the most recent addition to the SPoRT scoliosis management concept.

Dynamic Elastomeric fabric orthoses (DEFO) were first reported in 1960. The authors described the use of crepe bandages wrapped around a child with athetoid cerebral palsy. This caused reduction in the muscle tone in his arms and legs which then enabled more stability and less fatigue [26].

In 1995, an Australian paper describing the use of custom "UPsuit" Lycra® suits on children and young adolescents, with semi-rigid reinforcement to provide stability to the spine and to improve sitting balance [27]. Management of the scoliosis was provided by metal spiral boning stitched in fabric pockets to provide rigidity and apply resistance to stretch - providing areas of higher resistance to stretch [28]. However, there is limited scoliosis management using Second Skin suits (**Figure 9**).

In 2007, a study from the United States introduced a basic base Lycra® short and pants with shoulder straps called the "Stabilizing Pressure Input Orthosis" (SPIO) [29]. The study stated that significant functional improvements to balance, improved postural control and muscle readiness were found, however as an observational and discussion report, the only evidence provided was photographic pre and in-intervention images. It was postulated that there were deep sensory changes which could account for the reduction in athetoid movement and the improved stability of the spine in children presenting with low tone [30].

In 1999, Rennie et al., in a repeated measures study of 8 children (7 children had cerebral palsy and 1 with Duchennes muscular dystrophy), used laboratory gait analysis to report on the outcomes of a long arm, long legged suit made by Camp Ltd., in the United Kingdom (**Figure 10**). Five participants showed a reduced root mean square error (RMSE) scores indicating improved postural stability, confirming the findings of Blair [28] and Hylton [30]. However, the improved postural stability only positively affected the distal stability in three participants, which could have been due to the short 6-week duration of the trial.

Compression at the pelvis in DEFO shorts [31, 32] can reduce the pain experienced by adults with intellectual disabilities, who experience high rates of falls and have gait and balance issues. The reason for this may be because the DEFO suits and shorts reduce the amplitude and range of movement in the spine and pelvis,

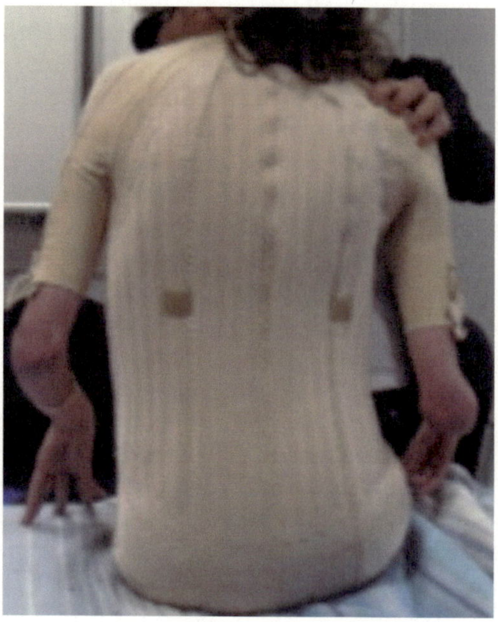

Figure 9.
Back view of a postural suit. https://www.secondskin.com.au/Products/postural_splint

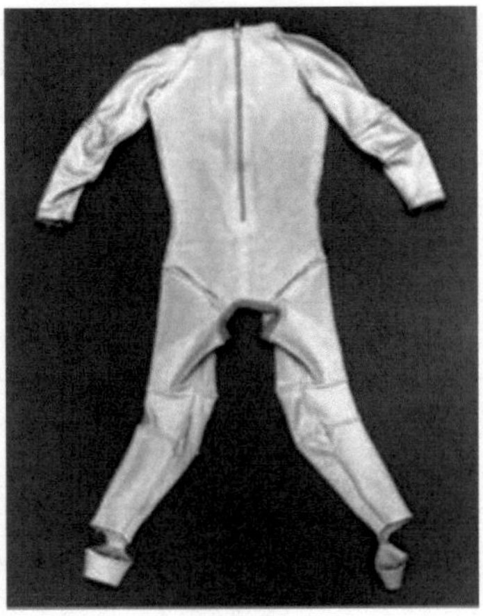

Figure 10.
The original basic Lycra® long legged and armed suit used in the Rennie study.

therefore providing pelvic stability [33] which consequently enhance the quality of life in both children and adults.

Scoliosis suits were first reported by Matthews and Crawford in 2004 [34] in a single case study using a DEFO to treat a child with a tumour on the spine. The tumour had previously been excised at the age of 7 yrs. The tumor extraction operation caused a 33-degree Cobb angle scoliosis to appear at the tumour site T9 (**Figure 10**). The child, did not want a rigid brace due to the rigid brace appearance [34]. The orthotist prescribed a non-invasive vest top suit to control the curve, based on experience, with children presenting with hypotonic cerebral palsy with scoliosis.

The suit applies a tight fit at the hips and thighs to prevents the suit from riding up and therefore a resistant force is applied to the shoulders. The suit uses the principle of pressure applied to the shoulders to facilitate an improved sitting posture, as seen when neurodevelopmental physiotherapists place their hands on the shoulders of children with low spinal muscle tone and retract the shoulders coupled with downward pressure to facilitate an extension of the spine in sitting. The compression of the suit also enables the patient to become more aware of their bodies position in space through heightened proprioception.

Elastomeric fabric sideways translation reinforcement panels, which were designed to reduce the scoliosis Cobb angle were added, using the patient pre-intervention x-rays and blue printing process (**Figure 11a** and **b**), as described in the Boston Brace clinical manual. The manual describes how to use the patient X-rays to identify the vertebra levels, position of the spinal curve and rotation [35] to guide prescription. The addition of, overlying a "V" shaped translation panel (see yellow arrows on **Figure 11b**) to the convex side of the curve ensured a lateral force was applied below the apical vertebra as close to midline as possible – this provided a long low pressure on the ribs which encourage the patient to move away from the pressure point into the comparative void of no reinforcement on the right side. A further shoulder compression panel (see red arrows on **Figure 11b**), extends upward posteriorly over the left superior border of the scapula and over the anterior shoulder, before continuing downwards until clear of the axilla and then continues diagonally anteriorly across the anterior ribs to finish at the right greater trochanter. The left shoulder compression, spinal derotation panels were so efficient, that the suit required the addition of touch and close fastening over the left shoulder to allow for the left shoulder to rise to accommodate the right compression, so assisting curve reduction.

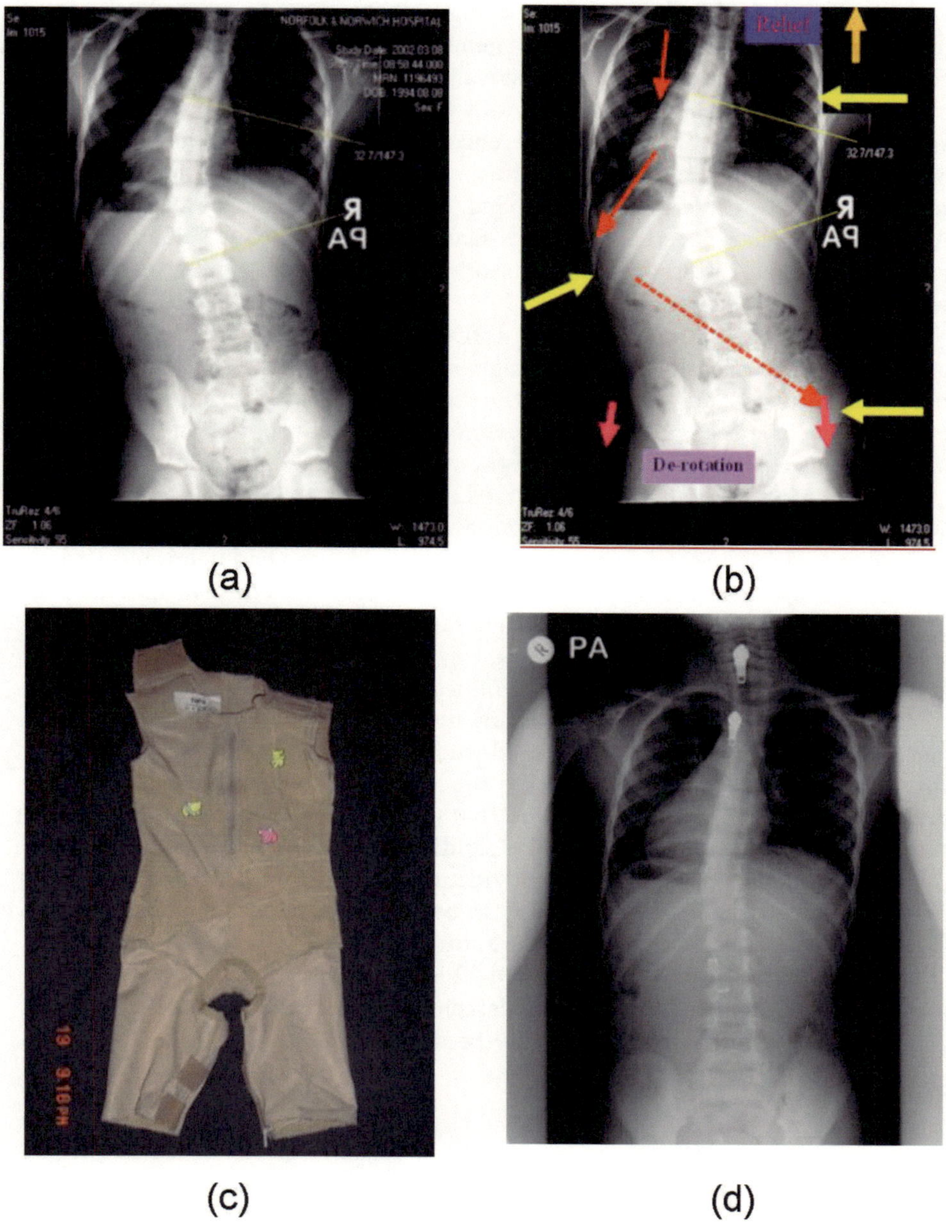

Figure 11.
(a) Before Suit X-ray shows 32.7° thoracic curve convex to the left. (b) The blueprinting which includes 3 point force (yellow) arrows, red full and dotted shoulder compression and de-rotation effect, and the upward shoulder movement (orange arrow) The two downward pink arrows indicate the counter force on the legs and hips that applies the pressure to the shoulders. (c) The scoliosis suit shows the lateral translation curve "V" shaped pane. The shoulder de-rotation and compression panel on the right of the photograph coupled with the touch and close over the shoulder pressure relief fastening. (d) In-suit X-ray shows 15° curve a reduction of 17.7 degrees, which was held for 2½ years. Note dual zips of suit.

The patient was provided with a 18 mm heel raise to accommodate the pelvic tilt, but this had no effect on the scoliosis. Throughout the next 2.5 years the patient was provided with three suits to accommodate natural growth. The suit was worn 23 hours a day. The in-suit x-rays (**Figure 11d**) showed that the curve was held at 15° Cobb angle, a reduction of 45%. The tumour re-occurred after 2 ½ year and was again removed, with additional surgery to staple the vertebrae above and below the tumor site to prevent a re-occurrence of the scoliosis.

Matthews & Bridges [36] reported a single case study of a 5-year-old child, presenting with myotonic dystrophy (a genetic disorder affecting muscle function), coupled with pectus carinatum (a chest wall deformity in which the breastbone pushes outward instead of being flat), and a left 70° Cobb angle thoracic curve, apex T8 with a vertebral rib angle difference greater than 20° and therefore very likely to worsen (**Figure 13a** and **b**). The x-ray provided the blueprint for a vest top scoliosis suit to be prescribed and supplied. One year later, routine x-rays showed that the curve had reduced to 35°, a 50% Cobb angle reduction in suit and the vertebral rib angle difference had reduced to under 20° and meaning that the curve was unlikely to get worse (**Figure 12**).

Although it is not normal to expect a 50% reduction in Cobb angle, this result proved that scoliosis suits could treat higher angle curves, than rigid braces successfully. This result also highlighted that the shoulder on the convex curve side should extend down over the upper arm to prevent the shoulder protraction (shoulder moving anteriorly) around the edge of the vest segment (**Figure 13c**).

In 2016, Matthews et al. [23] reported on an audit of 180 children and adolescents with, or at risk of developing scoliosis from five centres in the south of England, UK. The study reported on 121 subjects who had been supplied with DEFO suits and scoliosis suits within three centres. The centres used local protocols to use DEFOs to treat children identified as GMFCS Level 4/5, who were primarily wheelchair ambulators, starting to develop a small lateral body shift and were at risk of developing scoliosis prophylactically. Fifteen years of scoliosis suit management experience by the clinical team had indicated that patients with GMFCS level 4/5 had reduced surgical interventions due to early suit provision. The audit also reported the noncompliance in the use of rigid braces in this sample. It is understood that rigid brace use in neurological onset scoliosis is difficult to wear due to the rigidity and lack of movement within the orthosis. There is no convincing evidence in the recent literature to suggest that rigid spinal orthotic management in neurological onset scoliosis is effective [37], which was also confirmed in the audit data.

Over the years, the children who had DEFO scoliosis suits were followed through their peak growth rates as adolescents. As the scoliosis development was identified early, the clinical team were able to observe and develop an

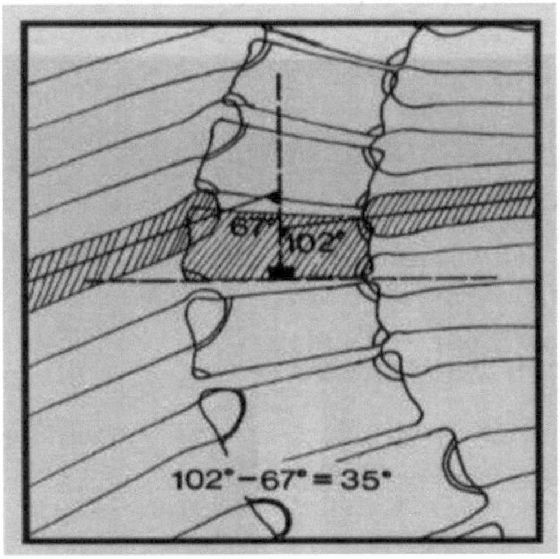

Figure 12.
This diagram shows the vertebral rib angle difference. If over 20° the curve is considered to get worse. https://boneandspine.com/rib-vertebral-angle-in-scoliosis/#how-to-measure-the-rib-vertebral-angle.

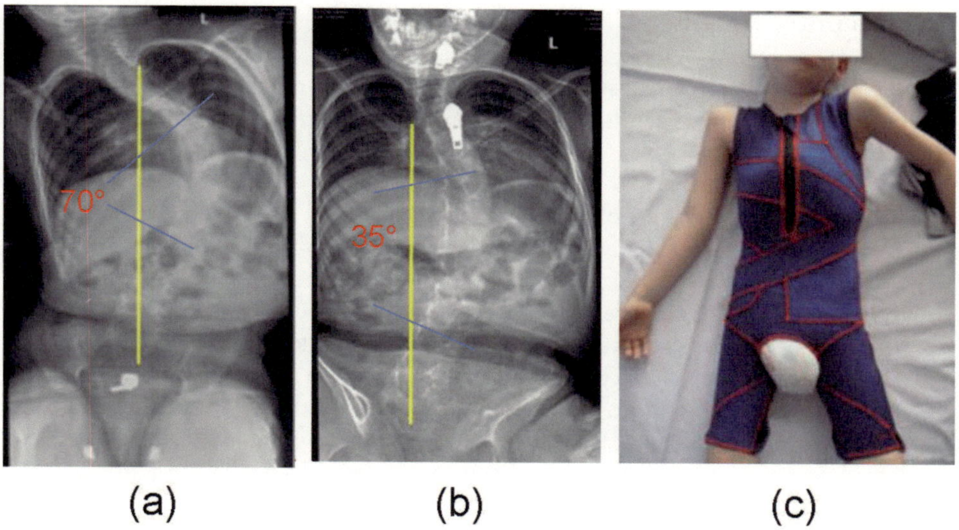

Figure 13.
(a) Pre suit X-ray. (b) X-ray in scoliosis suit. (c) The child in suit. "V" shaped translation panel is clearly seen originating from right hip to left waist and back to under right axilla. Note: shoulder protracting around the vest segment.

understanding of which scoliosis curves were at high risk of progressing. The clinical team understood that during growth, peak growth occurs during early adolescence and continued throughout adolescence. Scoliosis- specific DEFO suits were shown to maintain the corrections in Gross Motor Functional Classification Scale (GMFCS) level 4 and slow the curve progression for those patients in GMFCS level 5 throughout adolescence.

It is recognised that most of the research in this field is in paediatrics, however there are now papers in preparation on an adult male using the DEFO scoliosis suit management. The N = 1 single case study (currently in press) reports on the changes to an adult male with ataxia telangiectasia (a rare inherited disorder that affects the nervous and immune system resulting in difficulty with coordinating movement from early childhood) with poor head control and issues with poor control of posture and extrapyramidal movements. The design included baseline pre-intervention gait laboratory data collection of the patient sitting, carrying out a routine hand function, the quality-of-life task of taking a drink to his mouth and reach to touch function. This was repeated in a postural scoliosis design suit, which included bilateral enclosed shoulders and standard strength paneling, and then again in a stronger, higher specification paneled postural scoliosis suit with interesting outcomes [38].

Ehlers Danlos Syndrome (EDS), an inherited condition that affects connective tissue is characterised by hyper-elasticity of the joints and fragility of the skin [39]. There is anecdotal evidence of patients with scoliosis, where pain is a major problem due to the connective tissue lack of rigidity that allows joints to dislocate. Serious pain is often experienced in women with EDS caused scoliosis, often from the age of 30 years, preventing or making their activities of daily living difficult. They also have increased reliance on strong pain medication. The use of DEFO scoliosis suits for this client group has produced improved posture with similar results to the adult use of SpineCor brace. The effect on the scoliosis angle was minimal, but effective, because pain was reduced due to the improved positioning and stabilisation of joints [25]. Therefore, the improved quality of life often leads to reduced pain relief medication.

4. Concepts of treatment

The DEFO scoliosis suits use different mechanisms to correct scoliosis in comparison with rigid or semi-rigid braces and it is important to understand the fourteen concepts.

1. **Compression of the trunk** provides a bracing effect due to the circular support normally associated with a rigid brace. Circumferential pressure provides some compressive stabilisation to the spine [26] and can reduce pelvic pain due to pelvic force closure [40], resulting in an improved level of comfort and quality of life. The compression on the trunk is a maximum of 26.9 mmHg (2 layers of fabric) – well below the level required to risk skin damage caused by restriction of blood flow or ischemia. If additional elastomeric layer of material are added on top of two layers, the pressure applied is reduced due to the "bridging effect" seen were three layers of material do not expand and contract on a local basis, due to adhesion to the other overlaid layers [41].

2. **Upper body counter de-rotational reinforcement** panels applied to the base suit design to compress the thoracic curve [34]. This reinforcement panel enables containment of the shoulder complex (including the upper arm and distal clavicle) with downward pressure applied to the convex thoracic curve coupled with rotation to unwind the mobile scoliosis (See **Figure 11b** and **c**).

3. **Dampening effects on external dynamic forces** acting across joints may contain overshooting of specific movement and reduce unwanted movements due to restriction and compression of the orthosis. The use of compact compression orthoses show a reduction in uncontrolled movement-patterns [42]. This is often seen as extreme uncontrolled upper and lower limb movement in patient with spastic athetoid patients. Circumferential pressure applied to the trunk, arms and legs provide a heightened idea of body position in space via the sensory nerves which help the brain to understand where the body parts are. This can reduce the excessive movements seen in some cerebral palsy presentations.

4. **Enabling the brain to update the internal model of self** to formulate motor plans for movement is well recognised in patients with cerebral palsy, to predict the best muscle synergy to achieve the required motor goal [8]. Due to the brain damage in patients with cerebral palsy the brain's image of self is different to reality and is seen clearly in unilateral presentations (hemiplegia) or one affected side. Therefore, if a patient with unilateral upper arm involvement reaches out to reach an object, it is highly likely that they will miss the object by approximately 25 mm. If they carry out the same task but wearing a glove specifically designed to turn their hand upwards (to supinate), they will be more able to go reach out directly to the object without missing it. This is due to the change in sensory information going from the hand to the brain and the ability to alter the resultant movement **requirement to react to this sensation.**

5. **An Exoskeleton** provides reinforcement to weaker muscle and skeletal biomechanics as the support and dynamic panels enable clinicians to provide biomechanical assistance the weaker muscles, like supination to adult with cerebral palsy or strokes. For instance, patients who present with unilateral upper limb weakness due to the brain damage and cannot supinate their forearm (rotate their palm upwards). Diagonal panels are built into the arm section of the

glove which can put tension on the arm and resulting in derotation of the forearm to provide a functional position in supination rather than pronation (hand turning palm downwards). See **Figure 14** [43, 44].

A similar affect can be seen where DEFO suits will provide compression to stabilise the trunk and additional scoliosis specific panels can initiate lateral and/or rotational movement of the spine (See **Figure 15**).

6. **Improved motor control** treatments are valuable in improving long term outcomes such as seen in chronic low back pain [45].

7. **Low level continual pressure guides rather than forces positional changes** by encouraging movement or gradual muscular localized stretch of muscle sarcomeres [46]. Physiotherapists use a long low pressure stretch to gain movement in stiff limbs as this allows different muscle fibres to give and lengthen with the gentle pull. A hard pull would cause the body's damage limitations mechanisms to activate and resist the pull strongly as muscle damage might occur, which makes the outcome worse.

8. **Proprioception**, often referred to as (kinesthesia) and often thought of as the "six sense" [47] is the knowing of where your body is in space [48], when your eyes are shut. This is built up over a time of learning specific motor function patterns, utilising feedback from sensory receptors within the muscle, skin and joints (feedback) and central signals from the brain to the muscles (feedforward), which is related to motor output. This enables the individual to combine other sensory information to judge limb position and movements by learnt patterning and continues whatever the age [44].

9. **Reduction of pain** as seen in children with cerebral palsy [17], and chronic low back pain where pain impacts the quality of daily life [45].

10. **Reduction in time for sequential movement planning due to feedback/feed forward system** enables the improved ability to develop an effective motor plan for desired action [8], If you think about lifting your arm upwards with a weight, you will find your brain has to set several actions in progress prior to the movement. Firstly, the spinal muscles will be put under tension to stabilise the thorax before you can even extend your arm out to pick up the weight. Once you reach the weight you must further activate your spinal and now upper limb muscles to enable the weight to be lifted. If you failed to do this, you would find that the weight was not moving at all and there is a likelihood that you would already have fallen forwards due to the weight of your arm only. The process of preparation is a sequential movement. People with cerebral palsy therefore would find this task extremely difficult. Wearing compression orthoses again enables them to plan the task quicker.

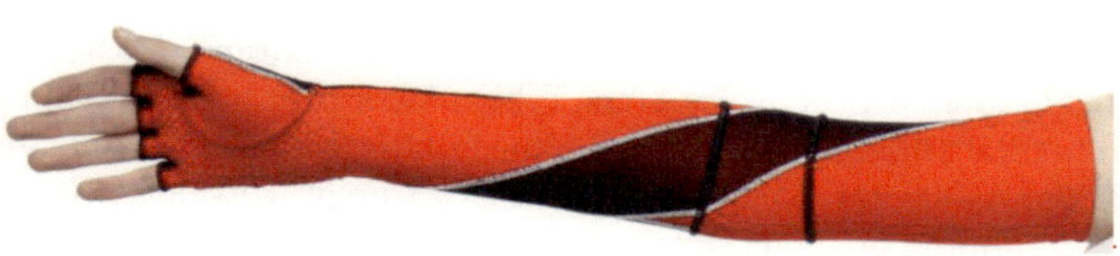

Figure 14.
Shows the diagonal reinforcement built into the DMO long sleeved glove to provide a supinatory in-built rotation causing the wrist to be held in supination.

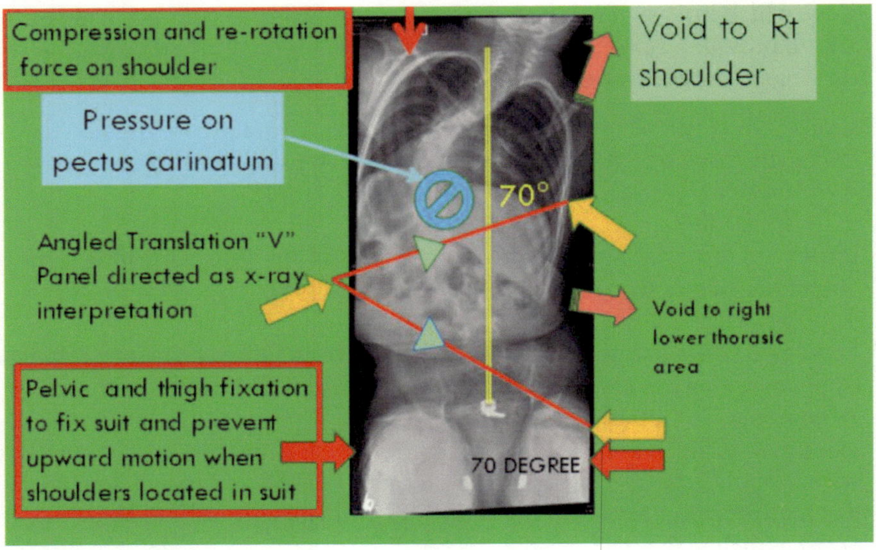

Figure 15.
The scoliosis blueprint for a scoliosis suit showing the translation panel with angulated yellow arrows on the left, representing the resultant force expected from the positioning of the two (upper and lower yellow arrows) on the right side of the image.

11. **Retraining of the motor control patterns** by repetition of sensation and movement have been used in rehabilitation of sports injuries particularly in patellofemoral pain and shoulder stabilisers, often after strength training has been unsuccessful in pain reduction [49, 50].

12. **Translatory reinforcement** to create a lateral shift to counter a lumbar or thoracolumbar curve [34].

13. **Truncal postural control is an important determinant of motor function** with a precise relationship between the control of the individual trunk segments and resultant effects on gross motor function and mobility [51]. In some very young children with cerebral palsy, they are unable to eat solid food as they are unable to move the food across their mouths due to the amount of energy, they have to use to hold their head ups as they are so floppy due to the cerebral palsy. However, if you stabilise them in a neonate suit or full height standing frame that allows the child to just concentrate on holding their head up and not the whole spine. They can often find that they are can start to eat solid foods after 6 weeks as they can learn to hold their heads up enough to move the food across their mouths so they can chew.

14. **Understanding the 3D nature of both idiopathic and neurological onset scoliosis** [11] is key to outcome expectation. The blueprinting principles (See **Figure 5**) used for the manufacture of the traditional Boston modular Brace and Boston 3D custom Brace apply to identify the correct vertebral level to treat and understand the vector forces required to reduce the curve and improve sagittal balance. The blue-printing process described in the clinical training manuals ensures the clinicians are totally focused on each vertebral level and fully understand the angle of inclination and the rotation of each vertebra.

5. Discussion

The criteria for using suits designed specifically for a person with scoliosis is like the use of rigid bracing, in that best outcomes are achieved in early intervention when children have good spinal mobility. When used in older adolescents and adults, it is sensible to encourage the patient to complete a course of physiotherapeutic scoliosis specific exercises (PSSE), which includes auto-correction in 3D, training in activities of daily living (ADL), stabilising the corrected posture and patient education. These exercise protocols have level II evidence, both for independent use and in conjunction with spinal bracing in patients with curves less than 45° Cobb angles and are also suggested prior to surgery to help improve outcomes [9].

In a testimonial, one patient reported improved balance, upright standing and patient confidence. The use of PSSE, combined with an enhanced power scoliosis DEFO suit provided a mechanism to ensure maximum vertebral movement, combined with the unique proprioceptive and long term low level force, known to be the most effective for muscle stretching [46]. When the suit was first applied the patient reported loss of balance, which indicated that the suit was having the desired effect and her mother reported a reduction in the pain she was experiencing [52]. After 3 years, the suit reduced the scoliosis progression and scoliosis surgery at the end of DEFO treatment was no longer required (**Figure 16**).

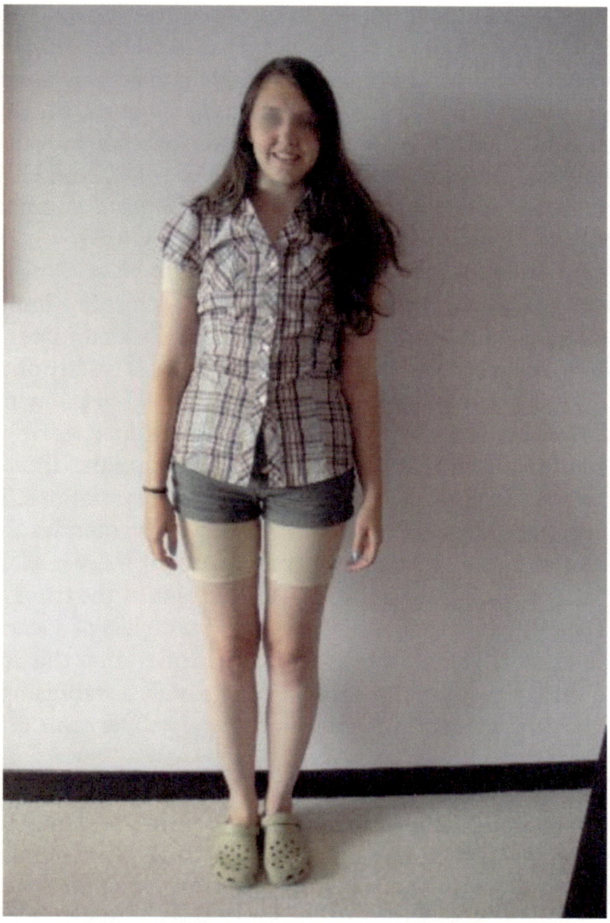

Figure 16.
Sixteen-year-old lady in structural scoliosis suit.

Improvements in walking have shown that improved proprioception and provision of a flexible supportive exoskeleton can improve image of self, reduced hip sway, hip force closure and to reduce the known mechanisms of increased lordosis to lock the spine, enabling smother movement [33, 40, 53]. People with scoliosis can learn a new sitting position by the mechanism of continual motor learning carried on throughout life. This can be initiated by external forces including poor sitting position, spinal injuries, strokes as well as left or right-handed wheelchair controls. The use of dynamic orthoses, therefore, have an important role to play in centralising the spine without the use of rigid force.

The mechanisms utilised in DEFOs dynamic orthotics became more objective than subjective, with more research and reports of use. It is important to understand the mechanism for the changes observed in the patients and their reaction to the intervention. For a number of years, the outcomes detected were put down to improved patient stability from the compressive forces on the hip and shoulder, coupled with the distraction of the shoulders as seen in proprioceptive neuromuscular facilitation (PNF) [54]. There is evidence that PNF on the trunk can reduce chronic low back pain in adult women, if applied in the sitting position [55]. There are two commonly used exercises. Rhythmic stabilisation training (RST) which uses isotonic (muscle working within normal contraction range) contraction of the agonistic (opposing) muscle patterns which results in co-contraction of the antagonists. The isometric contraction of the muscles is provoked into working by pushing or pulling an immovable object. This prevents muscles shortening in length and improves fitness and builds up strength. It is used where weakness is a primary factor. The combination of isotonic exercises (COI) is used to evaluate and develop the ability to carry out purposeful and controlled movements, involving alternating concentric (circular), eccentric (non-circular) and isometric movement to treat strength deficiency and range of motion. Four weeks of RST and COI proprioceptive neuromuscular facilitation have shown increased muscle endurance, decrease in back pain intensity, as well as improved functional ability.

There are several different mechanisms that appear to be working together to provide the DEFO's positive reported outcomes and therefore it is important to understand the different concepts of treatment. The orthoses initiate change where the effect is likely to be constrained by the linear range of elasticity of the fabric or "dynamic" [56]. The fabrics are designed to grip the skin while allowing air and moisture through without slippage. A DEFO uses these properties by griping onto the skin and therefore transfers the torsional resistance from the different reinforced fabric layers, which are designed to have different linear orientations. These forces are conveyed through the skin and soft tissue directly to the muscles and skeleton beneath with set movements expectations. For instance, if there is a long spinal curve to the right, set pattern options are applied to the left side of the trunk to resist stretch, therefore providing a stiffer area in the suit resulting with less of a lean to the right.

It is understood that slight compression of the trunk rather than distraction (as used in rigid and semi rigid spinal orthoses) can provide a stabilising effect on low core stability in children presenting with cerebral palsy. The same effect can be initiated in adults.

New innovations are signaling that the use of textile fabric materials can have positive spinal correction. Computer modeling has been developed to geometrically model scoliosis through finite element modeling (FEM). It is a numerical technique used to perform finite element analysis (FEA) of any given phenomenon (https://www.simscale.com/blog/2016/10/what-is-finite-element-method/). The use of 2D x-ray clinical data on appropriate textile materials, measuring physical and mechanical properties were used to determine the performance of the textile brace in terms of Cobb angle through FEM simulation. The results showed that textile materials with banded parallel fabric layers provide good softness and air permeability (key for compliance in hot climates). There was high capacity to provide a 14.4% Cobb angle improvement, when used on a teenage patient with adolescent idiopathic scoliosis presenting with a 62° typical double curve [57]. This provides some medical and biological engineering evidence of the orthotic effect.

This study also highlighted the need for cosmetic appearance and the effects on patient compliance. Rigid braces have been proven to be effective in reducing scoliosis progression [4], however there have been issues with compliance particularly from discomfort caused by the brace and psychological stress from the visual impact. Patient involvement in brace design and aesthetics have shown improved compliance [58], so the use of elastomeric fabrics will further enhance this patient based involvement and provide scoliosis suits which are more comfortable in both adolescents and adults alike thereby improving activities of daily life.

There is evidence for the use of DEFO scoliosis management in neuropathic onset scoliosis and early indicators that the same orthoses can be effective in adolescent idiopathic scoliosis. The key thing to remember is the need for flexibility of the spine to be able to use dynamic movement to facilitate a spinal scoliosis angle reduction, vertebral rotational control and improved cosmetic outcome. The most effective treatment plan would be to combine PSSE with the use of scoliosis specific DEFO suits to start the treatment early in the onset rather than wait for the 25° Cobb angle starting point, that has historically been suggested. This highlights the need for early intervention and further research on this specific scoliosis presentation.

6. Conclusion

The use of scoliosis DEFO suits have shown that specifically designed paneling can provide scoliosis curve reduction based on tried and tested clinical evaluation and design to provide cosmetic orthoses which are discrete and robust. The onset of dynamic elastomeric fabrics has provided both proprioceptive and mechanical means to change body movement and function for all age groups. The continuing research provides an insight into the future of orthotics and provision of patient involvement are assisting in improved outcomes offering new areas of use. The case study discussed earlier within this chapter, also shows the possibility of using DEFO structural scoliosis suits for adolescent idiopathic scoliosis, which provides a further orthotic option for treatment and research, particularly in the early stages of the disorder.

Compliance with the DEFO suits is presumed to be improved due to the less rigid orthotic structure and improved cosmesis, coupled with the use of low-level continual pressure to gradually encourage the patient to relearn motor pathways. These orthoses achieve improved sitting and standing posture, which results in the reduction of the scoliosis curve Cobb angles and pain for adolescents and adults. Dynamic elastomeric fabric orthoses have shown that orthotics do not need to be rigid to provide a lasting neurophysiological effect combined with the enhancement of continual motor learning and reprogramming of the brain and movement patterns.

Conflict of interest

Martin Matthews is employed as Chairman and United Kingdom state registered clinical specialist orthotist by DM Orthotics Ltd., UK in clinical roles, within the National Health Service hospitals. He is also an Honorary Associate Professor at the University of Plymouth.

James H. Wynne, CPO is employed as Vice President – Director of Education by Boston O&P, Boston, Massachusetts, USA. JIm Wynne and I worked as co authors and therefore although I fully acknowledge Jims involvement we worked closely together as dual authors.

Authors contributions

Both authors have contributed equally to the design and writing of this chapter and have over thirty years of personal experience in managing scoliosis in all age groups and presentations.

Acronyms and abbreviations

ARTbrace	asymmetrical rigid torsion brace
ADL	activities of daily living
Boston 3D	Boston three dimensional scoliosis brace
CADCAM	computer aided design and manufacturing
COI	combination isotonic exercises
CP	cerebral palsy
DEFO	dynamic elastomeric fabric orthosis
DMO	Dynamic movement orthosis
EDS	Ehlers Danlos syndrome
FEA	finite element anaylsis
FEM	finite element modeling
GMFCS	gross motor function classification scale
IOS	idiopathic onset scoliosis
NOS	neuropathic onset scoliosis
PNF	proprioceptive neuromuscular facilitation
PSSE	physiotherapeutic scoliosis specific exercises
QOL	quality of life
RMSE	root mean square error
RST	rhythmic stabilisation training
SPIO	stabilising pressure input orthosis
SPoRT	symmetric, patient oriented rigid three-dimensional

Author details

Martin Matthews[1*] and James Wynne[2]

1 Faculty of Health: Medicine, Dentistry and Human Sciences School of Health Professions, Peninsula Allied Health Centre, University of Plymouth, Plymouth, UK

2 Boston O and P, Avon, Massachusetts, USA

*Address all correspondence to: martin.matthews@plymouth.ac.uk

References

[1] Thomas A. Appliances for the spine and trunk. In: Edwards J, editor. Orthopaedic Appliances Atlas. 1. Ann Arbor, Michigan: The American Academy of Orthopaedic Surgeons, Inc; 1953. p. 179-250.

[2] Hall JM, ME; Cassella, MC. Manual for the Boston Brace Workshop. Boston: Boston: Children's Hospital Medical Centre; 1976.

[3] Emans JK, A; Bancel,P; Hall,J; Miller,M. The Boston Brace System for Idiopathic Scoliosis: Follow up results in 295 patients. Spine. 1986;11(8):792-801.

[4] Weinstein SD, LA; Wright,JG; Dobbs,MB. Effects of Bracing in Adolescents with Idiopathic Scoliosis. The New England Journal of Medicine. 2013;369:1512-1521.

[5] Terjesen T, Lange JE, Steen H. Treatment of scoliosis with spinal bracing in quadriplegic cerebral palsy. DevMedChild Neurol. 2000;42:448-454.

[6] Nakamura NU, M; Inaba,Y; Machida,J; Okuzumi,S; Saito,T. Use of dynamic spinal brace in the management of neuromuscular scoliosis: a preliminary report. Journal of Pediatric Orthopaedics. 2014;23(3):291-298.

[7] Leech KDR, R; Bastian,A. Movement and perception recalibrate differently across multiple days of locomotor learning. J Neurophysiology. 2018(120):2130-2137.

[8] Kurz MB, KM; Heinrichs-Graham,E; Wilson,TW. Neurophysiological abnormalities in the sensorimotor cortices during the motor planning and movement execution stages of children with cerebral palsy. DevMedChild Neurol. 2014;56(11):1072-1077.

[9] Negrini SD, S; Aulisa,AG; Caprowski,D; Schreiber,S; De Mauroy, JC; Diers,H; Grivas,TB; Knott,P; Kotwicki,T; Lebel,A; Martin,C; Maruyama,: O'Brien,J; Parent,E; Rigo,M; Romano,M; Stikeleather,L; Wynne,J; Zaina,F. 2016 SOSORT gudelines: orthotpadic and rehabilitation treatment of idiopathic scoliosis dring growth. Scoliosis and Spinal Disorders. 2016;2018(13.1):1-48.

[10] de Mauroy JJ, A; Gagaliano,F; Lecante,C; Barral,F; Pourret,S The new Lyon ARTbrace versus the historic Lyon brace: A prospective case series of 148 consecutive scoliosis with short time results after 1 year compared with a historical retrospective case series of 100 consecutive scoliosis: SOSORT award 2015 winner. Scoliosis. 2015;2015(10:26):1-15.

[11] Rigo MJ, M. Brace technology thematic series: the 3D Rigo Cheneau-type brace. Scoliosis and Spinal Disorders. 2017;12.10:1-46.

[12] Burger MC, W; PLessis,L; Geldenhuys,L; Joubert,F; Myburgh,E; Van Rooyen,C; Vermeulen,N The effecitveness of Schroth exercises in adolescents with idiopathic scoliosis: A systematic review and meta-analysis. South African Journal of Physiotherapy. 2019;75(1):1-9.

[13] Tsirikos AI. Development and treatment of spinal defromity in patients with cerebral palsy. Indian Journal of Orthopaedics. 2010;44(2):148-158.

[14] Wood E, Rosenbaum PL. The Gross Motor Function Classification System for Cerebral Palsy: a study of reliability and stability over time. DevMedChild Neurol. 2000;42:292-296.

[15] Alliance CP. Gross Motor Function Classification System (GMFCS) Australia: Cerebral Palsy Alliance; 2018 [cited 2018 26/01/2018]. Available from: https://cerebralpalsy.org.au/

our-research/about-cerebral-palsy/what-is-cerebral-palsy/severity-of-cerebral-palsy/gross-motor-function-classification-system/.

[16] Murans GG-F, EM; Saraste, H. Kinematic and kinetic analysis of static sitting of patients with neuropathic spine deformity. Gait & Posture. 2011;34(2011):533-538.

[17] Ramstad KJ, R; Skejeldal,O; Diseth,T. Characteristics of recurrent musculoskeletal pain in children with cerebral palsy aged 8 to 18 years. Developmental Medicine & Child Neurology. 2011;53(11):1013-1018.

[18] Medicine USNLo. Ehlers-Danlos syndrome. Your Guide to Understanding Genetic Conditions. Genetics Home Reference: USA.gov; 2020. p. https://ghr.nlm.nih.gov/condition/ehlers-danlos-syndrome.

[19] Henderson FA, C; Benzel,E; Bolognese,P; Ellenbogen,R; Francomano,C; Ireton,C; Klinge, P; Koby,M; Long,D; Patel,S; Singman,E; Voermans,N Neurological and spinal manifestations of the Ehlers-Danlos syndromes. American Journal of Medical Genetics. 2017;175(1):195-211.

[20] Coillard; Vachon VC, AB; Beausejour,M; Rivard,CH. Effectiveness of the SpineCor Brace based on the New Standardized Criteria proposed by the Scoliosis Research Society for Adolescent Idiopathic Scoliosis. Journal of Pediatric Orthopaedics. 2007;27(4):375-379.

[21] Will YSIQ, X; Walker,MR; Sanders,JO;. Cobb Angle Progression in Adolescent Scoliosis Begins at the Intervertebral Disc. Spine. 2009;34: 2782-2786.

[22] Gutman GB, M; Joncas,J; Beausèjour,M; Barchi,S; Labelle,H; Parent,S The effectiveness of the SpineCor brace for the conservative treatment of adolescent idiopathic scoliosis. Comparison with the Boston Brace. The Spine Journal. 2016;16:626-631.

[23] Zaina FD, F; Donzelli,S; Romano,M; Negrini,A; Lusini,M; Minnella,S; Negrini,S SpineCor vs rigid brace for Adolescent Idiopathic Scoliosis: end of growth results from a retrospective controlled study. In: SOSORT, editor. Scoliosis and Spinal Disorders; Chicago, USA: Springer; 2013. p. 1.

[24] Negrini SM, G; Tessadri,F. Brace technology thematic series- The Sforzesco and Sibilla braces, and the SPoRT (Symmetric, Patient oriented, Rigid, Three-dimensional, active) concept. Scoliosis. 2011;6(8):1-17.

[25] Marcotte L. SpineCor in the treatment of adult with scoliosis. In: Central B, editor. 7th International Conference on Conservative Management of Spinal Deformities; 25/2/2020; Montreal, Canada: Scoliosis; 2010. p. 1.

[26] Beaman P. Restriction, fatigue and motor capacity in athetoid children. In: Little Club Clinics in Developmental M, editor. Child Neurology and Cerebral Palsy. No2. London1960. p. 82-89.

[27] 2ndS. Second Skin Dynamic Lycra Splints for Neurological Dysfunction. 2000.

[28] Blair E, Ballantyne J, Horsman S, Chauvel P. A study of a dynamic proximal stability splint in the management of children with cerebral palsy. DevMedChild Neurol. 1995;37(6): 544-554.

[29] Hylton N. Deep Presure Sensory Input - SPIOFlexible Compression Bracing. NDTA Network. 2007:8-12.

[30] Hylton NA, C. The Use of Compression Stabilizing Type Bracing as an Adjunct to Therapy. Pediatric Rehabilitation. 1997;1(2):109-116.

[31] Finlayson JC, J; Shanmugam,S; Stansfield,B. Lycra splinting garments for adults with intellectual disabilities who fall due to gait or balance issudes: a feasibility study. Journal of Intellectual Disability Research. 2018:1-16.

[32] Snowdon NS, D; Potia,T; Wheat,J; McLean,S. Compression garments and fabric orthoses for rehabilitation and function: a systematic mapping review. International Journal of Therapy and Rehabilitation. 2018;25(12):655-664.

[33] Serrao MR, A; Casai,C; Mari,S; Conte,C; Draicchio,F; Sandrini,G; Pierelli,F. Use of dynamic movement orthoses to improve gait stability and trunk control in ataxic patients. European Journal of Physical and Rehabilitation Medicine. 2014;Edizioni Minerva Medica(January):1-4.

[34] Matthews MJ, Crawford R. The use of dynamic Lycra orthosis in the treatment of scoliosis. A treatment case study. Journal of International Society of Prosthetics and Orthotics. 2006;30(2):174-181.

[35] Emans JH, M; Hall,J; Hedequist,D; Karlin,L; Miller.J; Miller,R; Magin,M; McCarthy,C; Cassella,M; Ryan,K. The Reference Manual for the Boston Scoliosis Brace Boston, MA: Boston Brace International; 2003 16/09/2020. 46 p.

[36] Matthews MB, S, editor Does the use of dynamic elastomeric fabric scoliosis suits provide an improved and more user friendly options for early intervention in childhood scoliosis? SOSORT; 2011 19/05/2011; Barcelona: Scoliosis.

[37] Morris C. Orthotic Management of Children with Cerebral Palsy. Journal of Prosthetics & Orthotics. 2004;14(4):150-160.

[38] Hensiek A. Scoliosis Chapter for online book Reference N=1 scoliosis adult patient. In: Matthews M, editor. Agreed wording for pre publication outcome notification. ed. Spinal Deformities in Adolescents, Adults and Older Adults online book chapter: Intech Open; 2020. p. 1.

[39] Natarajan DS, D; Wong,Y; Luk,K; Cheung,K. Natural History of spinal deformity in a patient with Ehlers-Danlos syndrome: a case study with 20-year follow up. The Spine Journal. 2011;2011:e1–e4.

[40] Sawle LF, J; Marsden,J; Matthews,M. Exploring the effect of pelvic belt configurations upon athletic lumbopelvic pain. Prosthetics & Orthotics International. 2013;37(2):124-131.

[41] Attard J, Rithalia S. Physiological effects of Lycra pressure garments on children with cerebral palsy. Medical and Healthcare Textile. 2010: Woodhead Publishing Series in Textile; 2010. p. 300-308.

[42] Attard J, Rithalia S. Review of the Use of Lycra Pressure Orthoses for children with Cerebral Palsy - including two case studies. International Journal of Therapy and Rehabilitation. 2004;11(3):120-126.

[43] Matthews M. The use of dynamic lycra gloves in the treatment of the neurologically impaired hand and forearm. Book of Abstracts ISPO 2001 Glasgow. 2001;World Congress of the International Society for Prosthetics and Orthotitcs:TH03.5.

[44] Watson MM, M; Crosby,P;. An evaluation of the effects of a Dynamic Lycra Orthosis on arm function in a late stage patient with acquired brain injury. Brain Injury. 2007;21(7):753-761.

[45] Roshini PLA, PA;. Motor Control Training in Chonic Low Back Pain. Journal of Clinical & Diagnostic Research. 2019;13(April):YC 01-5.

[46] Pin TD, P; Chan,M. The effectiveness of passive stretching in children with cerebral palsy. DevMedChild Neurol. 2006;48:855-862.

[47] Wikipedia. Proprioception 2020 [cited 2020 16/4/2020]. Available from: https://en.wikipedia.org/wiki/Proprioception.

[48] Norris.CM. Chapter 5 Excercise therapy. 2011 16/042020. In: Managing Sports Injuries [Internet]. Elsevier; [84-110]. Available from: https://www.sciencedirect.com/science/article/pii/B9780702034732000095?via%3Dihub.

[49] Davis IT, AS; Neal,BS; Roper,JL; Willy,RW. Gait Retraining as an intervention for Patellofemoral Pain. Current Reviews in Musculoskeletal Medicine. 2020;13103-114.

[50] Chilgar LM, B; Gandhi,H; Mehta,A. Effect of Motor Control Retraining of Scapular Stabilizers versus Mullign Mobilisation with Movement in Shoulder Impingement Syndrome. International Journal of Physiotherapy and Research. 2020;8(1):3337-3349.

[51] Curtis DB, P; Saavedra,S; Bencke,J; Kallemose,T; Sonne-Holm,S; Woolacott,M. The central role of trunk control in the gross motor function of children with cerebral palsy: a retrospective cross -sectional study. DevMedChild Neurol. 2015;57:351-357.

[52] Matthews M. Meet Chloe [Website page]. DM Orthotics Ltd; 2014 [updated 20th October 2014 uploaded to website 20th October 2017; cited 2020 31/7/2020]. V2:[A testimonial about our Scoliosis Suit]. Available from: https://www.dmorthotics.com/scoliosis-testimonials.

[53] Matthews MB, S; Marsden,J; Freeman,J. The use of dynamic elastomeric fabric orthoses suits as an orthotic intervention in the management of children with neuropathic onset scoliosis: a retrospective audit of clinical case notes. Scoliosis and Spinal Disorders. 2016;11:14:1-10.

[54] Kim BL, H. Effects of propriocpetive nueromuscular facilitiation- based abdominal muscle strengthening training on pulmonary function, pain.and functiional disability index in chronic low back pain patients. Journal of Excercise Rehabiltiation. 2017;13(4):486-490.

[55] Kofotolis NK, E. Effects of Two 4-Week Proprioceptive Neuromuscular Facilitation Programs on Muscle Endurance, Flexibility, and Functional Performamnce in Women With Chronic Low Back Pain. Phys Ther. 2006;86:1001-1012.

[56] Senthilkumar MA, N; Hayavadana,J. Elastane fabrics- A tool for stretch applications in sport. Indian Journal of Fibre & Textile Research. 2011;36(September):300-307.

[57] Hui CP, J; Wong,MS; Chen,Z. Study of Textile Fabric Materials used in Spinal braces for scoliosis. Journal of Medical and Biological Engineering. 2020;40:356-371.

[58] Law DC, M; Yip,J; Yick,K; Wong,C. Scoliosis brace design: influence of visual aesthetics on user acceptance and compliance. Ergonomics 2017;60(6): 876-886.

Chapter 5

A Mixed Methods Study of the Experiences and Effectiveness of a Soft Brace for Adults with Degenerative Scoliosis

Adam Park, Josette Bettany-Saltikov and Jonathan Ling

Abstract

This chapter details a mixed-methods investigation of the experiences and effectiveness of a soft brace for adults with degenerative scoliosis. Study 1 explored patients' experiences of living with scoliosis, together with the pain and quality of life they experienced as a result of scoliosis. The secondary aims of the qualitative aspect of the study were to explore patient perceptions of wearing the soft brace together with the overall functionality and practicalities of the brace design. We found the main experiences of living with scoliosis in people over 50 were one of constant pain and limited activity. The interviews also identified the benefits of wearing the brace along with design issues associated with the comfort and practicalities of wearing the brace. Study 2 investigated the quantitative effects the brace had on adults with degenerative scoliosis. The quantitative questionnaire results were compared with those from the control group who did not receive the brace. Overall, we found that patients in interviews reported improvements in their quality of life, although these improvements were not reflected in the quantitative results. Implications of our findings for the treatment of adults with scoliosis by bracing, and directions for future work are discussed.

Keywords: scoliosis, degenerative, soft brace, experiences, quality of life, disability

1. Introduction

Surgery is the only form of treatment currently offered by the United Kingdom National Health Service (NHS) as standard care for adults who develop scoliosis. However, this treatment method has associated risks, such as trauma to the body, substantial blood loss and a high complication rate [1]. Operative treatment for adult lumbar scoliosis has a complication rate ranging between 56 and 75% with an 18–58% re-operative rate [2]. Compared to adolescents, adults and older adults who develop scoliosis have a greater risk of suffering from surgical complications due to age, as degenerative scoliosis predominantly develops in older adults.

An alternative method of treatment to surgery is bracing. There are several types of braces used to treat adults with scoliosis; the most frequently used brace is the thoracolumbar-sacral orthoses (TLSO). This type of brace is a two-piece plastic brace that is required to be worn full time [3]. One type of TLSO brace is the Boston brace. This brace is made from prefabricated polypropylene material and is used to treat deformities that range from spinal regions T5 to L4 [4, 5]. Most braces are made up from at least one rigid component that affects the overall comfort and hence the efficacy of the brace. Additionally, most braces require a wearing time in excess of 12 hours, which has the potential to have an impact on wearers' lives.

This mixed methods study evaluated both the subjective patients' views of the effectiveness of the soft brace as well as the objective results of brace effectiveness [6]. The brace encourages corrective movements in the spine through manipulation using soft flexible bands, which are altered on a regular basis depending on the progress of the individual. The brace is made up from three individual sections: pelvic shorts, a body jacket and elastic corrective bands. The pelvic shorts act as an anchor and attachment point for the elastic corrective bands with the jacket acting as the second attaching point. The bands are designed to encourage spinal correction by reactivating (pulling the muscles back into the correct position and training the muscles to stay in that position) the spinal muscles. Furthermore, the brace aims to improve the patients' coronal and sagittal plane balance through the use of the corrective elastic bands as past research has indicated that an improvement in the coronal and sagittal plane can lead to an improvement in pain and/or functionality [7, 8].

To our knowledge, this is the first study to explore the experiences of wearing a spinal brace in a group of older adults with degenerative scoliosis using a qualitative design as previously this type of brace has only been used on adolescents [9–12]. The practicalities of the brace design for adults were unknown. Therefore, the use of a qualitative data collection method allowed for this new information to be gathered. For these reasons, it was decided that semi-structured interviews would provide a deeper understanding of the issues faced by patients with scoliosis than quantitative data by providing a much richer in-depth account and would allow the participants to give detailed descriptions of their experiences of living with scoliosis and wearing the brace [13].

Only two previous studies have examined the views of patients regarding the impact of scoliosis on their lives. Schwab et al. [14] in 2003 reported a self-assessment of 49 patients, 22 of whom had adolescent onset scoliosis and 27 patients who had degenerative scoliosis. Participants had a mean age of 63. The main aim of their study was to investigate the impact scoliosis had on health. They found that when comparing the SF-36 questionnaire data between patients with adult scoliosis against adults who experienced lower back pain, those with scoliosis had significantly higher perceptions of their health than those who had lower back pain. One of the main limitations of this study was that 22 of the patients had adult idiopathic scoliosis and their analysis did not differentiate between the two groups.

The second paper investigated individuals' self-assessment of their health-related quality of life when living with scoliosis [15]. The scores on the SF-36 and the Walter Reed Visual Assessment Scale questionnaires (WRVAS) were collected on 71 individuals who had an age range of 17–66, with a mean age of 33. They concluded that on both the SF-36 and WRVAS, older adults reported more pain than younger ones. However, one of the main issues with the study was that no Cobb angle measurements were taken; this is a limitation as previous research [16] has shown that there are correlations between an individual's Cobb angle and self-assessment. The second limitation is related to the ratio of gender in the sample: of the 71 participants, only 13 were male.

All other papers we found focused upon adult idiopathic scoliosis or solely operative management methods to treat scoliosis and therefore were not relevant to this study. Although the two papers described above did not present qualitative accounts, they are based on the self-assessment of living with scoliosis. The primary aim of this study was to explore patients' experiences of living with scoliosis using a qualitative approach. The secondary aims of the study were to evaluate patient perceptions of wearing a soft spinal brace and to explore the functionality and practicalities of wearing this type of brace.

2. Study 1: qualitative investigation of patients' experiences of living with scoliosis and using a soft brace.

2.1 Method

2.1.1 Participants

For participants to be eligible for this part of the overall study, they were required to wear the brace for 6 months. This time period was selected as clinicians felt it would be where the most noticeable changes in the patients' health and pain scores would be observed. Furthermore, 6 months gave enough time for any initial teething problems with wearing the brace to be identified and resolved, as well as allowing the patients to reflect on their experiences of wearing the brace over a reasonable period of time. In total, eight participants, 1 male and 7 female, aged 55 and over were eligible for the semi-structured interviews.

2.1.2 Ethical approval

Ethical approval was granted by the NHS and the university research ethics committee of the first author. All participants were provided with a participant information sheet which provided a detailed explanation of the purpose of the study. A consent form asked participants to confirm that they had read the information sheet and fully understood what was being asked and whether they were happy to take part, if they met the inclusion criteria and did not match any of the exclusion criteria. Potential participants were also informed that the interview would be audio-recorded and that they had the right to withdraw their data up to 2 weeks after participating, after which time the data would be anonymised.

2.2 Interview schedule and procedure

2.2.1 Interviews

In this study, participants were asked about their experiences of living with scoliosis before they received the brace and once they had received the brace. From the overall larger themes that were generated from the participants' answers, sub-themes were then extracted [17]. Braun and Clarke [17] recommend that thematic analysis should be seen as the foundation method for all qualitative analysis. They describe thematic analysis as a method for identifying, analysing and reporting patterns and themes within data. No specific interview schedule was used when carrying out the interviews; however, a list of overall questions was used to ensure consistency throughout all the interviews.

Semi-structured interviews are a common technique used in qualitative research as the method allows flexibility for both the researcher and the participant in regard to the fluidity and structure of the questions [18]. For this study, the semi-structured interview transcripts were analysed using thematic analysis [17]. Thematic analysis was adopted as it allows flexibility with regard to how the participants' answers are organised, analysed and grouped [17]. Furthermore, the aim of thematic analysis is to obtain and extract themes from the written transcripts generated from the interviews.

An interview schedule was prepared at the beginning of the study. However, as the interviews were semi-structured, the schedule was only a guide, and based on the responses from the participants, further questions were also asked. The main areas covered by the interview schedule are related to the participants' lives before they received the brace and whether the brace had changed the individuals' quality of life. The questions were focused on gaining an insight into any changes to the participants' scoliosis that they thought were due to wearing the brace. The third set of questions focused on gaining an insight and understanding into the patients' feelings towards the brace. These questions asked the participants if they would change any aspect of the brace's design, and what if any problems they encountered (if any) whilst wearing the brace.

Participants who dropped out of the study were also interviewed, but with a slightly different interview schedule. Instead of the final set of questions focusing on satisfaction, the questions focused on the reasons why the participants dropped out and what could be improved in the future to stop this from occurring. Participants 1–6 continued with the trial, whilst participants 7 and 8 dropped out of the trial shortly after the interviews took place.

2.3 Results

2.3.1 Themes and sub-themes

From the interview transcripts, four major themes emerged as follows: the persistence of pain, the impact of the brace on pain and daily living, problems with the device and trial satisfaction.

2.4 Persistence of pain

The overall emerging theme reported by participants was the persistence of pain as a result of their scoliosis. This replicates earlier work that has found that for patients who have a form of degenerative scoliosis, lower back pain is the most common presenting symptom [19, 20]. Further work has found that older adults with degeneration believe they are in more pain than both younger adults and adults with standard lower back pain [7, 15]. This research study has highlighted the severity of pain that older people with degenerative scoliosis experience. When the researcher asked the participants questions about their pain and how much pain they were in, they reported a number of difficulties in carrying out everyday activities as a result of the severity of their pain as seen below:

> *Some days I cannot move the pain is that bad, it takes me over 40 minutes to do my hair. I wet it, I sit down, I put gel on, I sit down, I brush it and I sit down. (Patient 3)*

Further analysis indicated that the pain the participants were living with had substantial limiting effects on both their activity levels and the activities that they could participate in; these activities were virtually limited to home-based stationary activities such as watching TV. Furthermore, household tasks were also limited to very basic chores such as folding, washing or drying dishes:

> *No nothing, I can do nothing (P8)*

I cannot clean the floor and I cannot even stand to do my ironing (P6)

Participants also identified problems with sleeping before they received the brace, stating that the constant pain they experienced due to their scoliosis significantly disrupted their sleeping patterns.

I could not move, and I could not be touched, even the bed covers could not be on me (P4)

I did not sleep very well at all, because if I moved anywhere, I was, I was erm, I was woken up by the pain, I could not get really comfortable, the pain also had a huge impact on my social life, I ended up with no social life at all, people use to come and see me for a while, but you know, over a year that drops off (P5)

Other individuals also echoed that before receiving the brace, their activity levels were minimal as a result of their scoliosis.

I could not walk very far at all. It's affected my life a lot as I used to be dancing all the time, and now I cannot even stand up for a while let alone dance (P6)

It's cut off my social life a lot as I cannot play badminton like I used to (P4)

In essence, pain was a central theme of the patients' experiences of living with scoliosis: all participants explained that they were in constant pain as a result of their scoliosis. From the responses the participants made in relation to living with scoliosis, it was apparent that pain had a substantial effect on all aspects of their lives and on a daily basis. Upon further analysis, a sub-theme emerged which focused on how the pain limited participation in activities, with some reporting only being able to carry out essential household tasks (P6), to the basic challenges of sleeping (P5). Furthermore, the participants' answers to the questions also gave the researcher a base for comparison before they started the trial and once they received the brace.

2.5 The impact of the brace on pain and daily living

The next theme that emerged from the researcher's questions indicated that the patients experienced a small reduction in pain whilst wearing the brace, which in turn led to a positive impact on their activity levels. When the participants were asked if the brace had allowed them to be able to participate in any additional activities or participate longer in activities they could already do, the participants gave answers such as:

Well I can walk further with my walkie frame (P1)

If anything, it's helped me going up and down the stairs as it keeps me more upright, I used to go up and down stairs on my hands and knees but the brace keeps me more upright instead of crawling (P4)

Further quotes revealed the brace reduced the level of pain that participants reported whilst walking or carrying out everyday tasks.

My pain has improved yes, especially when I'm sleeping or doing household chores (P5).

Yea, it helps, it really helps, it helps to get me out, it gets me moving. (P6)

I have got totally active again since receiving it. (P4)

However, it emerged a reduction in pain was not the belief or views of all the participants, as other participants did not believe they received any benefits from the brace, to the extent that one participant even believed wearing the brace was leading to an increase in their pain.

Yea my back has started to get worse. (P7)

It's affected my sleeping; my sleeping has got worse it feels as if it pulls me into painful positions. (P8)

In summary, the participants generally indicated that the brace was having a positive impact in terms of improving their quality of life and their overall activity levels. With regard to participants 7 and 8, both dropped out of the trial shortly after this interview.

2.6 Problems with the brace

Patients reported several design problems with the brace that limited the amount of time the participants were able or willing to wear the brace. This was particularly problematic as previous research has shown that bracing is only effective when worn for the recommended time (Rowe et al. and Maruyama et al.) [21, 22]. Participants indicated that they were not adhering to the 8 hours a day, 7 days a week, minimum recommended wearing time that was required to achieve maximum efficiency. They gave a number of reasons for this. When asked how long they were wearing the brace, the participants answered:

Well approximately 4 days a week, but it really depends on what I'm doing. (P6)

I wear it when I'm in the house, but I cannot wear it whilst I'm out as I cannot get it off. (P2)

Further probing revealed the main reason the participants were not keeping to the recommended wearing time was the brace's practicality and functionality with regard to using the toilet, due to the design of the shorts.

I find it's really difficult to take it off so I do not when I'm going out. (P2)

Because I find the use of the toilet very difficult if we are going to the theatre or places like that. (P5)

It's a bit awkward to get it off, if you were to need the toilet. (P6) The only problem is going to the toilet. (P3)

Furthermore, additional problem participants identified, as a reason for not fulfilling the recommended wearing time, was the cosmetic appearance of the brace under their clothes.

You know, I cannot wear my clothes properly because of that bump in my shoulder from the shoulder strap, in fact it's not the strap, it's the back of the jacket thing that comes across the back of my neck, well it always shows, no matter what I wear. (P4)

In summary, participants reported several design issues with the brace, which limited the amount of time they could wear the brace for. As a result of these problems, the optimum recommended wearing time was not achieved, which would have reduced any benefit of the brace. The main reason reported for this noncompliance wearing the brace was toileting as a result of the design of the brace shorts, a problem that was exacerbated by the fact that several participants could not remove or fit the brace independently.

2.7 Trial satisfaction

From the final set of questions, the theme that emerged was that participants were happy with the format of the brace trial. This was in regard to the frequency and duration of the clinical visits and the questionnaires the participants had received.

No, I think they the questionnaires ask the right thing really, they are simple to answer, I have not found them simple to answer as I've been in a lot of pain last month with my IBS but normally, I'm ok with them. (P4) The questionnaires are simple really; they ask sensible questions and the number of visits is fine also. (P2)

The answers from the remaining participants who reached the 6-month treatment point also indicated they were happy to continue with the trial. Participants gave generally brief responses to these questions; they did not expand or give any extra information to the questions asked. Participants indicated they were happy with the format of the trial and felt the questionnaires were appropriate; they also indicated they were happy to continue with the trial.

2.8 Interviews with the participants who had withdrawn from the trial

The interviews with the participants who had dropped out of the trial were carried out over the telephone and recorded with their permission; consent forms were sent out in the post prior to the interview. The interview schedule followed the same progression as the treatment group, with the initial questions focused on the participants' life before they received the brace. The participants indicated the primary complaint of living with scoliosis was their persistent pain.

Erm, very bad, well to my mind it was very bad, but I'm sure there must be people who are worse. (P7)

Yes, yes I cannot, I can no longer go shopping for example, Christmas shopping for example is an absolute nightmare really, erm, you know the weekly shop, my husband has to do it now, the only time that I'm alright is if I'm pushing the trolley, it's almost like I can run then. (P8)

The next set of question focused on why the participants dropped out of the trial. Participants provided answers identifying the primary reasons being the fitting of the brace.

> *I could not wear it because I take diuretic tablets and I could not get the brace off and I kept needing to go to the loo all of the time. If something like that could be devised and designed with erm, with easier fittings because I need to have somebody to help me get in and out and quite often, they could not understand it either. (P7)*

Furthermore, one participant indicated the reason they dropped out of the trial was due to the bracing causing them even more pain.

> *I did not wear the brace for any length of time because it hurt my body, that might sound silly but it actually hurt; it hurt my stomach for example, it just seemed altogether too tight and pulling me, although when it was on for a short length of time it was quite good. (P8)*

In summary, it was apparent the design of the brace and its practicalities were the main factors for these participants dropping out. Furthermore, the brace also led one participant to believe their pain increased; however, as stated earlier in this study, this participant was only included due to the small study numbers and at the specific request of the consultants.

2.9 Discussion

The primary aim of this study was to use a qualitative approach to explore the patients' experiences of living with scoliosis. Furthermore, the secondary aims of the study were to obtain rich and in-depth qualitative information with regard to how the brace affected the scoliosis, together with the functionality and practicalities of the brace design. The results and themes generated from the semi-structured interviews indicated that the primary experience of living with scoliosis is one of persistent pain and limited activity, with all participants who were interviewed identifying these two factors as the main issues. Furthermore, the results from the interviews also identified and highlighted design problems and limitations with the brace shorts that were previously unknown. As the brace has previously only been used on adolescents [9, 23, 24], the problems experienced by adults with regard to the design of the shorts were previously unknown. It is unclear why older women had a problem with the design when this issue has not to our knowledge been reported elsewhere.

An additional result from this study was the identification that the literature on adults' experience of living with scoliosis is very sparse. The data obtained from this study contributes significantly to the gap in knowledge with regard to the experiences of living with scoliosis and its effectiveness. From the responses participants gave, the brace did offer a reduction in the participants' reported pain and allowed them to take part in a wider range of activities. However, for a more definitive conclusion and indication as to how successful the brace has the potential to be, this study would need to be carried out on a larger sample size. Furthermore, the participants would need to be willing and able to wear the brace for the recommended time and would need to fully match the study criteria.

Furthermore, as the interviews provided a greater reflection of the experiences of living with scoliosis, it is suggested that each participant should receive a minimum of three interviews in any future trial. The first interview would be scheduled at the beginning of the trial, one in the middle and one at the end of the study. The implementation of three interviews would also allow for a more in-depth comparison to be obtained, as the interviews would be more frequent and the participants would be able to give more detailed descriptions of their experiences of living with the brace.

The information obtained from the qualitative interviews allowed for a greater understanding of patients' experiences of living with scoliosis that the questionnaires failed to capture, such as problems with the brace and the extent to which the brace was helping with their pain and activity levels. Furthermore, Participant 4's answer to the set of questions regarding trial satisfaction also showed how some patients found it difficult to that they experienced was due to IBS or scoliosis. This qualitative study also revealed that patients' experiences of pain had a limited effect on the amount of activity they could do due to their degenerative scoliosis.

3. Study 2: exploratory (pilot) randomised control study (RCT)

3.1 Research design

The study was initially going to be carried out as a randomised control trial (RCT) for 24 months. The RCT study design is considered to be the highest level of scientific testing as it minimises patient control bias [25]. However, halfway through the recruitment process, it became apparent that the numbers required to achieve an RCT would not be met due to a number of factors that were out of the control of the research team. These factors included a drop in patient referrals due to a reform in the referral process from primary care into secondary care, a lack of engagement by treatment centres in terms of not fully understanding which healthcare professionals could refer patients into the trial and a small number of eligible participants who matched the study inclusion criteria. Therefore, after the discussions with the consultants, brace clinicians and research team, it was decided that the best solution to these problems would be to continue the trial as a prospective study with a control group for 6 months. There are several reasons for the reduction in the trial time scale. Firstly, it took over 13 months to gain NHS ethics; secondly, the participant referrals dramatically decreased after the first 12 months due to NHS reforms, and therefore any new entries into the trial would not have finished their treatment program before the scholarship of the primary author concluded. Therefore, recruitment was halted after 18 months. As a result of this, the data presented in this work are from 6 months of data collection.

3.2 Recruitment of participants

The participants for the study were recruited and identified by consultants, physiotherapists and spinal nurses when they attended their regular orthopaedic clinics. When attending these appointments, the patients were screened by their consultants to ensure they were suitable and matched the study criteria. Participants for the study were initially going to be recruited from three different treatment centres; however, only one referred any participants into the trial. Once a participant was referred into the trial, they were randomised into either the treatment or control group; this was done through a computer randomisation program. Participants in the treatment group received the soft brace in addition to the standardised assessment tools described below.

3.3 Participant inclusion/exclusion

To ensure that appropriate patients were recruited for the trial, after a number of discussions amongst the research team, brace manufacturers, surgeons and physiotherapists, a set of inclusion and exclusion criteria was drawn up. This was to ensure that the participants would be able to fully partake in the trial without having any additional problems or issues placed upon them as a result of participating.

3.4 Inclusion criteria

Patients were included from the study if they had any of the following:

- Patients were required to be 50 years old or over, of either gender, to ensure the scoliosis was that of a degenerative origin and not a missed case of adolescent idiopathic scoliosis.
- Patients whose scoliosis had a Cobb angle of ≥20° with associated vertebral rotation, previously confirmed on a full spine standing posterior anterior X-ray. The reason for this was because it was thought if the brace could reduce the pain in patients with a large Cobb angle, it should be able to ease the pain in patients with Cobb angles of over 20°.
- The curve needed to have an apical vertebra (situated at the apex) level at T12 or below (this included double and triple curves) to ensure the scoliosis was degenerative.
- Participants were required to have an ODI score of ≥32 to allow minimal changes in ODI scores to be detected.

3.5 Exclusion criteria

Patients were excluded from the study if they had any of the following:

- Leg pain that was linked to lumbar spine pain, as a number of additional health problems could have led to the development of leg pain
- If the participants were unable to fit the brace on their own or did not have someone to help with this process
- If the participants were not ambulant, as the brace was designed to treat patients who were not confined to bed
- If the participant had already received instrumental thoracic or lumbar surgery as the brace was designed to delay the need for surgery

3.6 Study instrumentation used in this study

The following study questionnaires were used to measure and monitor the effectiveness of the brace. Three questionnaires were used. The first questionnaire that was used to assess pain was the Oswestry Disability Index Questionnaire v2.1a (ODI) [26]. The second questionnaire that was used to assess the patients' quality of life was the EQ5D-5L [27]. The final questionnaire was used to assess the patients' mental and physical health, the Short Form-36 Version 2 (SF-36v2) [12]. The participants in the control group received the questionnaires together with the standard NHS treatment; this comprised a yearly follow-up appointment with their regular consultant to assess whether the curve had progressed to the point where a surgical approach was required.

3.7 Oswestry Disability Index (ODI v2.1a)

The ODI v2.1a questionnaire is one of the most commonly used questionnaires to assess lower back pain. The ODI is one of the most valid and reliable outcome measures with regard to the patient's perception of the 'pain they feel today' [28]. The ODI comprises of 10 sections; each section has six statements (see example below; **Table 1**). Responses are made on a five-point scale. As shown in the example below, the first statement is marked 0, and the last statement is marked 5. All additional statements are scored according to rank, with the highest score being taken if more than one box is marked in each section. Once the questionnaire is complete, the score is then calculated using the following formula: ODI % = Total score/5 × number of questions answered × 100. Therefore, if the ODI score is 40 based on the participant answering 4 for all 10 sections, the percentage of disability is determined: 40/5 × 100 = 80% disability. Since the initial publication, the ODI has been widely validated [29] and deemed to be a reliable measure for detecting small reductions in pain and disability before and after treatment [30].

The ODI correlates positively with the SF-36 and EQ5D questionnaires. In essence, a reduction in pain attained from the ODI correlates with an improvement in mental and physical health on the SF-36 questionnaire and an improvement in quality of life from the EQ5D for patients who had lower back pain [31, 32]. Wittink et al. [32] compared the outcomes of 424 patients with chronic pain who had been referred to a multidisciplinary pain centre where each patient was required to complete the SF-36, Multidimensional Pain Inventory (MPI) and the ODI before or on the date of their first appointment. They found that the MPI, SF-36 and ODI had good psychological measurements. The study also concluded that the ODI had the least amount of respondent burden and was easier to score, although the questionnaire does not provide as much detail as the MPI or the SF-36.

3.8 EQ5D-5L

The EQ5D-5L is a widely used generic measurement of health-related quality of life that requires patients to self-report problems with regard to five elements: mobility, self-care, usual activities, pain/discomfort and anxiety/depression [33]. The questionnaire is split into two parts with the first part containing five questions that explore different elements of health, with each of the five questions containing three levels of severity, no problem, some problem or extreme problem, allowing patients to be classified into 1 of 243 states [34, 35]. An example question (see **Table 2**) from the EQ5D questionnaire is seen below:

Section 2: personal care	**Score**
I can look after myself normally without causing extra pain	0
I can look after myself normally but it causes extra pain	1
It is painful to look after myself and I am slow and careful	2
I need some help but manage most of my personal care	3
I need help every day in most aspects of self-care	4
I do not get dressed, wash with difficulty and stay in bed	5

Table 1.
Example ODI questions.

Please mark accordingly
I have no problems in walking about
I have slight problems in walking about
I have moderate problems in walking about
I have severe problems in walking about
I am unable to walk about

Table 2.
Example EQ5D questions.

From these 243 health states, a time trade-off (TTO) is calculated; this TTO is used to represent a person's quality of life. A value of 1 represents full health and a value of 0 represents being dead [36]. For this research study, the TTO scores were calculated using the software provided by EuroQual who designed the questionnaire. The second part of the EQ5D-5L requires the patient to indicate how 'good' or 'bad' their perception of their own general health is by marking a visual analogue scale (VAS). A VAS is a measurement tool that aims to measure an attribute of health that is believed to be on a continuous range across a continuous value. The scale ranges across a horizontal line that starts at 0 representing no pain and moves gradually to 100 representing extreme pain. The line is 100 mm in length and words are placed at the start of the continuum (0) representing no pain, and at the end of the line a100mm line representing extreme severe pain (see **Figure 1** below).

The validity and reliability of the EQ5D questionnaire have previously been confirmed by Brazier et al. [37] who compared the results of the EQ5D to the SF 6D (a development from the SF-36). Brazier's research study [37] found that on a data set of 2436 patients with a wide range of medical conditions ranging from lower back pain, chronic obtrusive pulmonary disease and irritable bowel syndrome, the questionnaire showed signs of being sensitive to change and having a strong coefficient of internal consistency.

3.9 SF-36v2

The last questionnaire used in this study was the SF-36v2. This questionnaire is a multidimensional, non-diagnostic-specific measure of pain that consists of eight health scales: physical functioning (10 items), role limitations—physical (4 items), bodily pain (2 items), general health (5 items), vitality (4 items), social functioning (2 items), role limitations due to emotional problems (3 items) and mental health (5 items) [38]. The scale is directly transformed into a 0–100 scale based on the assumption that each question carries equal weight. The lower the score, the greater the disability; in essence, a score of 0 is equivalent to a maximum disability, and a score of 100 is equivalent to no disability. The SF-36v2 has been reported to be both a reliable and valid measurement of health and has been shown to be sensitive to changes in health conditions [39].

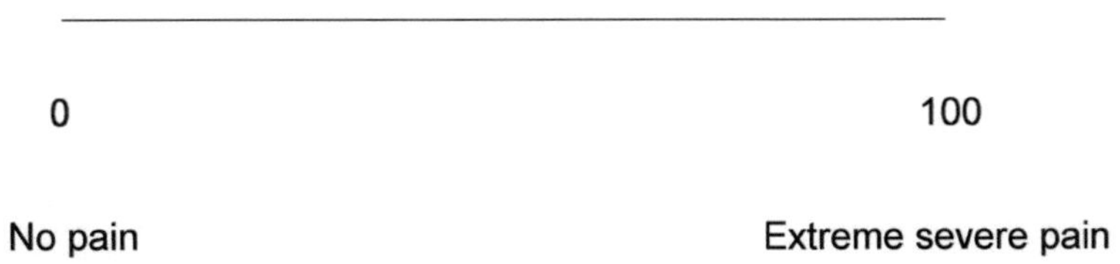

Figure 1.
Example of a visual analogue scale.

3.10 Procedure

Medical staff including consultants, physiotherapists and spinal nurses were the primary recruiters for participants for the study. Participants were recruited when they attended their regular orthopaedic clinics. Once consent was attained, the participants were then randomised into either the treatment or control group by a computer randomisation program. As part of the standard NHS procedure, on arrival the participants received a routine clinical examination. This included the measurement of the Cobb angle and pelvic/shoulder tilt, in addition to a posterior/anterior X-ray using the soft brace X-ray protocol. The soft brace X-ray protocol was used for all clinical visits as it provided a standardised foot position, which in turn kept the patient's posture natural and standardised from visit to visit. The protocol also allowed for direct comparison of frontal and lateral X-rays and increased the inter-session reliability. If the participant fulfilled the study criteria, they were offered the opportunity to participate in the trial; if they declined, they then continued along the standard NHS treatment pathway.

If the patient chose to participate in the study, they were given the participant information sheet (PIS) together with the series of questionnaires described above to complete (ODIv2.1a, EQ5D-5 L and SF-36v2). Further information about the trial and details of future clinical appointments were also included in the PIS. The information sheet gave details about future clinical appointments, how the trial would run and what was expected of the individual with regard to their participation (such as being able and willing to attend the clinical appointments, adhere to the 8 hours wearing time and complete the questionnaires on time). The lead researcher then explained to the patients that they would be randomly allocated by a computer program into either the treatment group where they would receive the brace and questionnaires or the control group where they would follow the standard NHS treatment and also receive the study questionnaires. If participants were placed in the treatment group, they were given an appointment where the brace was fitted by a trained soft brace clinician.

The baseline questionnaire data were then administrated and collected by the lead researcher. A follow-up appointment was also made 1 month into treatment where an additional in-brace X-ray was taken as specified by the study protocol. This additional X-ray was not part of the standard NHS treatment; however, it was deemed necessary to assess whether the brace was having any immediate effect on the shape and position of the spine. This extra dose of radiation that the patients received as a result of the additional X-ray was deemed to be acceptable by the research ethics committee. Patients were also informed that they would be required to attend future appointments at 1, 3 and 6 months. This was in addition to their standard clinical appointments to see their regular consultant at 12 months to assess the long-term effects of the brace. Upon attending these routine clinic visits, the brace was adjusted by the soft brace clinicians if it was deemed to be too loose or ill-fitting as a result of any changes in their shape and/or posture.

The brace is recommended by the manufacturer to be worn for 8–12 hours per day for the first 3 months and then adjusted to the individual's requirements after this. These adjustments included changing the wearing time and/or adapting the position of the bands if they had become loose or ill-fitting. Apart from the first appointment, which lasted approximately 90 minutes, each follow-up clinical visit lasted no longer than 40 minutes. The first appointment was slightly longer as this was where the participants were fitted and measured for their brace, whilst also providing them with the opportunity to ask the chief investigator (CI) or clinicians any further questions regarding their participation in the trial.

The participants in the control group received the ODIv2.1a, EQ5D-5L and the SF-36v2 questionnaire at home at months 1, 3 and 6 months, in addition to their standard treatment pathway. A follow-up yearly X-ray together with an appointment with their consultants was also made to see if surgery would be required due to curve progression. Both groups of participants were asked to complete and return all documents to the first author's University in a prepaid envelope. If individuals decided they did not want to participate in the trial or if they decided to have surgical treatment, they were followed up at 12 months by their consultant with an X-ray to assess if any curve progression was apparent.

If patients chose to enter the trial, they were told that they could withdraw at any stage without giving a reason and it would not affect their future treatment. Participants were then provided with a participant information sheet and offered the opportunity to discuss the study with their consultant or a member of the research team. If patients agreed to participate in the trial, the consultants obtained signed consent. These completed forms were then passed on to the researcher who contacted the individual to verify they were still interested in participating in the trial (with at least a 24-hour gap after completing the slip). Once the patients confirmed they were still interested in participating, it was at this stage of the trial that they were informed which group they had been randomised into. At this point if the participants decided not to participate in the trial, it was explained they would follow the standard NHS treatment pathway. Each participant was also informed that if they did participate, all data they provided would be kept confidential and anonymised.

3.11 Sample size

A sample size of 102 for this study was originally calculated based on literature from previous back pain studies. An attrition rate of 10% was also added to the sample size [40], meaning a total sample size of 112 participants was required. Due to recruitment issues, this number of participants was not achieved. In total only 15 participants were recruited to the study. However, as randomisation took place before the research team had the opportunity to meet and screen the potential participants, two participants who were included by the consultants did not meet the inclusion criteria and were therefore not eligible, ultimately resulting in only 13 participants being involved. Given the low sample size, it is important to establish that the appropriate analyses (and therefore appropriate conclusions) were applied to the data. Research [41] has shown that even with a sample size of two people in a series of fake t-tests, the Type 2 error that occurred did not surpass the acceptable value of 5%; this has also been confirmed in studies by [42, 43]. Therefore, the small numbers in this study should not have any effect on the validity of the results generated from the questionnaires, although of course the small study numbers must be recognised in the interpretation of the results, as it is possible that the participants may not form a typical cross section of patients with degenerative scoliosis.

3.12 Statistical analysis

All study data were anonymised and analysed using a two-way repeated measure analysis of variance in SPSS [44]. The two-way analysis of variance (ANOVA) was used as it allows the differences between group means and their treatment methods to be compared over several time points [45]. The treatment group was compared against the mean data from the control group for each of the three time points to determine whether any significant differences were present. In-group comparisons were also calculated for both groups to see if any significant in-group changes occurred.

Any missing data or data belonging to participants who withdrew from the study were analysed based on an intention-to-treat (ITT) basis. It was important to use ITT as the main problem researchers find when using an RCT study design is that participants do not always follow the instructions or they drop out of the trial [46]. The benefits of using ITT are that the analysis still reflects clinical situations and it gives unbiased estimations on the effectiveness of the proscribed treatment [47]. Furthermore, the use of ITT maintains the original sample size; if dropouts were excluded from the overall data set, a reduction of statistical power may occur.

3.13 Outcome measures

The primary outcome measure for this study was a change in the participants' ODI scores over the 6-month duration. Secondary outcome measures were any changes in the EQ5D-5L and SF-36v2 scores.

3.14 Results

3.14.1 Oswestry Disability Index

The baseline data in **Table 3** show that the treatment group had a higher mean ODI than the control group upon initial consultation, although this difference was not statistically significantly different. Furthermore, a greater standard deviation was also present which indicated that a larger variation from the mean score was present within the treatment group. After 3 months, the mean ODI calculated from the treatment group's data showed a reduction of 9% in the 'pain they feel today' from baseline, in comparison to a 6.25% increase from the control group, although the standard deviation remained similar for both groups.

At the 6-month stage of the trial, the treatment groups' mean ODI decreased by a further 1.6%; this indicated a decrease in pain. This is in contrast to the control group, who as a group had a mean ODI change from data collected between months 3 and 6 of the study of 19%. The scores represent an overall decrease of 10.6% from the treatment group over the 6-month trial compared to an overall increase of 25.25% over the course of the 6-month trial from the control group.

Group	Mean	Std Deviation	N	+/-
Treatment	52.50	16.39	8	-
ODI Score M0 Control	41.60	12.97	5	-
Treatment	47.75	5.66	8	-9%
ODI Score M3 Control	44.20	10.83	5	+6.25%
Treatment	47.0	14.12	8	-1.6%
ODI Score M6 Control	52.60	22.32	5	+19%

1M0 represents the baseline mean ODI scores, M3 represents month 3 mean scores and M6 represents month 6 mean ODI scores. The +/- column represents score changes between months. Treatment represents the treatment group and control represents the control group

Table 3.
Analysis of ODI scores over 6 months.

1M0 represents the baseline mean ODI scores, M3 represents month 3 mean scores and M6 represents month 6 mean ODI scores. The +/− column represents score changes between months. Treatment represents the treatment group and control represents the control group. Furthermore, there was no significant difference between the treatment and control group over the course of the 6-month study (see **Table 3**). Also, there was no significant difference or in-group interaction amongst the groups between the treatment time points.

3.14.2 EQ5D

The data presented in **Table 4** show that at baseline, the control group's reported health state appeared worse than the treatment group. As the score gets closer to 0, the closer the individual feels to a state of death. The control group had an initial TTO 22.2% higher than that of the treatment group even before receiving the brace, which means that they felt less well than those in the treatment group. The mean TTO data from month 3 showed that both groups' health state changed, with a 21.4% increase coming from the control group, and the treatment group's mean TTO score improved by 10.62%.

Data from the 6-month collection point presented a further increase for the treatment group with an improvement in score of 7.69% and with an overall increase in score of 18.31% over the duration of the study with regard to their TTO health state. Furthermore, although no change in score was found for the control group in the final 3 months, over the full duration of the study, a total improvement of 22.2% was calculated. From the EQ5D questionnaire, it was also found that over the course of the 6-month study period, no statistically significant differences were found between the groups' TTO scores or in-group interaction.

3.14.3 SF-36 mental health scores

The results from the initial month's questionnaires show that both groups of patients had similar mean scores in terms of their mental health (see **Table 5**). After 3 months in the brace, the treatment groups reported mental health score decreased by 8.26%. However, this change in reported mental health was smaller than that of the decrease calculated from the control group questionnaires whose mean score decreased by 11.84%. The results from the month 6 time point indicated that both

	Group	Mean	Std Deviation	N	+/-
TTO MO	Treatment	.35	.35	8	
	Control	.28	.14	5	
TTO M3	Treatment	.39	.18	8	10.62%
	Control	.34	.54	5	22.2%
TTO M6	Treatment	.42	.17	8	7.69%
	Control	.34	.49	5	0

Note: [1]M0 represents the baseline mean scores, M3 represents month 3 mean scores and M6 represents month 6 mean TTO scores. The +/- column represents score changes between months. Treatment represents the treatment group and control represents the control group

Table 4.
EQ5D health states over 6 months.

	Group	Mean	Std Deviation	N	+/-
MHS M0	Treatment	45.38	11.60	8	
	Control	48.2	9.8	5	
MHA M3	Treatment	41.63	12.32	8	-8.26%
	Control	40.20	11.95	5	-11.84%
MHA M6	Treatment	46.50	12.54	8	+4.87%
	Control	42	10.61	5	6.94%

Note. [1]MHS M0 represents the baseline mean scores, M3 represents month 3 mean scores and M6 represents month 6 mean mental health scores. The +/- column represents score changes between months

Table 5.
SF-36 mental health scores.

groups' mental health increased between the months of 3 and 6. The treatment groups' mean scores increased by 4.87%, whilst the control group's score increased by 6.94%.

3.14.4 SF-36 physical health scores

The initial month's mean SF-36 physical health scores show that the treatment group had an inferior physical health score of 25% compared to the control group, as the closer the score to 0, the lower the individuals' physical health. Data collected from 3 months into the study show that wearing brace for 3 months leads to the treatment group having an increase in their scores of 16.95%. This was in comparison to the control group, whose scores showed signs of their physical health decreasing by 3.31%. The scores calculated from data collected between the months of 3 and 6 show the treatment group's mean physical health decreased by 3.67%.

	Group	Mean	Std Deviation	N	+/-
PHS M0	Treatment	22.63	5.18	8	
	Control	30.20	10.01	5	
PHS M3	Treatment	27.25	3.69	8	+16.95%
	Control	29.20	6.14	5	-3.31%
PHS M6	Treatment	26.25	4.65	8	-3.67
	Control	31.80	9.18	5	+8.18

Note: [1]PHSM0 represents the baseline mean scores, M3 represents month 3 mean scores and M6 represents month 6 mean physical health scores.

Table 6.
SF36 physical health scores.

The results also demonstrated that no significant differences or group interactions were found between the treatment group's physical health score and the control group's physical health score at 6 months (**Table 6**).

4. Discussion

4.1 Aims of the study

The primary aim of this study was to obtain both patients' quantitative experiences of living with scoliosis together with developing an understanding of the pain they experienced and their quality of life. The secondary aims of this study were to investigate the effects the soft brace had on adults with degenerative scoliosis. Another aim of the study was to compare the questionnaire results from the treatment group against the questionnaire results from adults who did not receive the soft brace.

4.2 Summary of main results

The study inclusion and exclusion criteria were designed to recruit individuals who were at the end of the non-operative treatment pathway. For these participants the next stage of treatment would be surgery. However, as discussed previously, due to the complications and difficulties of the procedure, the need for a surgery should if possible be delayed or avoided especially in those patients who have additional underlying health conditions such as irritable bowel syndrome (IBS) and arthritis. These dangers are further highlighted as the complication rates of surgery in older adults range from 20% to as high as 80% [48].

The anthropometric data of nine patients (8 female, 1 male) in the treatment group and six (all female) in the control group were as follows: the female patients in the treatment group had an average weight of 75.3 kg with an average height of 155.4 cm; the one male participant had a height of 165.2 cm and weight of 84.7 kg. This is in comparison to the six female participants recruited into the control group, who had an average weight of 77.6 kg and average height of 153.8 cm. In comparison to the average healthy individual who has an ODI score of 10.19 [49], the mean ODI score of the individuals in this trial was 47. Moreover, the mean ODI score of 47 was also substantially higher than the minimum ODI score of 32 outlined in the initial study inclusion criteria. In comparison the control group showed an 8.18% increase in ODI in comparison to the data collected between the initial month and month 3.

The results further demonstrated that there were no significant differences or interactions between the treatment group's physical health score and the control group's. The average healthy individual has an ODI score of 10.19 [49], whilst the mean benchmark ODI score of the individuals in this trial was 47. Moreover, the mean ODI score of 47 was also substantially higher than the minimum ODI score of 32 outlined in the initial study inclusion criteria. In addition to a higher mean ODI score than the average healthy individual, participants also had a lower mean score in terms of SF-36 MH and SF-36 PH than the average healthy individual. A healthy individual's SF-36 MHS score is on average 50.17 and PHS 50.1 [50].

The mean baseline mental and physical health scores of the patients in this trial were 45.5 and 26.4, respectively. Additionally, a mean health TTO score of the average healthy individual is 0.94 [51] compared to the mean TTO score of 0.32 obtained from those in this trial. Furthermore, the inclusion criteria required participants' Cobb angle to be a minimum of 20. The average Cobb angle measurement of patients in this trial was 43° (+/−12), again highlighting the severity of the degenerative scoliosis our participants had. The questionnaire data showed that over the course of 6 months, patients treated with a soft brace had a reduction in their ODI score regarding the 'pain they felt today'. However, no significant differences or interactions were observed over the 6 months of the trial. In addition to the change in the ODI scores, changes in the TTO and mental and physical health scores were also calculated from the treatment group's data. However, again no significant differences were found between questionnaire scores.

Like the treatment group, participants in the control group also showed no significant changes over the course of the 6-month study period. Furthermore, as seen in the tables above, the participants in the control group had a lower baseline ODI, EQ5D and SF-36 scores than the average healthy individual. It was difficult to compare the results of this study to previous work as little research has compared braced patients with patients who received no or standard NHS treatment. Furthermore, although several studies have been published [9, 52], these investigated the effectiveness of bracing on adolescents which has a different aetiology to adult scoliosis.

5. Discussion

In this study, the treatment group's data showed no significant difference in changes over the duration of the trial for all questionnaires. This contrasts with research [53, 54] which found a significant difference between the effectiveness of a surgical approach and a non-operative method of treatment. Research from Grubb et al. (1994) [53] examined the effectiveness of a surgery on 28 adults with idiopathic scoliosis and 25 adults with degenerative scoliosis. In comparison to the 10.6% change in scores over the 6-month treatment period for the present study [53], Grubb et al. found that patients who had degenerative scoliosis and were treated operatively reported a decrease in their pain scores of 70% whilst patients with adult adolescent scoliosis reported an 80% reduction. Furthermore, both sets of patients reported improvements in their health-related quality of life in addition to improvements in standing and walking over the 2–7 year follow-up period.

Li et al. [54] compared self-reported outcome scores from patients treated operatively to those treated non-operatively. They found that patients who received operative treatment reported significantly better self-outcome scores in the EQ5D VAS and SRS-22, but not in the ODI or the SF-12. Although the results from our quantitative work showed no significant difference over time for braced patients, discussions between patients and clinicians gave insight into the benefits of the brace. Patients spoke about how the brace reduced their pain, allowing their participation in new activities or longer participation in activities that they could already carry out. Some participants discussed how for the previous few weeks their pain levels were low, but when the time came to complete the questionnaires, they were having a 'bad week', due to their scoliosis pain or pain from other underlying health conditions. With a small sample size, the effect of 'bad weeks' would have a substantial effect on the results obtained, with potentially a Type 2 error where actual differences between groups may not have been detected. Furthermore, from the questionnaire results, it would appear that the questionnaires may not have been sensitive enough to assess small changes for patients who received the brace.

6. Conclusions

In conclusion this small pilot study has demonstrated that a soft brace has a potential as a treatment for degenerative scoliosis. In interviews, patients who were given the brace reported an improved quality of life, although such improvements were not detected in the questionnaire data. A larger, sufficiently powered, quantitative study is required to provide a clearer understanding of the effect of a soft brace on pain and quality of life for older people with degenerative scoliosis.

Author details

Adam Park[1], Josette Bettany-Saltikov[2*] and Jonathan Ling[1]

1 School of Health Sciences and Wellbeing, University of Sunderland, Sunderland, UK

2 Teesside University, Middlesbrough, UK

*Address all correspondence to: j.b.saltikov@tees.ac.uk

References

[1] Bettany-Saltikov J, Weiss HR, Chockalingam N, Taranu R, Srinivas S, Hogg J, et al. Surgical versus non-surgical interventions in people with adolescent idiopathic scoliosis. Cochrane Database of Systematic Reviews. 2015;**4**:CD010663. DOI: 10.1002/14651858.CD010663.pub2

[2] Akbarnia BA, Ogilvie JW, Hammerberg KW. Debate: Degenerative scoliosis: To operate or not to operate. Spine. 2006;**31**(19S):S195-SS20. DOI: 10.1097/01.brs.0000234732.43489.0f

[3] Clin J, Aubin CÉ, Parent S, Labelle H. A biomechanical study of the Charleston brace for the treatment of scoliosis. Spine. 2010;**35**(19):E940-E947. DOI: 10.1097/BRS.0b013e3181c5b5fa

[4] Watts HG, Hall JE, Stanish WM. The Boston brace system for the treatment of low thoracic and lumbar scoliosis by the use of a girdle without superstructure. Clinical Orthopaedics and Related Research. 1977;**126**:87-92

[5] Périé D, Aubin C-E, Petit Y, Beauséjour M, Dansereau J, Labelle H. Boston brace correction in idiopathic scoliosis: A biomechanical study. Spine. 2003;**28**:1672-1677. DOI: 10.1097/01.BRS.0000083165.93936.6D

[6] Coillard C, Leroux MA, Zabjek KF, Rivard C. Soft brace a non-rigid brace for the treatment of idiopathic scoliosis: Post-treatment results. European Spine Journal;**12**(2):141-148. DOI: 10.1007%2Fs00586-002-0467-x

[7] Schwab FJ, Smith VA, Biserni M, Gamez L, Farcy JPC, Pagala M. Adult scoliosis: A quantitative radiographic and clinical analysis. Spine. 2002;**27**(4):387-392. DOI: 10.1097/00007632-200202150-00012

[8] Glassman SD, Berven S, Bridwell K, Horton W, Dimar JR. Correlation of radiographic parameters and clinical symptoms in adult scoliosis. Spine. 2005;**30**(6):682-688. DOI: 10.1097/01.brs.0000155425.04536.f7

[9] Lonstein JE, Winter RB. The Milwaukee brace for the treatment of adolescent idiopathic scoliosis. A review of one thousand and twenty patients. The Journal of Bone & Joint Surgery. 1994;**76**(8):1207-1221

[10] Nachemson AL, Peterson LE. Effectiveness of treatment with a brace in girls who have adolescent idiopathic scoliosis. A prospective, controlled study based on data from the Brace Study of the Scoliosis Research Society. The Journal of Bone & Joint Surgery. 1995;**77**(6):815-822. DOI: 10.2106/00004623-199506000-00001

[11] Asher M, Min Lai S, Burton D, Manna B. The reliability and concurrent validity of the Scoliosis Research Society-22 Patient Questionnaire for Idiopathic Scoliosis. Spine. 2003;**28**:63-69

[12] Coillard C, Vachon V, Circo AB, Beauséjour M, Rivard CH. Effectiveness of the Spinecor brace based on the new standardized criteria proposed by the scoliosis research society for adolescent idiopathic scoliosis. Journal of Paediatric Orthopaedics. 2007;**27**(4):375-379. DOI: 10.1186%2F1748-7161-5-25

[13] Bryman A. Social Research Methods. 5th ed. Oxford: OUP; 2015

[14] Schwab F, Dubey A, Pagala M, Gamez L, Farcy JP. Adult scoliosis: A health assessment analysis by SF-36. Spine. 2003;**28**(6):602-606. DOI: 10.1097/01.BRS.0000049924.94414.BB

[15] Tones MJ, Moss ND. The impact of patient self-assessment of deformity on HRQL in adults with scoliosis. Scoliosis. 2007;**2**(1):14. DOI: 10.1186/1748-7161-2-14

[16] Sanders JO, Polly DW Jr, Cats-Baril W, Jones J, Lenke LG, O'Brien MF, et al. Analysis of patient and parent assessment of deformity in idiopathic scoliosis using the Walter Reed Visual Assessment Scale. Spine. 2003;**28**(18):2158-2163. DOI: 10.1097/01.BRS.0000084629.97042.0B

[17] Braun V, Clarke V. Using thematic analysis in psychology. Qualitative Research in Psychology. 2008;**3**(2):77-101. DOI: 10.1191/1478088706qp063oa

[18] Coolican H. Research Methods and Statistics in Psychology. East Sussex: Psychology Press; 2004. ISBN: 978-1-4441-7011-5 (pbk); ISBN: 978-0-203-76983-6 (ebk)

[19] Kostuik JP, Bentivoglio J. The incidence of low-back pain in adult scoliosis. Spine. 1981;**6**(3):268-273. DOI: 10.1097/00007632-198105000-00009

[20] Jackson RP, Simmons EH, Stripinis D. Incidence and severity of back pain in adult idiopathic scoliosis. Spine. 1983;**8**(7):749-756. DOI: 10.1097/00007632-198310000-00011

[21] Rowe DE, Bernstein SM, Riddick MF, Adler F, Emans JB, Gardner-Bonneau D. A meta-analysis of the efficacy of non- operative treatments for idiopathic scoliosis. The Journal of Bone & Joint Surgery. 1997;**79**(5):664-674. DOI: 10.2106/00004623-199705000-00005

[22] Maruyama T, Grivas TB, Kaspiris A. Effectiveness and outcomes of brace treatment: A systematic review. Physiotherapy Theory and Practice. 2011;**27**(1):26-42. DOI: 10.3109/09593985.2010.50398

[23] Asher MA, Burton DC. Adolescent idiopathic scoliosis: Natural history and long term treatment effects. Scoliosis. 2006;**1**(1):2. DOI: 10.1186/1748-7161-1-2

[24] Moher D, Schulz KF, Altman DG. The CONSORT statement: Revised recommendations for improving the quality of reports of parallel- group randomised trials. The Lancet. 2001;**357**(9263):1191-1194

[25] Frost H, Lamb SE, Stewart-Brown S. Responsiveness of a patient specific outcome measure compared with the Oswestry Disability Index v2. 1. 2008

[26] Frost H, Lamb SE, Stewart-Brown S. Responsiveness of a patient specific outcome measure compared with the Oswestry Disability Index v2. 1 and Roland and Morris Disability Questionnaire for patients with sub-acute and chronic low back pain. Spine. 2008;**33**(22):2450-2457

[27] Herdman M, Gudex C, Lloyd A, Janssen MF, Kind P, Parkin D, et al. Development and preliminary testing of the new five- level version of EQ-5D (EQ-5D-5L). Quality of Life Research. 2011;**20**(10):1727-1736

[28] Fairbank J, Couper J, Davies J. The Oswestry Low Back Pain Disability Questionnaire. Physiotherapy. 1980;**66**: 271-273

[29] Kopec JA, Esdaile JM, Abrahamowicz M, Abenhaim L, Wood-Dauphinee S, Lamping DL, et al. The Quebec back Pain Disability Scale: Conceptualization and development. Journal of Clinical Epidemiology. 1996;**49**(2):151-161

[30] Fisher K, Johnston M. Validation of the Oswestry Low Back Pain Disability Questionnaire, its sensitivity as a measure of change following treatment and its relationship with other aspects of the chronic pain experience. Physiotherapy Theory and Practice. 1997;**13**(1):67-80

[31] Grönblad M, Hupli M, Wennerstrand P, Järvinen E, Lukinmaa A, Kouri JP, et al. Intel-correlation and test-retest reliability of the pain disability index (pdi) and the

Oswestry disability questionnaire (odq) and their correlation with pain intensity in low back pain patients. The Clinical Journal of Pain. 1993;**9**(3):189-195

[32] Wittink H, Turk DC, Carr DB, Sukiennik A, Rogers W. Comparison of the redundancy, reliability, and responsiveness to change among SF-36, Oswestry Disability Index, and Multidimensional Pain Inventory. The Clinical Journal of Pain. 2004;**20**(3): 133-142

[33] Rabin R, Charro FD. EQ-SD: A measure of health status from the EuroQol group. Annals of Medicine. 2001;**33**(5):337-343

[34] EuroQol. EuroQol–a new facility for the measurement of health- related quality of life. Health Policy (Amsterdam, Netherlands). 1990;**16**(3):199

[35] Dolan, P. Modelling valuations for EuroQol health states. Medical Care. 1997;**35**(11):1095-1108

[36] Tijhuis GJ, Jansen SJT, Stiggelbout AM, Zwinderman AH, Hazes JMW, Vlieland TV. Value of the time trade off method for measuring utilities in patients with rheumatoid arthritis. Annals of the Rheumatic Diseases. 2000;**59**(11):892-897

[37] Brazier J, Roberts J, Tsuchiya A, Busschbach J. A comparison of the EQ-5D and SF-6D across seven patient groups. Health Economics. 2004;**13**(9): 873-884

[38] Ware JE Jr, Sherbourne CD. The MOS 36-item short-form health survey (SF-36): I. Conceptual framework and item selection. Medical Care. 1992;**6**:473-483

[39] Beaton DE, Bombardier C, Hogg-Johnson SA. Measuring health in injured workers: A cross-sectional comparison of five generic health status instruments in workers with musculoskeletal injuries. American Journal of Industrial Medicine. 1996;**29**(6):618-631

[40] Cairns MC, Foster NE, Wright C. Randomized controlled trial of specific spinal stabilization exercises and conventional physiotherapy for recurrent low back pain. Spine. 2006;**31**(19):E670-E681

[41] De Winter JCF. Using the Student's t-test with extremely small sample sizes. Practical Assessment, Research & Evaluation. 2013;**18**(10):2

[42] Box JF. Guinness, Gosset, Fisher, and small samples. Statistical Science. 1987;**2**:45-52

[43] Lehmann EL. "Student" and small-sample theory. In: Selected Works of EL Lehmann. US: Springer; 2012. pp. 1001-1008

[44] IBM Corp. IBM SPSS Statistics for Windows, Version 22.0. Armonk, NY: IBM Corp; 2013

[45] Day RW, Quinn GP. Comparisons of treatments after an analysis of variance in ecology. Ecological Monographs. 1989;**59**(4):433-463

[46] Hollis S, Campbell F. What is meant by intention to treat analysis? Survey of published randomised controlled trials. British Medical Journal. 1999;**319**(7211):670-674

[47] Wertz RT. Intention to treat: Once randomized, always analysed. Clinical Aphasiology. 1995;**23**:57-64

[48] Russo A, Bransford R, Wagner T, Lee MJ, Chapman JR. Adult degenerative scoliosis insights, challenges, and treatment outlook. Current Orthopaedic Practice. 2008;**19**(4):357-365

[49] Kankaanpää M, Taimela S, Laaksonen D, Hänninen O,

Airaksinen O. Back and hip extensor fatigability in chronic low back pain patients and controls. Archives of Physical Medicine and Rehabilitation. 1998;**79**(4):412-417

[50] Maglinte GA, Hays RD, Kaplan RM. US general population norms for telephone administration of the SF-36v2. Journal of Clinical Epidemiology. 2012;**65**(5):497-502

[51] Burström K, Johannesson M, Diderichsen F. A comparison of individual and social time trade-off values for health states in the general population. Health Policy. 2006;**76**(3):359-370

[52] Goldberg CJ, Moore DP, Fogarty EE, Dowling FE. Adolescent idiopathic scoliosis: The effect of brace treatment on the incidence of surgery. Spine. 2001;**26**(1):42-47

[53] Grubb SA, Lipscomb HJ, Suh PB. Results of surgical treatment of painful adult scoliosis. Spine. 1994;**19**(14):1619-1627

[54] Li G, Passias P, Kozanek M, Fu E, Wang S, Xia Q, et al. Adult scoliosis in patients over sixty-five years of age: Outcomes of operative versus nonoperative treatment at a minimum two-year follow- up. Spine. 2009;**34**(20):2165-2170

Chapter 6

Living with a Severe Spinal Deformity: An Innovative and Personal Patient Account of Self-Management Using a Corset, Postural Correction, and Exercises

Andrej Gogala

Abstract

Conservative treatment of scoliosis using brace and exercises usually ends when growth stops. Scoliosis may, however, deteriorate in adulthood especially when curves are larger. The author decided to try to help himself when he was 43 years old. He had been diagnosed with juvenile idiopathic scoliosis when he was 7 years old, but his treatment with a Milwaukee brace ended when he was 11 years old. When his growth ended, the author had a severe scoliosis with a thoracic curve of around 100° Cobb. In adulthood, a corset from fabric with steel reinforcements was used for part of the day intermittently which also included days without wear. To derotate the rib cage, pressure to the rib hump was applied from behind. After some years it was obvious from photo documentation that some derotation had been achieved. The rib hump is smaller; ribs can now be seen on the concave side where they were not seen previously, and a skin mark which was located laterally before moved to the front side. Curves to the side as seen in anteroposterior X-ray images, however, did not improve. But the therapy proved helpful as marked cosmetic improvement was achieved and curve increase was most likely prevented.

Keywords: self-management, conservative treatment, juvenile idiopathic scoliosis, adult with scoliosis, derotation

1. Introduction

In the human being, the spine is curved in the form of two S letters because of upright posture, if seen from the side. It is bent back in the thorax and sacrum and forward in the lumbar and neck regions. If you look from behind, the spine is usually straight when the body is upright. This is true for most healthy people, but asymmetric growth in children can lead to bending of the spine in a sideways manner. This state or condition is called scoliosis [1–4]. The name is of Greek origin, meaning curvature, and was already used by Hippocrates centuries ago [5]. Galen narrowed the meaning to a sideways curvature. Most often and seen from the back, the backbone is curved to the right in the thoracic spine and to the left in the lumbar part. Vertebrae are also twisted, turned in their axis, causing a rib hump to develop in the back [1–4].

Guidelines of the SOSORT Society for the treatment of idiopathic scoliosis from 2011 [1] and 2016 [2] indicate that the goal of conservative treatment is to halt curve progression at puberty (or possibly even reduce it). Bracing is recommended to treat patients with curves above 20 ± 5° Cobb which are still growing. It is recommended that braces should be worn until the end of vertebral bone growth.

Weinstein et al. [6] recently found that wearing a brace prevents curve progression in people with adolescent idiopathic scoliosis, if it is worn for up to at least 13 h a day. Results are better, however, when the brace is worn over a longer time. 90% of children who wore a brace for at least 13 h a day reached the end of the growth period without the need for surgery. Further Aulisa et al. [7] reported that the brace is also very effective in the treatment of juvenile scoliosis. Curve correction was accomplished in 79% of patients, the curve stabilized in 16%, and only in 6% of children did it progress. Juvenile scoliosis starts at the age of 3–9 years and can lead to larger curvatures than adolescent scoliosis which starts between 10 and 17 years of age [1]. Lusini et al. [8] further found that wearing a brace can reduce the curvature even in patients with curve magnitudes over 45° Cobb, who had refused to have surgery.

After maturity, most adult patients are left without any prescribed therapy. But their scoliosis may worsen over time. Usually the curvature progresses slowly also in adulthood. The linear rate of progression is about 1° Cobb per year, and this has been demonstrated to occur in progressive adult scoliosis [9]. Curves larger than 50° are associated with a high risk of continued deterioration or progression throughout adulthood and thus usually indicate the need for surgery [6].

Scoliosis fusion surgery is generally considered the only means to stop the progression of the spinal deformity in patients with adult idiopathic scoliosis. However, when patients with adult scoliosis progress, scoliosis-specific exercises can be effective in order to obtain stability and in some cases to reduce the Cobb angles in degrees. In highly progressive curves, exercises appear to slow down the progression of the curvature [10]. Using traction and massage, Brooks et al. [11] were able to improve chest expansion and decrease thoracic curvature in an adult with idiopathic scoliosis. Negrini et al. [12] hypothesized that the improvement of adult scoliosis that was achieved by one of their patients is a consequence of recovery from a postural collapse without any changes in bone structure. The structural bony component of scoliosis cannot be improved with a cast or other corrective measures and can be seen in a radiograph of a person in the correction with a cast or a brace. The postural collapse component of scoliosis can be seen as the difference between the curvature on a radiograph taken while standing and the one taken while lying down.

For adult patients with late-onset idiopathic scoliosis, cosmetic concerns and pain are the main reasons for seeking treatment. Daily exercise and part-time bracing can also potentially reduce pain in the adult scoliosis population [13].

Rigid braces for the treatment of scoliosis were first used by Ambroise Paré (1510–1590). They were made out of metal. Among other things, he wrote that bracing does not help when the skeleton matures and growth stops [14]. This assertion has rarely been contradicted in the literature and is considered the "truth" up to this day. Brodhurst [15] describes and provides figures of a fairly successful treatment of an 18-year-old girl with his supporting device, which was the precursor of today's rigid braces and acted in the same way. It put pressure on the convex side of the curve and lifted the shoulder in the concave side, just like a modern

Chêneau brace made of plastic. His instrument (**Figure 1**), as he called it, consisted of a frame made out of a pelvic hoop, upright crutches, and connecting dorsal band placed at the superior extremity of the primary curve. The shoulder sling or loop was placed on the shoulder which corresponded to the concavity of the primary curve and was connected to the lever. The convexity of the primary curve was supported by a large pad. The effectiveness of a combination of Schroth and SEAS exercises together with wearing a brace in adult patients with scoliosis was reported by Papadopoulos [16].

My scoliosis was discovered when I was around 7 years of age when I was treated with a Milwaukee brace in the orthopedic hospital in Valdoltra. But when I was 11 years old, I experienced acute renal failure. The inflammation that followed left lasting effects on my kidneys, and since 1978 when I was 16 years old, I had to attend hemodialysis regularly. As this was a life-threatening condition, my parents decided to stop the therapy of scoliosis which unfortunately was left unmanaged since then. For a few years, I still grew and unfortunately over the years the back curvature increased.

In 2005 I decided to finally do something about my scoliosis. I was 43 years old at that time, and the predominant view was that after growth is completed, the correction of scoliosis without surgery is no longer possible. The risk of complications in surgery in adults is very high, and long-term effects are questionable [17]. So I decided to take action by my own method.

From the archives of the Department of Dialysis of the Ljubljana Medical Centre, I got X-ray images showing my spine. I was able to measure Cobb angles, which are used to measure the curvature and to estimate the severity of deformation. In the images from the years 1997 and 2005, only the thoracic curvature is seen which is equal in both images, so it did not deteriorate over this time period before the

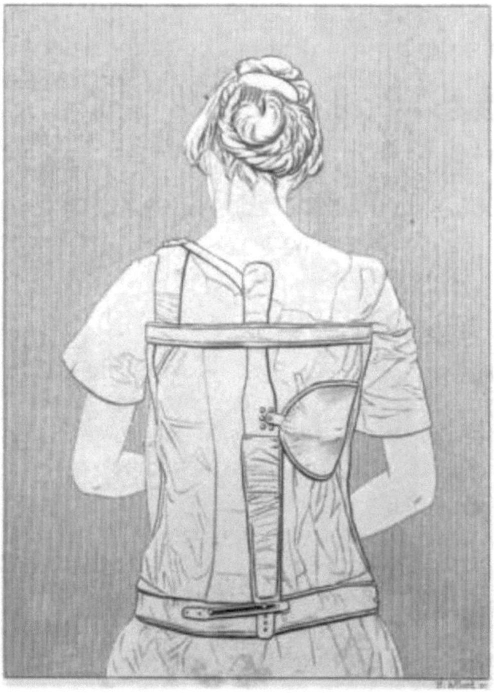

Figure 1.
Brodhurst's instrument for the treatment of scoliosis (Brodhurst, 1855).

treatment. The image from 2010 shows both curves. The upper thoracic curve is larger and measures 104°, while the lower lumbar measures 57°. Curves over 60° are considered a very severe form of scoliosis, and in curves over 80°, it affects lung function which is impaired. The vital capacity of my lungs measured 1380 ml in 2010, a value which is only 40% of the value that is estimated for a man without scoliosis, for my height.

Early-onset scoliosis like mine can result in larger curves than more common adolescent scoliosis because the unbalanced growth of the spine lasts longer. If untreated, juvenile scoliosis can cause serious cardiopulmonary complications and premature death [18]. In comparison untreated late-onset scoliosis causes little physical impairment other than back pain and cosmetic concerns [19]. The prognosis for most patients with more than 100° curvature of the spine is generally death in their 40s or 50s due to respiratory or heart failure, although there are exceptions to this [20].

2. The therapy

I found that my spine is not bent forward in the lumbar area as found in the lordosis of a person without scoliosis. It was only bent sideways. I assumed that the sideways curvature would diminish, if I managed to bend the spine forward, as is correct. I thought that this would also have a beneficial impact on the higher parts of the spine. I decided to buy an elastic bodice from a shop that sold medical equipment. I then stitched longitudinal metal braces to it, which I twisted to the form of my own body. The one that crossed the hump had to be bent almost at right angles to fit. With this corset I then carried out my activities of daily living; I also slept in it and went for walks in the bodice. Three months later, in the spring of 2006, I ordered an underbust corset of the waist cincher type on the Internet, otherwise used by ladies to constrict their waists (Axfords C225, the firm ceased trading since). It forced me into an upright posture and created a lumbar lordosis. I had to take it off before lunch so I could eat, but then I put it on again before I go to sleep. After some months I ordered a longer underbust corset, which grasped the pelvis and ribs better, but since it was not custom made, it did not fit perfectly (Axfords C229). When I received it by post, my mother showed me hers that was very similar, only it was laced by the side, not the rear. She had scoliosis at a young age too, and in that time (the 1950s) scoliosis was treated with corsets made from fabric, like the one I was using. I walked a lot wearing the corset, also in the mountains.

Flat back often accompanies scoliosis [1]. It has the same shortcomings as a flat foot, so it does not allow much flexibility. The spine should ideally be slightly curved, so the creation of a correct lordosis is very important. When the spine is curved in the sagittal plane, curves to the sides may be reduced [21]. In people without a lordotic curve, the head is not positioned above the pelvis, but in front of it. The center of gravity outside the body axis then causes overload of the back muscles causing pain.

When I lost hope that I would achieve anything with the corset that I had used for a couple of years, I then stopped wearing it. After a few days, however, I was surprised to find that there has been an improvement. Thus it was necessary to interrupt my treatment with the corset. I found that I needed a corset that would stretch all the way from the armpits to the pelvis and press the hump in order to reduce it. It needed to be custom made, and I found a website where I could order an overbust corset (reaching above the bust), made to my measures without too much additional charge (Corsetcurves Venus, the website does not exist anymore).

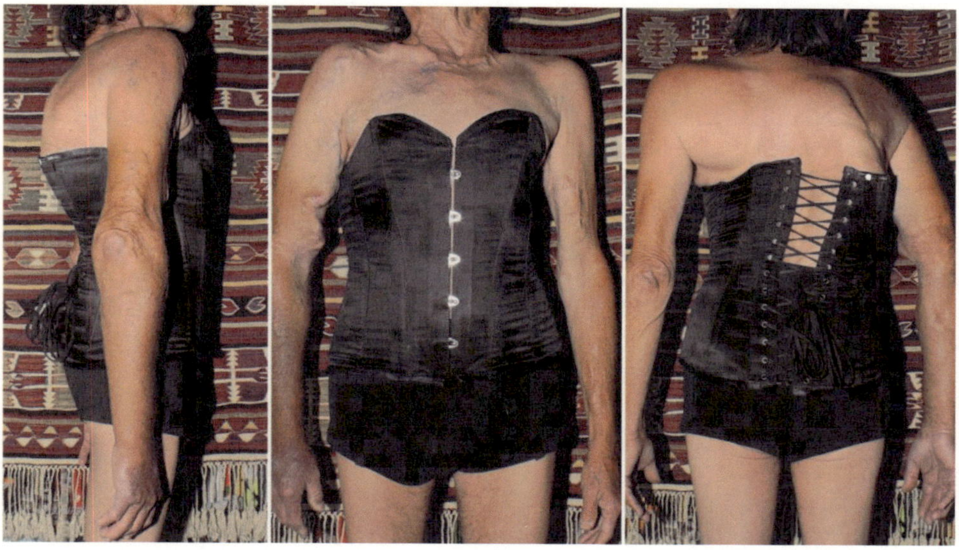

Figure 2.
Overbust corset used from September 2008 to October 2016. View from the side, front, and rear in July 2011.

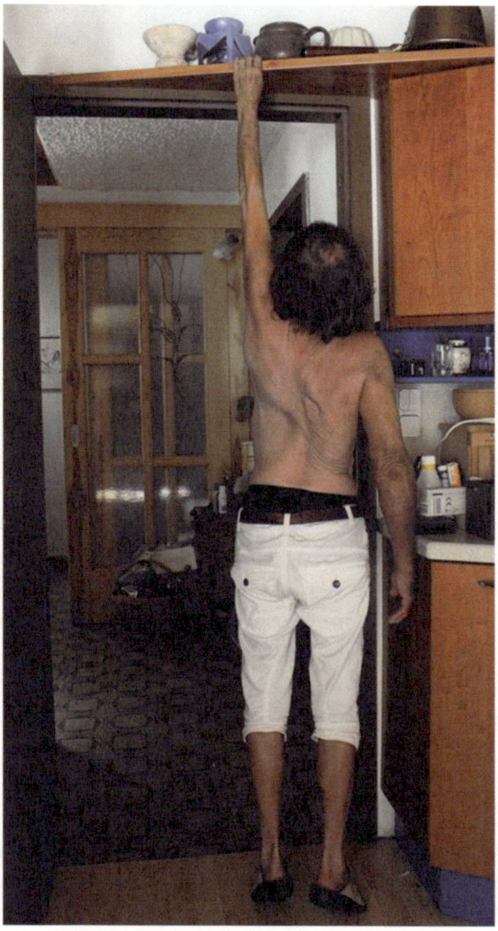

Figure 3.
Extending to and hanging with the left hand on barely accessible holds has proven to be the most effective exercise for stretching the spine. If a right convex scoliosis is caused by the predominant use of the right hand, it may possibly be improved by the frequent use of the left hand in normal work and exercise.

It fitted me much better, but behind the hump it lay sideways; this was inevitable due to my rib hump (**Figure 2**). It was made from three layers of fabric with steel reinforcements. I wore it from September 2008 to October 2016.

To successfully derotate my chest, I used additional manipulation and physiotherapy. I pressed on the hump from behind and stretched muscles on the concave side by improvements and overcorrections of my posture. My walks with a backpack in nature were not intended to be part of the therapy; they were part of my job as a biologist, but they proved to be just that: therapy. The straps were forcing my shoulders to be at the same height when wearing a backpack with photo camera equipment. I also found that correcting my posture many times during the day was also very important as this eliminated any unbalanced loading of my skeleton [3]. I added occasional pressure to the hump from behind. This is similar to the treatment recommended also when applying plaster cast as an effective treatment for scoliosis in young children [22]. In order to stretch the spine and reduce side curvature, I also included stretching exercises for the left side of the body into the therapy in 2013. With my left hand, I pushed at the hip while standing or at the thigh while sitting and stretched the left side. I lifted the body with my hands holding the handles of a chair, and the spine stretched due to gravity. With my left hand, I stretched out to reach a shelf above the door. The last exercise in particular has proven to be effective, since the hump reduced during the exercise and the spine straightened significantly (**Figure 3**).

3. Results

3.1 July 2011 until January 2012

From July 2011 to January 2012, I continued to alternate the days when I wore the corset and days when I did not as I found this to be more effective than continuous wear as far as derotation was concerned. The corset improved the position of the ribs and arched my back, but it could not decrease the vertebral rotation and therefore did not reduce the hump immediately. But after I have taken off the corset, by pressing the hump from behind against the floor when lying or against the backrest when sitting and with contractions of the back muscles, I could decrease the hump slightly, moving the vertebrae slightly toward the correct position.

The comparison of images taken in July 2011 and January 2012 documents a substantial improvement. In side view from July, the hump was of a semicircular shape and at a right angle to back. The skin of the chest and abdomen in the front was loose and wrinkled as it was not supported by the ribs. On 10 January 2012, the back was evenly narrowing toward the waist in side view. At the front, the ribs supported the skin of the chest and abdomen. A skin mark which was located laterally in the earlier image moved to the front (**Figure 4**).

3.2 March 2012

I photographed myself again on 23 March 2012. The view from the rear, in comparison with the image taken in January, showed improvement on the left concave side where previously the ribs were hidden as they were shifted forward because of the rotation of the spine and chest (**Figure 5**).

If a line is drawn from the extremity of the curve to its upper and lower end, and the angle measured that is formed by these lines, we find that the angle was 140° in January and 150° in March: the apparent curve on the surface was reduced. In an upright spine, this angle would measure 180°; a smaller angle thus means a larger

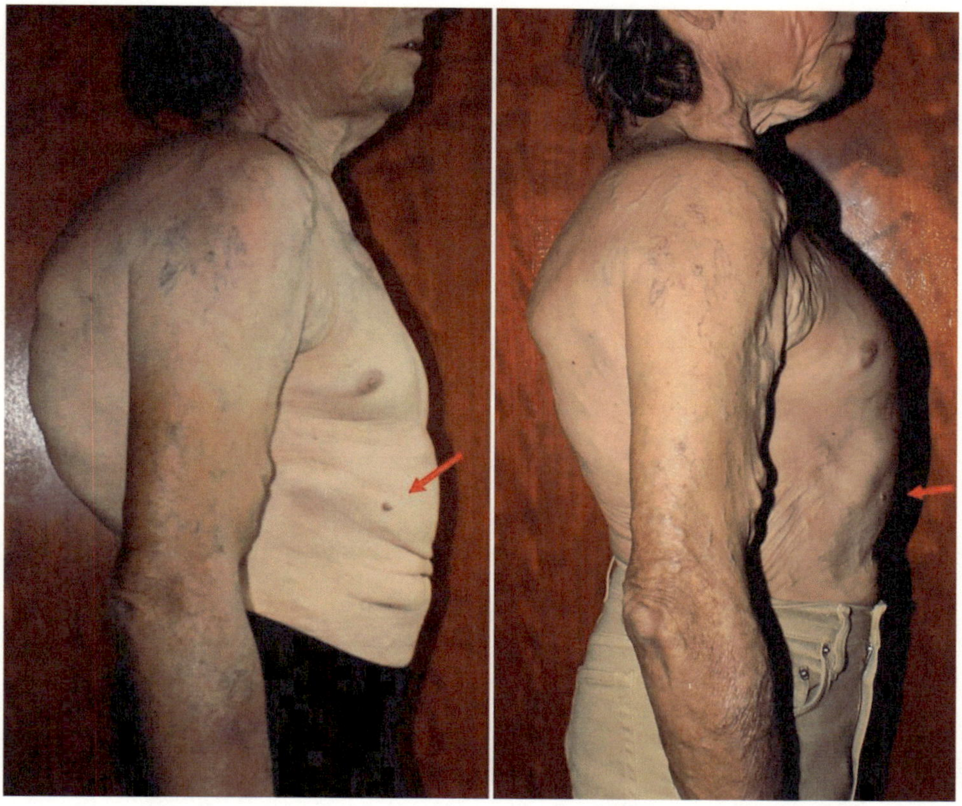

Figure 4.
The left image was taken on 1 July 2011. The hump is of a semicircular shape and connects with the back at a right angle. The skin of the chest and abdomen at the front is loose and wrinkled, because it is not supported by the ribs. The right view was created on 10 January 2012. The difference is obvious. From the side the blade down the back is evenly narrowing toward the waist. At the front, the ribs support the chest and skin of the abdomen. A skin mark (pointed by the arrows), located laterally in July 2011, moved to the front side in January 2012.

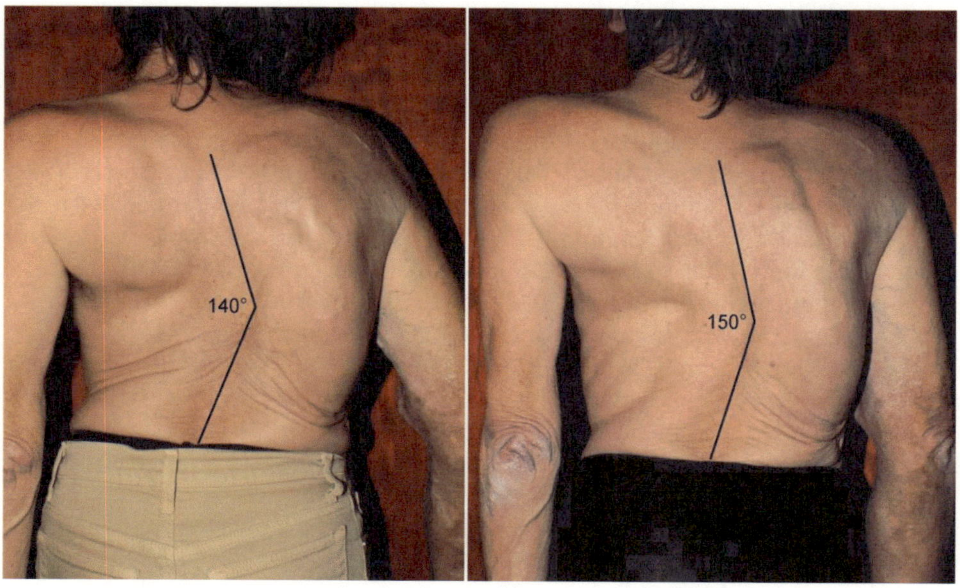

Figure 5.
Comparison of the back, photographed in January 2012 (left) and March 2012 (right). The apparent curve has been reduced in March, and on the left side of the body we see the ribs, which were not seen in January (left) as they were shifted forward because of rotation of the spine in its axis. We can only see the wrinkled skin in the place of ribs seen in the march image.

curvature. Digital photographs can be taken without limitations as the body is not exposed to radiation like in X-ray imaging. To measure the angles, the lines from the photos were transferred to a picture of a protractor in the Adobe Photoshop program. The apparent curve on the surface does not correspond with the curvature of the spine, however. It is just a simple indicator used in monitoring the development of the curve and is dependent of several factors. As proven in my case, it was an indicator of the degree of rotation.

In side view, in comparison with January, the hump seemed to have increased again at first sight. But a closer examination revealed that the scapula, which was previously raised by the hump, was lowered. The ribs, which previously had raised it, formed the curve of the hump. But the chest and abdomen at the front were supported well and were not loose, as they have been in July 2011. This means that the derotation, achieved between July 2011 and January 2012, was preserved.

3.3 April 2012

To find out the cause for a benefit of alternating days when wearing a corset or not, I wore the corset for 5 days in a row during the day and then had my back photographed on 6 April 2012. I found that in lateral view, the hump was reduced and the scapula was lifted. The view from behind showed that the apparent curve sideways measured 144°. Thus, it was more pronounced than in the previous image taken on 27 March 2012 (151°). The next day, the curve measured 151° again. I found that the corset could therefore temporarily increase rotation, but this was rapidly corrected when corset wear was interrupted. The chest easily rotates to a certain degree when the corset is tightened too much because of pressure to the ribs, diminishing the circumference of the chest. Then it derotates again when the corset is taken off. When this happens often, therapy should be discontinued for a longer time to allow ligaments to stiffen and prevent rotation. Care must also be taken not to tighten the corset too much.

3.4 June 2012

The apparent curvature (rotation) diminished over time during the therapy. The exceptional case of the 6th of April cannot be considered because it was not documented under the same conditions. On 10 January 2012, the curve was 140°; 23rd of March, 150°; 27th of March, 151°; and 14th of April, 154°. If a graph is drawn on these data points, a straight line can be drawn through. However, on the 4th and 22nd of May and on the 9th of June 2012, the curve remained the same as in the 14th of April. The limits of any possible derotation had probably been reached.

The imaging on the 9th of June 2012 showed an important change from the previous state, however. My pelvis was no longer tilted as much as before, and the analysis of the photographs showed a significant difference. The pelvic obliquity may be the consequence of unequal leg length, but the pelvis could also be shifted due to rotation in the lumbar part of the spine that is present in scoliosis. Scoliosis can develop because of pelvic obliquity, but scoliosis also causes or increases pelvic tilt. It is difficult to determine what occurred first. I linked the iliac crests on the photos with a line and drew a line along the middle of the body (**Figure 6**). Then I measured the angle between these lines. It would measure 90° if the pelvis was not inclined as in a healthy person. In me, the angle at the right side of my body measured 96° on 4 May 2012, but only 92.5° on June 9. A mistake due to changes in posture was possible, so I waited for the imaging of June 22. The angle was the same, so the pelvic tilt was actually reduced.

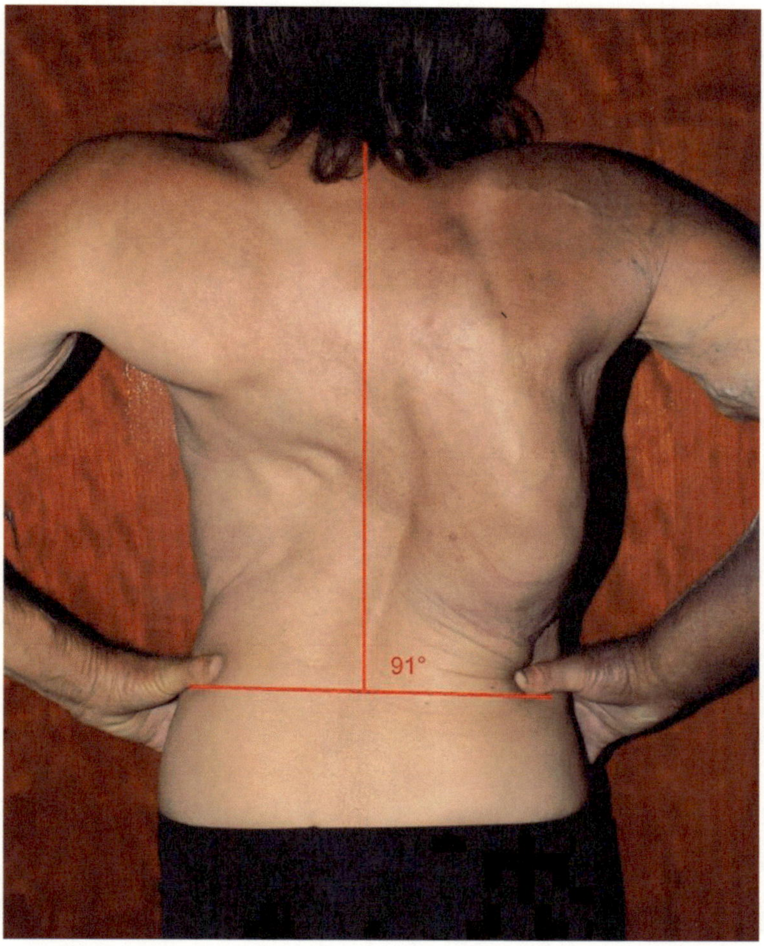

Figure 6.
Pelvic tilt measured on 17 August 2012. Thumbs are put to the iliac crests of the pelvis to mark them. The angle at the right side was 91°.

3.5 October 2012 and further

According to appearance, the scoliosis improved substantially since the beginning of treatment. The hump was markedly reduced. However, it is important to note that only X-rays can show the true state of the curves, so I was X-rayed on 8 October 2012. The comparison with X-ray image from 2010 showed that there was almost no change in spinal curvature (**Figure 7**). I have achieved derotation of the chest and improvement of the shape of the ribs as well as the lumbar lordosis. This reduced the hump and led to better rib support of the right side of the chest in front and left side in the rear (concave side). The changes had a positive effect on breathing and possibly prevented further deterioration of the curves. Lung volume reduction, which can be life-threatening, is not caused by curvature of the spine, but by the rotation of the rib cage which becomes flattened. Radiographs from 4 March 2015 also showed that the curvature did not improve. In years to come, I was still using the corset for at least some hours a week. I obtained a better corset in October 2016, which was much stiffer acting almost like a true brace (Vollers Eye Candy: https://www.vollers-corsets.com/eye-candy-made-in-england). But without reduction of the curve, additional derotation and rib hump reduction were not possible either.

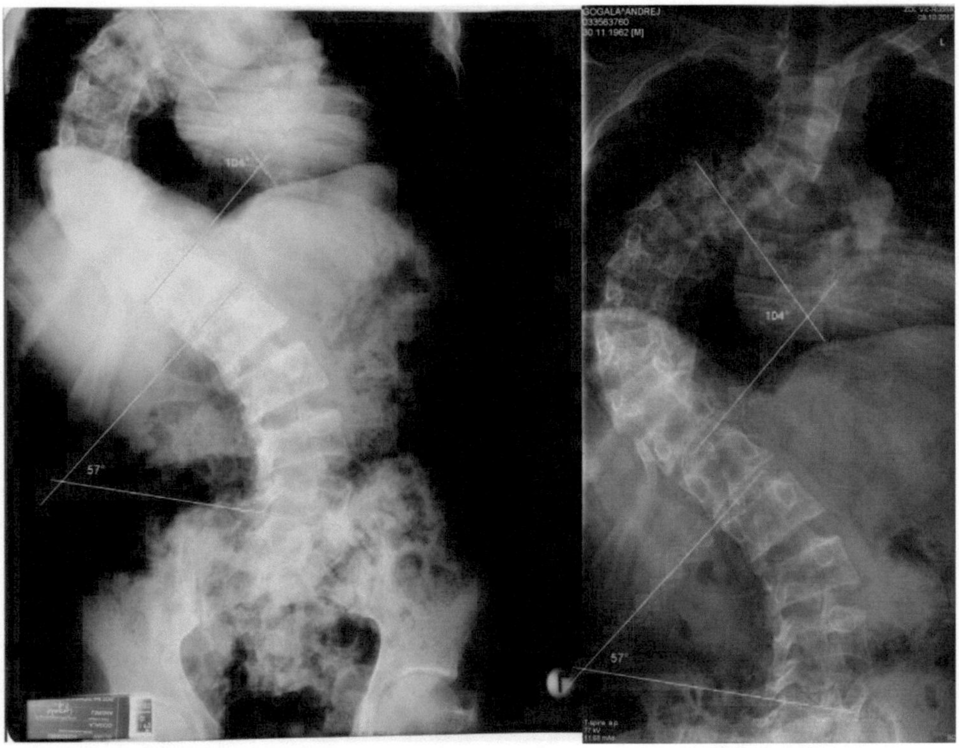

Figure 7.
At the left an X-ray image from 2010 with cobb angles measured. The thoracic curve measured 104° and lower lumbar 57°. At the right the X-ray image of the spine from 8 October 2012. The same angles are inserted as on the left image; there is almost no change.

I have never experienced back pain. Only when I started going on walks without the corset after I wore it almost every day for some time that a muscle started to ache on the left (concave) side of the back, which was shortened due to scoliosis and weakened during corset wear. But I persisted. If the pain was severe, I stopped for a rest and then went on. When the muscle strengthened again, the pain no longer occurred. The curves of my spine seem to be quite stiff and not mobile as they do not change between imaging sessions. But I do not have any problems with spine mobility during my activities. I have reduced lung capacity, however, and was never able to run over longer distances. With a long walk I had no problems; only when walking uphill, I was slower than others.

4. Discussion

Although corsets from textiles in the nineteenth and the first half of the twentieth century were sometimes used to treat or at least alleviate scoliosis, they were not accepted by the leading physicians at the time. Albee [23] published a picture of a textile corset for the treatment of scoliosis, but he recommended it only for the immobilization of the spine after spine surgery. A textile corset is more comfortable than a rigid brace as it adapts to the shape of the body. Since it is made of cloth, it is permeable to the air and moisture. Also the feeling of a hug given by the bodice is pleasant.

The corset should absolutely not be tightened too much, however. If it starts to pinch, then this means the grip must be released by loosening the lace at the back. This allows one to constantly adapt the corset to ones' body state. The body changes its circumference with food intake and the degree of hydration. If the corset is tightened too much, it forces the ribs to rotate the vertebrae and diminish the chest circumference. It needs to be tightened only as much as is needed for good support and pressure to the prominent angles of the ribs; it should not press on the concave sides of the chest. Excessive tightening of the corset known as tightlacing or waist training was probably the cause of the bad reputation of wearing corsets as stated by medical experts in the Victorian times. The doctors cited corset wear in young women of the higher social classes as one of the main causes of scoliosis.

Textile corsets embrace the whole body, but the strongest pressure needs to be directed at the most prominent angles of the ribs to push them forward and inward posteriorly and backward anteriorly. Since the bodice acts with the same force on the ribs from the other side also, the ribs slowly get a more rounded shape, thus gaining a better form. Consequently the deformation of the chest is reduced. However, since the corset does not have empty spaces where the chest can expand into, treatment with a textile corset needs to be periodically interrupted.

After the corset is taken off, derotation forces directed to the back of the rib hump forward can then be applied to the thorax to derotate it, pushing the ribs in the opposite direction to the rotating forces. The hump needs to be pressed from behind, not laterally as this flattens the rib cage. A similar type of manipulation was performed to correct spinal deformities by Hippocrates and Galen millennia ago. While extending the body, they pressed the hump with the leg, whole body or with a plank, attached to the wall for leverage [5]. But pressing against the chair backrest or the hard floor when lying is sufficient. In the days when the corset is not worn, the chest can expand, and the muscles are more active and can be strengthened.

Corset wear also has an important effect on learning how to correct the erect posture. Patients with scoliosis have a distorted feeling of upright posture. When the corset forces them into it, they learn to keep an upright posture even when they are not braced.

While partial derotation was achieved with the help of a textile corset, the corset was not effective in diminishing the side curvatures of the spine as it is symmetrical. Modern rigid braces are far better at in-brace curve reduction, necessary for long-term improvement. But rigid braces for side curves of about 100° Cobb do not exist yet. In such cases we should be satisfied when deterioration is prevented.

The side curvature of the spine is always accompanied by rotation of the vertebrae and rib cage. Ribs are connected by intercostal muscles and cannot spread apart on the convex side when the spine bends. The curvature of the spine in the thoracic region is not possible without rotation of the vertebrae and deformation of the ribs. The ribs at the apex of the curve are pulled inward toward the vertebrae. Intercostal muscles under stress pull them up and down, but the composite force is directed toward the spine because the ribs at the apex of the curve are shifted further from the midline than other ribs [24]. The side curvature of the spine stretches the intercostal muscles like an archer pulls a bow string and the taut muscles push the ribs like the bow string pushes the arrow.

With rotation of the vertebrae at the apex of the curve, which are compressed between the ribs, the thoracic circumference diminishes, and the tension in the chest wall is alleviated. The deformation becomes irreversible if new growth or bone resorption and remodeling change the shape of the ribs and vertebrae or if the ligaments are not firm enough. When the rib cage and vertebrae become structurally rotated, the vertebrae lose the balanced support from the ribs from both sides. Shear forces from the ribs turn the vertebrae further and push the vertebral bodies toward the convexity (**Figure 8**). Continuous progression of scoliosis starts. With therapy one is able to diminish only the excessive rotation, while some rotation is

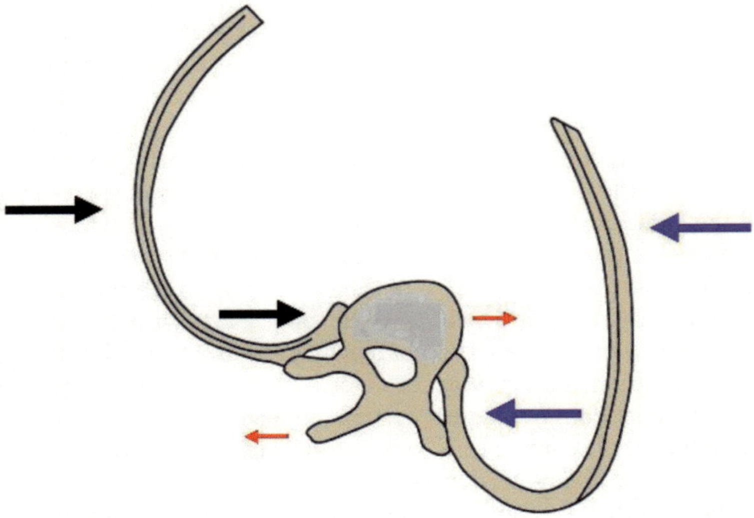

Figure 8.
In a rotated chest, forces transmitted by the ribs turn vertebrae and bend the spine sideways. Ribs on one side of the vertebrae are not opposed by equal support from the ribs on the contralateral side, so ribs on the concave side push vertebral bodies toward convexity, bending the spine [24].

necessary at a given curvature. The side curvature in the frontal view must be reduced for further improvement.

5. Conclusion

Although the reduction of spine curvature developed in scoliosis is unlikely during adulthood, therapy in this period of life is not without benefits. We can achieve partial derotation of the chest leading to a significant improvement of appearance. Deterioration of scoliosis may probably be prevented. Textile corset may be more acceptable than a rigid brace for active adult patients as it is more comfortable and not noticeable under clothing. Corset wear should be complemented with other therapies, like postural correction, exercises, and physical manipulation.

Conflict of interest

The author declares that he has no competing interests. The study was not supported by funding.

Author details

Andrej Gogala
Slovenian Museum of Natural History, Ljubljana, Slovenia

*Address all correspondence to: agogala@pms-lj.si

References

[1] Negrini S, Aulisa AG, Aulisa L, Circo AB, de Mauroy JC, Durmala J, et al. 2011 SOSORT guidelines: Orthopaedic and rehabilitation treatment of idiopathic scoliosis during growth. Scoliosis. 2012;7:3

[2] Negrini S, Donzelli S, Aulisa AG, Czaprowski D, Schreiber S, de Mauroy JC, et al. 2016 SOSORT guidelines: Orthopaedic and rehabilitation treatment of idiopathic scoliosis during growth. Scoliosis and Spinal Disorders. 2018;**13**:3. DOI: 10.1186/s13013-017-0145-8

[3] Lehnert-Schroth C. Three-Dimensional Treatment for Scoliosis. A Physiotherapeutic Method for Deformities of the Spine. Palo Alto, California: The Martindale Press; 2007. 276 p

[4] Cheng JC, Castelein RM, Chu WC, Danielsson AJ, Dobbs MB, Grivas TB, et al. Adolescent idiopathic scoliosis. Nature Reviews Disease Primers. 2015;**1**: 15030

[5] Vasiliadis ES, Grivas TB, Kaspiris A. Historical overview of spinal deformities in ancient Greece. Scoliosis. 2009;**4**:6

[6] Weinstein SL, Dolan LA, Wright JG, Dobbs MB. Effects of bracing in adolescents with idiopathic scoliosis. New England Journal of Medicine. 2013; **369**:1512-1515

[7] Aulisa AG, Guzzanti V, Marzetti E, Giordano M, Falciglia F, Aulisa L. Brace treatment in juvenile idiopathic scoliosis: A prospective study in accordance with the SRS criteria for bracing studies—SOSORT award 2013 winner. Scoliosis. 2014;**9**:3

[8] Lusini M, Donzelli S, Minnella S, Zaina F, Negrini S. Brace treatment is effective in idiopathic scoliosis over 45°: An observational prospective cohort controlled study. The Spine Journal. 2014;**14**(9):1951-1956. DOI: 10.1016/j.spinee.2013.11.040

[9] Marty-Poumarat C, Scattin L, Marpeau M, Garreau de Loubresse C, Aegerter P. Natural history of progressive adult scoliosis. Spine. 2007; **32**:1227-1234

[10] Negrini A, Negrini MG, Donzelli S, Romano M, Zaina F, Negrini S. Scoliosis-specific exercises can reduce the progression of severe curves in adult idiopathic scoliosis: A long-term cohort study. Scoliosis. 2015;**10**:20. DOI: 10.1186/s13013-015-0044-9

[11] Brooks WJ, Krupinski EA, Hawes MC. Reversal of childhood idiopathic scoliosis in an adult, without surgery: A case report and literature review. Scoliosis. 2009;**4**:27

[12] Negrini A, Parzini S, Negrini MG, Romano M, Atanasio S, Zaina F, et al. Adult scoliosis can be reduced through specific SEAS exercises: A case report. Scoliosis. 2008;**3**:20

[13] Weiss H-R, Moramarco K, Moramarco M. Scoliosis bracing and exercise for pain management in adults —A case report. Journal of Physical Therapy Science. 2016;**28**:2404-2407

[14] Fayssoux RS, Cho RH, Herman MJA. History of bracing for idiopathic scoliosis in North America. Clinical Orthopaedics and Related Research. 2010;**468**:654-664

[15] Brodhurst BE. On Lateral Curvature of the Spine, its Pathology and Treatment. London: John Churchill; 1855. 67 p

[16] Papadopoulos D. Adult scoliosis treatment combining brace and exercises. Scoliosis. 2013;**8**(Suppl 2):O8

[17] Weiss HR, Goodall D. Rate of complications in scoliosis surgery—A systematic review of the Pub Med literature. Scoliosis. 2008;**3**:9

[18] Mohar J. Untreated early onset scoliosis—The natural progression of a debilitating and ultimately deadly disease. In: Grivas TB, editor. Recent Advances in Scoliosis. London: IntechOpen; 2012. pp. 311-328. DOI: 10.5772/2497

[19] Weinstein SL, Dolan LA, Spratt KF, Peterson KK, Spoonamore MJ, Ponseti IV. Health and function of patients with untreated idiopathic scoliosis. A 50-year natural history study. JAMA. 2003;**289**:559-567

[20] Rom WN, Miller A. Unexpected longevity in patients with severe kyphoscoliosis. Thorax. 1978;**33**:106-110

[21] van Loon PJ, Kühbauch BA, Thunnissen FB. Forced lordosis on the thoracolumbar junction can correct coronal plane deformity in adolescents with double major curve pattern idiopathic scoliosis. Spine. 2008;**33**: 797-801

[22] D'Astous JL, Sanders JO. Casting and traction treatment methods for scoliosis. Orthopedic Clinics of North America. 2007;**38**:477-484

[23] Albee FH. Orthopedic and Reconstruction Surgery, Industrial and Civilian. W. B. Saunders Company: Philadelphia and London; 1919. 1138 p

[24] Gogala A. Role of the ribs in the onset and progression of idiopathic scoliosis. Zdravniški vestnik. 2017;**86**:404-413. DOI: 10.6016/ZdravVestn.2483

Chapter 7

Conservative Treatment of Degenerative Lumbar Scoliosis

Shu Yan Ng

Abstract

Degenerative lumbar scoliosis (DLS) is commonly seen in people over the age of 50 years. The prevalence increases with age. Patients with DLS often complain of low back pain and radiculopathy. Neurological complaints are rare. Current treatments are generally targeted at pain relief. Effects are temporary; this is understandable as the spinal deformities which are the cause of the pain are not addressed. A few studies have shown that scoliosis specific exercises and lordotic bracing stabilize or reduce the rate of curve progression in patients with DLS. Patients should also be instructed in performing corrective movements in daily activities. In the presence of sarcopenia or decreased bone mineral density (BMD), resistance exercises and nutritional supplements should also be prescribed, as reduction in paraspinal muscle mass and BMD are risk factors of DLS. In the presence of neurological involvement or when the symptoms are refractory to conservative treatment, referral for surgery is required.

Keywords: degenerative lumbar scoliosis, adult scoliosis, scoliosis-specific exercise, spinal brace, sarcopenia, osteoporosis

1. Introduction

Adult scoliosis includes adult idiopathic scoliosis as well as degenerative lumbar scoliosis (DLS). DLS is a de novo scoliosis. It is defined as a lateral curvature of the spine in excess of 10° and a sagittal vertical axis (SVA) of more than 50 mm. in an adult over 50 years of age [1]. The sagittal vertical axis is the horizontal distance from the vertical plumbline dropped from the centroid of C7 to the posterosuperior corner of the sacral end plate.

The prevalence of DLS varies with different studies. The reported rate ranges from 8.3–68% [2–5]. The marked variation in prevalence reported is possibly a result of the differences in inclusion criteria of the different studies. Kilshaw et al. [6] evaluated the prevalence of lumbar scoliosis using abdominal and kidney–ureter-bladder radiographs on patients over the age of 20 years [6]. The study showed that lumbar scoliosis is more prevalent in women and increases with age [6]. At the ages of between 60 and 69 years, the prevalence was 6%, whereas at the age of 90 years, the prevalence was over 30% [6]. It has, however, to be noted that the study did not differentiate between adult idiopathic scoliosis and DLS and that the radiographs employed were supine films, which might underestimate the Cobb angle and thus the prevalence of lumbar scoliosis. Xu et al. [7] evaluated 2395 Han Chinese over 40 years of age for the presence of DLS, using dual energy X-ray absorptiometry (DEXA) images. They reported a prevalence of 13.3%, with females more commonly affected than males. Also, the prevalence increased with age [7]. Prevalence was reduced with increasing curve severity; over 80% of the patients with DLS had curves in between 10° and 20° [7].

2. Etiopathogenesis

The causes of adult scoliosis are many. Aebi [1] classified adult scoliosis into four different groups, based on their etiologies. Type 1 refers to primary or de novo degenerative lumbar scoliosis. Type 2 refers to adult idiopathic scoliosis (ADIS), and type 3 refers to adult curves with other primary causes. The last type includes two subgroups. Type 3a refers to adult scoliosis caused by spinal or extra-spinal factors, while type 3b refers to those caused by metabolic bone diseases [1]. Thus adult scoliosis patients are not a homogeneous population group. Our present discussion would focus on DLS which is more prevalent than other types of adult scoliosis.

The pathomechanisms of DLS have not been entirely elucidated, though vertebral instability has been proposed to play a role in its pathogenesis [8, 9]. Kobayashi et al. [4], in a study of the prevalence of DLS, proposed that lateral osteophytes present at the endplate which are in excess of 5 mm together with an asymmetric tilt of disc space >3° are risk factors for the development of DLS [4].

The factors initiating the vertebral instability, however, are unknown. Lumbar paraspinal muscle atrophy; facet tropism, which is defined as the angular asymmetry between the left and right facet joint orientation; and osteoporosis have all been implicated in the pathogenesis of the condition [7, 10, 11].

Lumbar multifidus muscle atrophy (LMA) has also been postulated to contribute to vertebral instability [10]. The multifidus muscle is the deepest and most medial paraspinal muscle, adjacent to the facet joint. LMA is common in DLS, particularly on the concave side of the lumbar scoliosis (**Figure 1**) [12, 13]. Conversely, hyperplasia of the multifidus muscle is evident on the convex side of DLS [14]. Sun et al. [10] investigated the relationship between LMA and various coronal and sagittal radiographic parameters in 144 patients with DLS [10]. They showed that the LMA in the upper and lower vertebral levels adjacent to the apex on the concavity of the lumbar scoliosis correlated positively with the Cobb angle [10]. Conversely, the LMA on the convex side correlated negatively with the lumbar Cobb angle [10]. Sun et al. [10] postulated that LMA may cause vertebral instability and subsequent degenerative changes of lumbar facet joints. Remodeling of articular processes, which includes cartilage degeneration and bone erosion, generally lags behind LMA [10].

Facet tropism has also been postulated to increase the risk of vertebral rotatory olisthesis (VRO) and degenerative lumbar scoliosis [11, 15, 16]. Vertebral rotatory olisthesis refers to lateral and rotatory vertebral translation. Facet joints were found to be more angled in a coronal plane on the convex side of VRO than those of the control subjects without VRO [11]. More severe facet tropism is associated with a higher incidence of VRO [11]. The asymmetric facet orientation causes uneven stress distribution across the zygapophyseal tissues and brings about degenerative changes and segmental instabilities [11]. An intraoperative biomechanical study demonstrated that facet tropism contributed to lumbar vertebral instability [17].

The role of osteoporosis in DLS has been controversial, with some studies showing that osteoporosis contributed to DLS, a number showing that DLS caused the osteoporosis, with others showing no correlation between the two [7]. The lumbar scoliosis brought about by vertebral instability may stabilize or progress [8, 9]. In the presence of marked scoliotic wedging of one disc in the early phase of DLS, adjacent discs may compensate by wedging in the other direction to maintain balance, with resultant stabilization or even regression of the lumbar scoliosis (**Figure 2**) [8].

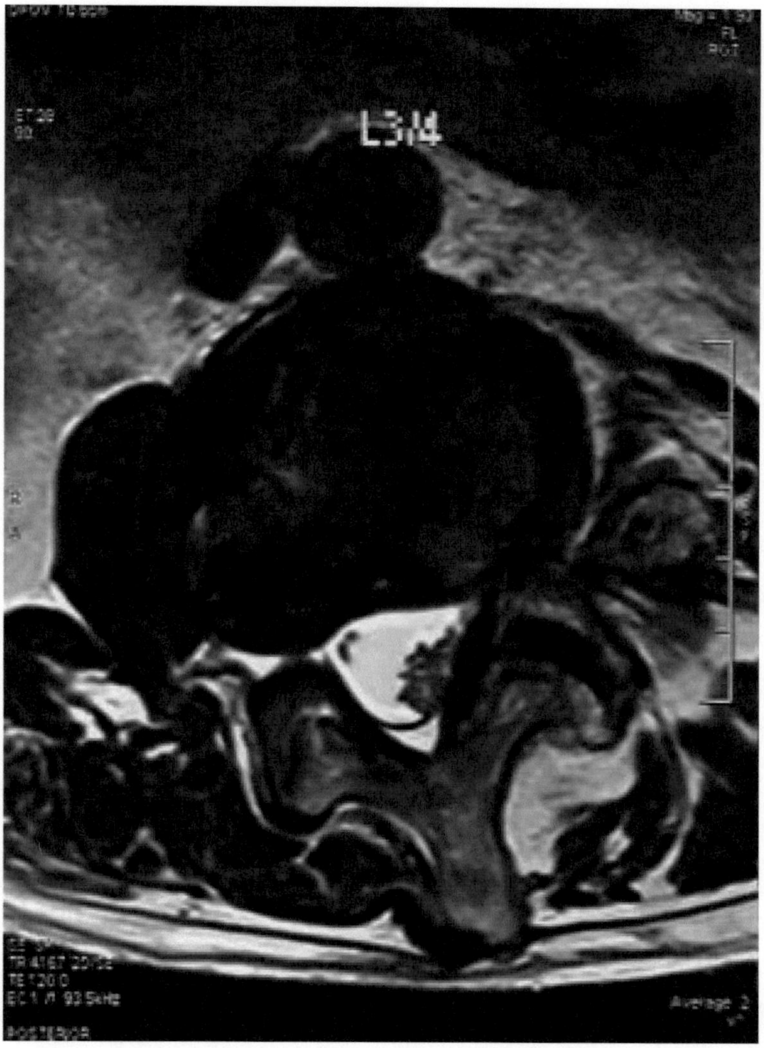

Figure 1.
Lumbar multifidus atrophy. From the MRI, it is evident that there was marked asymmetric lumbar multifidus atrophy at the level of L3/L4. The fatty infiltration area in the left multifidus was significantly larger than that in the right multifidus.

In other cases, degenerative scoliosis may progress. The increased pressure and shear stress on the facet joints cause alterations within the synovial surfaces of the articular processes with subsequent facet hypertrophy, capsular degeneration, and ligamentous hypertrophy [18]. Also, asymmetric loading of the lumbar facet joints and intervertebral discs may result in spinal deformities occurring in three planes [19, 20], particularly in the presence of decreased bone density. Depending on the number of segments involved, this can also cause segmental or multi-segmental vertebral instabilities. Further instability in the sagittal and coronal planes may result in degenerative spondylolisthesis and rotatory olisthesis, respectively [21]. It has to be noted that rotatory olisthesis is present even in mild lumbar scoliosis of less than 20° [21].

Lumbar VRO is prevalent in L3–L4, followed by L2–L3 and L4–L5. Of all the VRO, L3–L4 laterolisthesis contributes around half of the prevalence [11, 22, 23]. Wataruki et al. [24] proposed that this was related to the mechanical stress at the L3–L4 levels, as the lower lumbar levels are more fixed and the upper lumbar

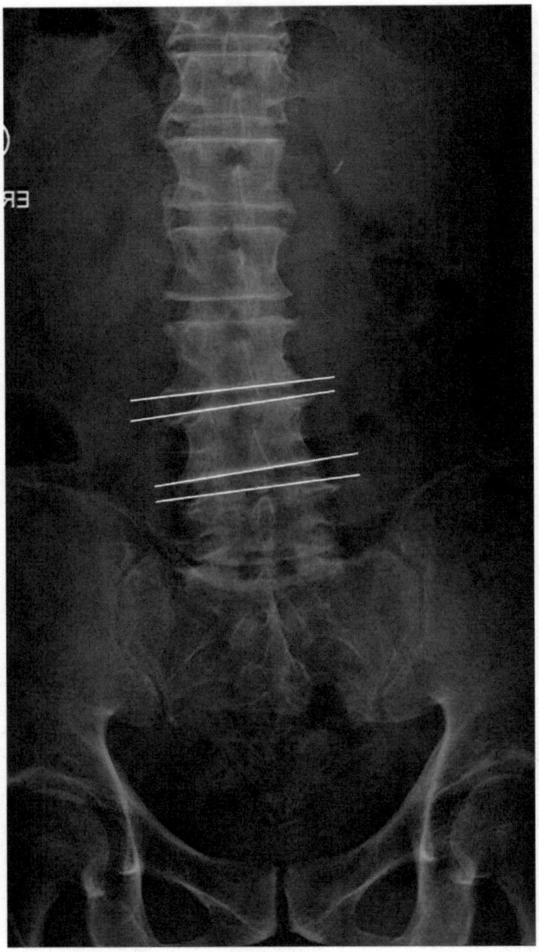

Figure 2.
Mild intervertebral disc wedging in one level is compensated by wedging in the opposite direction to maintain coronal balance. Mild disc wedging was evident in L4/L5 level. The wedging was compensated by disc wedging above (L3/L4) in the opposite direction, balancing the spine.

segments are more mobile [24]. The smaller size of the L4 vertebral body may also contribute to the higher incidence of laterolisthesis at L3–L4, as a reduction of 25% of the vertebral cross-sectional area increases mechanical stress by 30% with an applied load, contributing to vertebral instability [25].

To reduce the instability, the body reacts by growing osteophytes (**Figure 3**). The spondylosis (osteophytes by the end plates) and the spondyloarthritis (degenerative changes of the facet joints) that result, together with the ligamentous hypertrophy, compromise the central spinal canal and the lateral recess and may bring about claudication and nerve root compression symptoms [1].

Apart from bone and articular involvement, paraspinal muscle atrophy is prevalent in DLS. Sarcopenia, which is a reduction in skeletal mass, is commonly seen in patients with DLS. Eguchi et al. [26], using DEXA scans to assess the appendicular and trunk skeletal muscle mass, showed that sarcopenia was present in 46.6% of the DLS patients [26]. Sarcopenia is defined as the appendicular skeletal mass index of less than 5.46 kg/m^2 [27]. The appendicular skeletal mass index (ASMI) is the sum of the arm and leg lean mass (kg) divided by square of the height (m^2) [27]. Studies have also shown that ASMI negatively correlated with pelvic tilt [26], whereas trunk skeletal mass index (Trunk SMI) which is defined as trunk lean mass

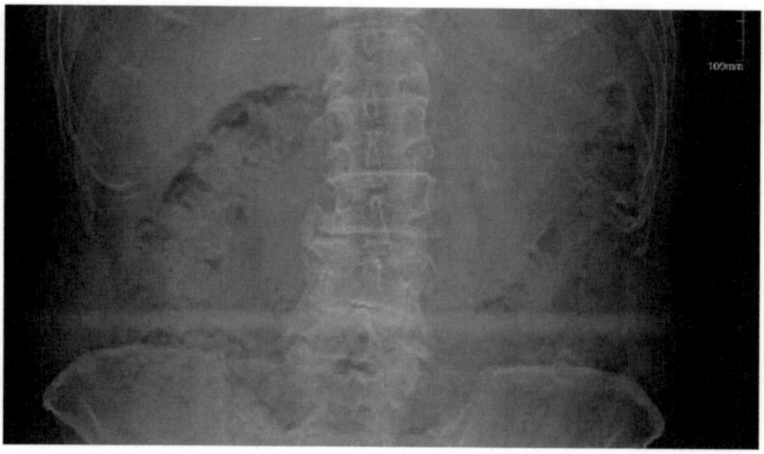

Figure 3.
The osteochondrosis at L4/L5 intervertebral level, together with the bridging osteophyte in the left of L3/L4, stabilized the mild scoliosis curve and maintained coronal balance in this man aged 63 years.

divided by height^2 (m^2) significantly correlated with the sagittal vertical axis, pelvic tilt (PT), and lumbar scoliosis [26]. Moreover, trunk SMI correlated positively with bone mineral density (BMD), suggesting that reduction in trunk muscle mass was associated with osteoporosis and sagittal imbalance [26], which is prevalent in patients with DLS.

3. Clinical presentation

Patients are generally over 50 years of age. Clinical presentation is variable. Onset is generally gradual, though it can be sudden, after a day's work, repetitive bending of the low back, poor sitting posture, or prolonged standing.

Most of the patients complain of low back pain, radiculopathy, and claudication [28]. Liu et al. [28], in a study of the clinical features of 112 patients with DLS treated surgically, found that 77% of them complained of low back pain, 90% complained of radiculopathy, and 48% complained of neurogenic intermittent claudication. Only 3% of them had neurological symptoms [28]. The symptoms can present singly or in combination [28].

3.1 Low back pain

Low back pain is generally diffuse. It is often located in the apex and concavity of the curve and at the junction between two curves [28]. The severity of the pain varies with different curve types, with thoracolumbar, lumbar, and lumbosacral curves being more painful than thoracic curves. A compensatory hemicurve is the least painful, except for the left compensatory lumbosacral hemicurve [29–31]. Pain is also localized on the iliac crest and the coccyx, where the tendons of the lumbar paraspinal muscles insert [1]. Rarely, the lowest ribs impinge on the iliac crest and cause pain [1]. In the presence of a reduced lumbar lordosis or a complete loss of the natural lumbar curve, the muscle pain is generally greater. This is not unexpected as the lumbar paraspinal muscles have to contract continuously to maintain coronal and sagittal spinal balance.

Whether the extent of the pain is related to the magnitude of the curve and coronal balance has not been clearly elucidated as yet [29, 32]. A number of studies have shown that Cobb angles in excess of 45° are associated with more pain [33].

Other studies, however, have shown that the magnitude of the curve was not related to the pain [29, 34].

The impact of coronal balance on low back pain is likewise controversial. Some studies showed that a coronal imbalance in excess of 4–5 cm. is associated with more pain and reduction in function in un-operated scoliosis patients [32, 35]. Further trunk shift is a predictor of surgery in patients with DLS [35]. Other studies, however, did not show such an association [36].

3.2 Radiculopathy

Radiculopathy is common in patients with DLS. Many studies have attempted to investigate the relationship between the scoliosis curve, VRO, and the nerve roots involved [28, 37, 38]. In a study evaluating 47 male and 65 female DLS patients with a mean age of 54.7 years, Liu et al. [28] showed that L3 and L4 nerve roots are generally compressed on the concave side of the scoliosis [28]. Conversely, L5 and S1 nerve roots are more commonly afflicted on the convex side of the scoliosis [28].

Liu et al. [37] evaluated the site of nerve root irritation in 22 DLS patients [37]. They identified three zones (**Figure 4**) where the nerve root could be compressed or irritated. These included the lateral recess zone, the foraminal zone, and the extra-foraminal zone [37]. The lateral recess zone refers to the zone where the nerve root passes from the thecal sac to the entrance of the foramen; the foraminal zone refers to the interval canal beneath the pedicle, and the extra-foraminal zone refers to the zone outside the lateral border of the pedicle [37]. They found that the L3 and L4 nerve roots are more commonly compressed in the foraminal and extra-foraminal zones in the concavity of the scoliosis curve. Conversely, L5 and S1 nerve roots are more commonly affected by a lateral recess stenosis on the convex side [37].

Gardner et al. [38] evaluated different patterns of lumbar spinal stenosis with lateral subluxation in patients with DLS and had similar findings [38]. They showed that the pattern of nerve root compression varies with the types of lateral subluxation, viz., the open subluxation and closed dislocation. Open subluxation refers to subluxation where the disc is open on the side where the vertebra above is slipping. The wedge is open on the convexity of the curve (**Figure 5**). Conversely, closed dislocation is present when the disc is closed on the side where the vertebra above is slipping [23]. Gardner et al. [38] showed that open subluxation commonly affects L3 and L4 levels. When present, it causes contralateral lateral recess and foraminal

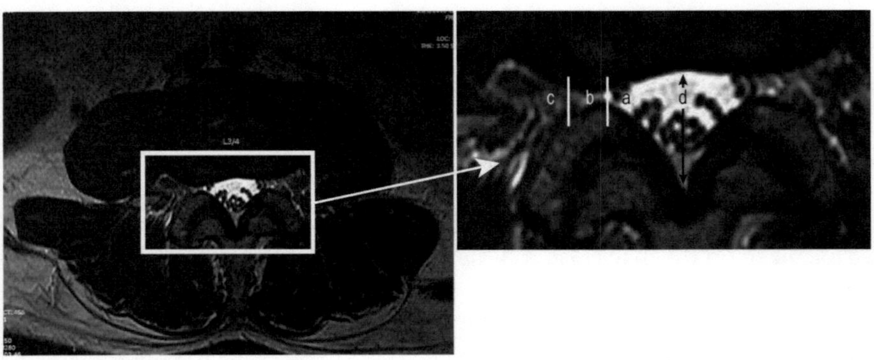

Figure 4.
The magnified view of the spinal canal and the intervertebral foramina. Nerve root irritation can occur in (a) the lateral recess zone, (b) the foraminal zone, and (c) the extra-foraminal zone; (d) is the sagittal diameter of the spinal canal. Spinal stenosis can result from narrowing of the sagittal diameter of the spinal canal or that of the lateral recess, when they are known as lumbar spinal stenosis and lateral lumbar spinal stenosis, respectively.

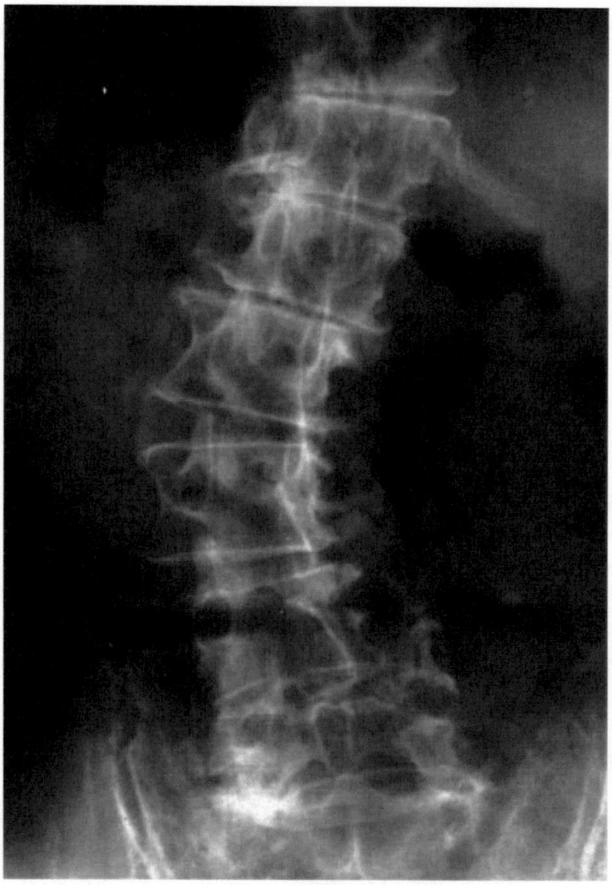

Figure 5.
VRO was evident at Ll, L2, and L3 levels. L1 translated tangentially to the right, with no disc wedging. L2 similarly translated to the right though to a smaller extent, with disc closing on the right, which was the concavity of the lumbar curve. This is defined as closed dislocation. L3, on the other hand, slipped to the left. The disc wedged open on the side of curve convexity. This is termed open subluxation.

stenosis. Closed dislocation, on the other hand, is generally seen on the concavity of the curve, causing an ipsilateral pattern of stenosis [38, 39]. L1 and L2 are the most frequently involved [38].

In a study of a cohort of 78 patients with DLS and spinal canal stenosis, Ferrero et al. [39] demonstrated that foraminal and lateral stenosis were most frequently observed on the concavity of the distal lumbosacral curve. L5 radicular pain was significantly more frequent in the presence of compensatory lumbosacral hemicurve [39].

In view of the different patterns of vertebral instability and compensatory curve patterns, it is understandable that the clinical presentation of DLS varies. Nerve root irritation may be single or multilevels, causing pain in different dermatomes [40, 41].

It is interesting to note that the side of radicular pain frequently corresponded to the side of coronal shift. Patients with right truncal coronal shift more frequently present with right radicular pain; similarly, patients with left coronal shift more commonly present with left radicular pain [39]. The mechanism involved was not clear, though it was found that in 69% of the cases, the truncal coronal shift was associated with the side of the lumbosacral counter-curve (i.e., C7 is shifted to the convex side of the main lumbar curve) [39].

3.3 Claudication

With progression of the condition, pain generally involves the buttock as well as the leg, causing neurogenic claudication symptoms which are worse with standing and walking and are relieved with sitting or stooping. The condition is a result of lumbar spinal stenosis brought about by impingement of nerves emerged from the spinal cord. Studies have shown that the symptoms vary over time in different patients. Symptoms tended to improve in 15% of the patients. In 40% of the patients, the condition tended to deteriorate during the initial 2–3 years of follow-up, and in 45% of the patients, the condition remained stable [42, 43].

3.4 Neurological symptoms

Compression of nerve roots is common, with reported incidence varying from 47–78% [44, 45]. The incidence of cauda equina compression with apparent bladder and rectal sphincter problems, however, is low [1].

Central spinal stenosis is generally seen at the junction between two curves. In the study by Ferrero et al. [39], 70% of the cohort had central stenosis at the junction between the main lumbar curve and the lumbosacral hemicurve. Central spinal stenosis also occurs in the concavity of the main lumbar curve and at the junction between the main thoracic curve and the lumbar curve [39].

3.5 Curve progression

Many studies have shown adult scoliosis tends to progress, with the rate of progression higher in DLS than ADIS [46].

DLS tends to progress irrespective of the magnitude of the curve (**Figure 6**) [46]. A study reported the rate of progression of scoliosis in patients with DLS to be 1.64° per year (0.77–3.82°) [7], while another study reported an increase of 3° per year in a cohort of 200 people over the age of 50 years [47]. The radiographic risk parameters are similar to that of ADIS and include apical vertebral rotation ≥ III, a Cobb angle >30°, lateral vertebral translation >6 mm., and L5 above the intercristal line, which is the line joining both iliac crests [9, 47].

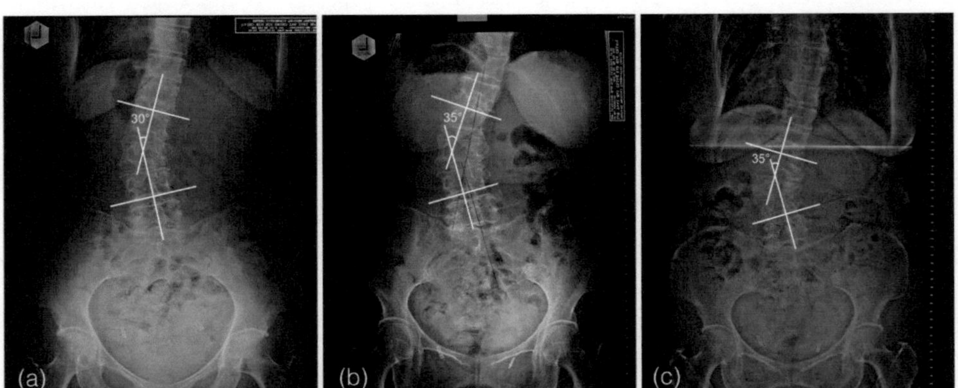

Figure 6.
Progression of degenerative lumbar scoliosis in a postmenopausal woman 70 years of age. In the year 2003 (a), the left lumbar scoliosis measured 30°. It increased to 35° in year 2009 (b). After the patient was prescribed Fosamax by his medical practitioner, the curve stabilized, as can be seen in the radiograph in 2017 (c).

4. Physical examination

The physical evaluation aims at the differential diagnosis of the condition as well as to identify the nerve root(s) involved. The findings depend on the severity of the condition and if there are signs of neurological involvement. In the presence of neurological claudication, patients generally walk with an antalgic gait (gait to avoid or reduce pain), with the trunk listing forward to widen the spinal canal and to reduce the compression on the nerve roots. In more severe cases, the patients may walk with flexed hips and knees [48]. With progression of the condition, the walking distance reduces. Not uncommonly, the patient reports a reduction in height, which averages 4–24 cm. in 1–22 years [49].

Inspection from the back generally shows a hump in the low back with the concavity on the opposite side. Generally pelvic obliquity occurs; Radcliff et al. [50] reported a pelvic tilt in 87% of patients with DLS [50, 51]. Patients with a single lumbar curve were more likely to have a higher pelvis contralaterally (79%), as a compensatory mechanism to maintain coronal trunk balance [50]. Patients with a lumbar curve and a compensatory lumbosacral hemicurve did not display consistent pelvic obliquity compensatory patterns [50].

In the presence of marked pelvic obliquity or pelvic tilt, apparent leg length discrepancy becomes evident, with the leg ipsilateral to the lumbar convexity appearing shorter [50] and the posterior superior iliac spines being unlevel. The coronal spinal imbalance can be determined by measuring the distance from C7

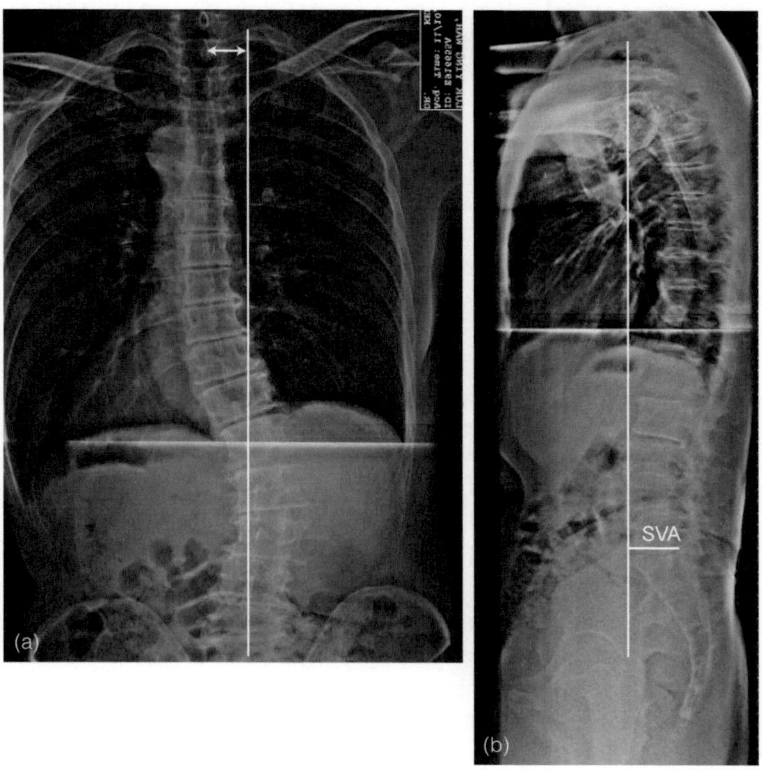

Figure 7
Coronal imbalance and sagittal imbalance are evident in this man aged 62 years old. He complained of radiculopathy localized to the right anterior thigh. The radiograph (a) showed a right lumbar scoliosis with a mild compensatory left thoracolumbar scoliosis. Though the sagittal imbalance was not significant (b), there was a reduction in sacral slope and thoracolumbar lordosis.

to the vertical line extended from the gluteal cleft. The distance measured in mm. represents the coronal shift (**Figure 7**). In the presence of a single thoracolumbar or lumbar curve, the spine is generally decompensated to the side of lumbar convexity.

In patient with DLS, sagittal imbalance is more significant clinically than coronal imbalance [52]. Loss of lumbar lordosis is generally evident with patients leaning forward [48]. In cases with spinal stenosis, patients may flex their hips and knees to compensate for the sagittal spinal imbalance. In long standing cases, contracture of the hips may result, which can be assessed by the Thomas leg raise test [53].

The physical examination can also be used to identify the pain driver. Tenderness is generally elicited at the junction between two major curves, including the junction between the thoracic and lumbar curves and between the lumbar curve and the compensatory lumbosacral hemicurve. Also, pain can be elicited at the apex of the thoracolumbar or lumbar curves [33] and on the iliac crest where the tendons of the lumbar paraspinal muscles attach [1]. A neurological examination which consists of the assessment of motor strength, reflexes, sensation, and gait also needs to be performed, to assess the extent of neurological involvement and to rule out other possible causes of back pain.

5. Radiographic examination

Radiographic examination usually involves taking erect posteroanterior and lateral full spine radiographs. This enables the evaluation of the regional spinopelvic parameters as well as global spinal balance. Sagittal spinal balance has been reported to be positively associated with health-related quality of life (HRQOL) [32, 35].

5.1 Frontal spinal radiograph

A frontal radiograph generally depicts a thoracolumbar or lumbar scoliosis, which is generally shorter than that seen in ADIS, involving only a few vertebral segments. Additionally, vertebral body deformities are less severe than that of ADIS [54]. Of interest is that the majority of lumbar curves with a convexity to the right had apexes above L2 and those with convexities to the left had apexes below L2 [55]. The authors, however, did not offer any explanation for the findings [55].

Depending on the degree of the DLS, radiographic features differ. In the early stages, mild lumbar intervertebral wedging may be present, and compensation in the form of wedging to the opposite direction may be seen in the upper vertebral levels [8].

With progression of the condition, vertebral instability in the form of a translatory shift may be evident [39]. Very often, lateral vertebral translation or laterolisthesis is accompanied by vertebral rotation, when it is known as VRO. VRO most often affects the L3 and L4 levels and less commonly L2–L3 and L4–L5. Of note is that 50% of the VRO occurs at the junction between the main lumbar curve and the compensatory lumbosacral hemicurve [39]. VRO also occurs at the apex of the main lumbar curve and at the junction between the thoracic curve and the lumbar curve [39]. Open subluxation tends to occur on the convexity of the main curve, while closed dislocation tends to occur at the junction between the scoliosis curves [39].

In late stage DLS, osteophytosis may be seen in the vertebral end plates in the concavity of the lumbar scoliosis. Large bridging osteophytes provide stability to previously unstable vertebrae. Also evident are signs of disc degeneration, facet arthrosis, and spinal stenosis [4]. The possibility of lateral recess stenosis and central spinal stenosis may also be discerned from the frontal radiographs. The Cobb angle and the apical vertebral rotation need to be measured, as they are related to the risk of curve progression and back pain. A lumbar scoliosis in excess of 30°, an apical vertebral rotation in excess of 33%, and lumbarization increase the propensity for curve progression and the incidence of back pain [34].

Pelvic obliquity is common in DLS [50]. From the radiograph, the coronal balance may also be determined. It is the distance between the vertical lines extended from the mid sacrum (central sacral line, CSL) to mid C7. When it is in excess of 4 cm, it is associated with deterioration of pain and function scores in adult scoliosis patients [32, 35]. Of importance is that Ferrero et al. [39] reported that the side of radicular pain corresponded to the side of coronal shift in 70% of the subjects [39].

5.2 Lateral spinal radiograph

Lateral spinal radiography generally reveals a reduction of lumbar lordosis and sagittal imbalance. This is important as regional spinopelvic parameters and global spinal balance have been found to be associated with clinical outcome. A study showed that pelvic incidence-lumbar lordosis (PI-LL) mismatch ≥10° and pelvic tilt ≥22° were reported to correlate with disability [56].

Sagittal spinal imbalance is common in patients with DLS. One of the commonly used parameters is the sagittal vertical axis, which is the distance between the vertical line dropped from C7 and the posterosuperior angle of the sacrum. It is noteworthy that a SVA ≥7 cm. is associated with clinical symptoms [32]. The finding was supported by other studies [36, 56]. In mild and moderate spinal malalignment, patients with DLS tend to incline the trunk forward and tend to develop a posterior pelvic shift to maintain balance and to provide relief from neurologic symptoms, especially in the presence of concomitant degenerative spondylolisthesis [48].

6. Advanced clinical imaging

In the presence of claudication and neurological symptoms, computed tomography and magnetic resonance imaging (MRI) may be indicated for diagnosis, monitoring, and follow-up. When decreased BMD is suspected, bone density measurement using a DEXA scan or radiofrequency echographic multi spectrometry (REMS) method is indicated. Computed tomography generally shows signs of facet arthropathy and spinal stenosis, including central spinal stenosis, lateral recess stenosis, and foraminal stenosis.

Magnetic resonance imaging of the lumbar spine is used to assess the soft tissues of the spine, including the spinal cord and tissues within the spinal canal. It is also useful for the assessment of the degenerative changes of disc and facets as well as to assess the extent of spinal stenosis. Recent studies have shown that bone marrow edema was associated with low back pain [57, 58]. In a study of 120 DLS patients, Nakamae et al. [57] found that bone marrow edema was associated with low back pain (**Figure 8**) and that the bone marrow edema score was positively associated with low back pain severity [57]. Bone marrow edema was often seen in the concavity of the curve [57]. Buttermann et al. [58] found that the painful scoliosis which was located at the apex of the scoliosis curve or at the lumbosacral junction was associated with a higher frequency of end plate inflammatory changes [58]. The study showed that the end plate changes demonstrated a bimodal distribution, with peaks at L2–L3 and L5–S1 [58].

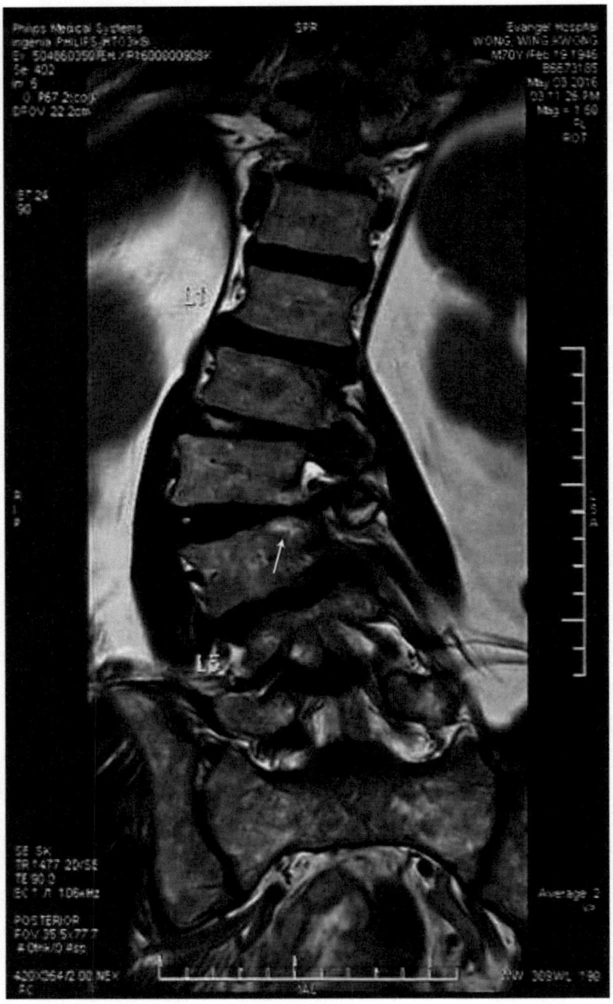

Figure 8.
Bone marrow edema is evident just below the inferior end plate of L2 and superior end plate of L3 in the left.

MRI may also reveal a reduction in muscle mass in the lumbar paraspinal muscles in patients with DLS [59, 60] as paraspinal muscles are involved in the stability of the lumbar spine; Barker et al. [59] suggested that their atrophy was associated with lumbar instability [59]. The percentage of fat infiltration areas in paraspinal muscles was significantly higher on the concave side than the convex side. Further the asymmetry of the multifidus muscle change is positively correlated with the lumbar curvature, lateral vertebral translation, and apical vertebral rotation [60].

Studies showed that BMD was lower in DLS patients than normal controls [7]. Also, BMD was found to correlate negatively with the Cobb angle [61]. Patients with DLS and Cobb angle ≥20° had lower BMD than those with curves less than 20° [7]. A low BMD was associated with increased risk of curve progression. Thus assessment of BMD is of importance in DLS patients.

BMD can be assessed using either the DEXA or the REMS methods. Though DEXA is the gold standard in the assessment of BMD, it has to be noted that DEXA is prone to errors, which includes wrong inclusion of vertebrae and positioning of patient [62]. In the presence of DLS, the spinal BMD could be falsely elevated [62], as the degenerative changes, such as aortic calcification, vertebral osteophytes, facet degeneration, end plate sclerosis, and vertebral rotation, may all have artificially elevated readings obtained from a standard anteroposterior lumbar DEXA scan [63], causing errors in clinical management. A study by Pappou et al. [62] study showed that the falsely elevated scores increased with Cobb angles in excess of 22.5° [62]. The viable alternative for conducting a BMD evaluation of patients with DLS are the hip DEXA values [62]. Alternately, REMS measurement can be used. It relies on a machine algorithm and takes into consideration the entire bony profile including the vertebral microarchitecture, compact bone to trabecular bone mineral density ratio, and collagen index, thus reducing the many errors that are associated with the DEXA measurement [64, 65].

7. Body composition assessment

The body composition of the patient needs to be evaluated, when sarcopenia or loss of muscle mass with aging is suspected. Recent studies have shown that 46.6% of patients with DLS had reduced muscle mass involving the extremities and the trunk [26]. The trunk SMI was found to be significantly negatively correlated with sagittal vertical axis, pelvic tilt (PT), lumbar scoliosis, and apical vertebral rotation, suggesting that the reduction in trunk muscle mass was related to the stooped posture, pelvic retroversion, and lumbar scoliosis [26].

8. Treatment

Patients with DLS generally seek treatment for pain and disabilities, instead of deformities [52]. Conservative treatment is generally indicated, and this often involves methods to control or relieve pain, such as epidural injection, non-steroidal anti-inflammatory drugs, analgesics, traction, electrotherapies, dry needling, manipulation, mobilization, and deep tissue massage. These methods can generally provide relief, though temporarily [66, 67]. A systematic review concluded that there was only level IV evidence in support of the effectiveness of physical therapy, chiropractic care, and bracing in the treatment of adult scoliosis patients and level III evidence for steroid injection [66]. The long-term successful rate of conservative treatment of symptomatic adult scoliosis was only 27% [68, 69].

The poor outcomes of the above interventions are not unexpected, as the treatments were directed towards pain relief, but not the deformities and the global imbalance that are causing the symptoms [69]. Treatment approaches that target spinal deformities yielded better results in terms of reduction in pain and disability ratings in ADIS patients [70–76]. Yet, it has to be noted that many of the studies targeted younger cohorts who suffered from ADIS rather than DLS. Further for patients who are in pain or have difficulties performing exercises, a spinal brace may be indicated. It stabilizes the spine, improves the sagittal imbalance, and reduces the load in the lumbar spine. de Mauroy et al. [77] have shown that a spinal brace is able to stabilize progressive curves in 80% of the adults with scoliosis [76].

8.1 Scoliosis-specific exercises

Many case reports and case series studies have reported that scoliosis-specific exercises (SSE) and multi-modal rehabilitation reduce pain, disability, and curves in patients ADIS [70–76]. Yet, only a few studies have targeted patients with DLS. Daily side plank exercises on the side of curve convexity for 3–22 months were reported to reduce the curves significantly in 30% of the patients with ADIS and DLS [70]. The study, however, did not evaluate the impact of the exercises on pain and disabilities [70]. A prospective pilot study by Ng et al. [72] showed that 9 months of scoliosis-specific exercises at home reduced the thoracolumbar or lumbar curves in over 30% of the ADIS and DLS subjects [72]. Also, our unpublished study showed that 6 weeks of SSE reduced pain and disability ratings of subjects with ADIS and DLS.

While many studies have addressed the coronal curves in ADIS and DLS patients, very few studies have addressed the impact of SSE on the sagittal profile of patients [72]. The effects of SSE on the sagittal profile of this group of patients are thus uncertain. Additionally while SSE may be indicated in the management of patients with DLS, our experience has shown that many older patients had difficulties in mastering the Schroth exercises or the scientific exercises approach to scoliosis (SEAS). They had difficulties in coordinating breathing together with the corrective movements needed. A number of patients encountered problems holding the spine in an erect position, while other patients had increased low back pain soon after the exercises, despite normal spine DEXA scores. This was possibly a result of the DEXA over-estimating the spinal BMD scores when the patient was actually osteopenic. Instead of focusing on corrective exercises, the patients may need to be instructed to adopt corrective postures during daily activities as they are easier to master.

In the presence of a left lumbar curve, the patient can stand, with his or her right knee flexed to lower the right pelvis. Alternately, the patient can raise the left heel. This raises the left pelvis [78]. Either way, this lowers the right sacrum, in relation to the left, and reduces the lumbar scoliosis. This may enable the patient to stand longer. To further reduce the left lumbar curve or reverse the curve, the patients could side shift to the left [78]. Conversely, in the presence of a right lumbar curve, the patient should reverse the above postures.

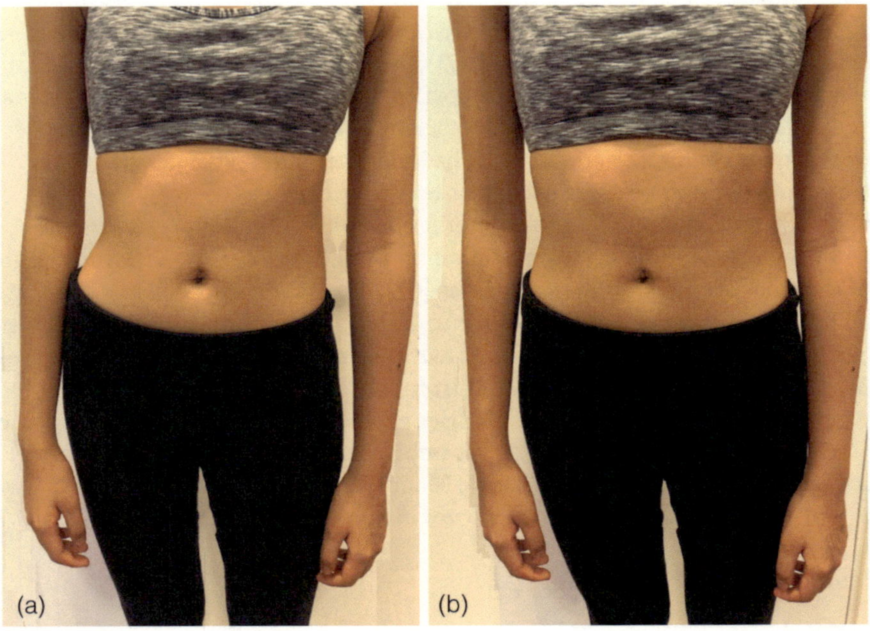

Figure 9.
Contraction of the gluteus medius would level the pelvis. (a) The patient was standing naturally. The right pelvis can be seen shifted to the right and was higher, with pelvis obliquity. (b) Contraction of the right gluteus medius leveled the pelvis. The patient was instructed to learn walking in this corrected position.

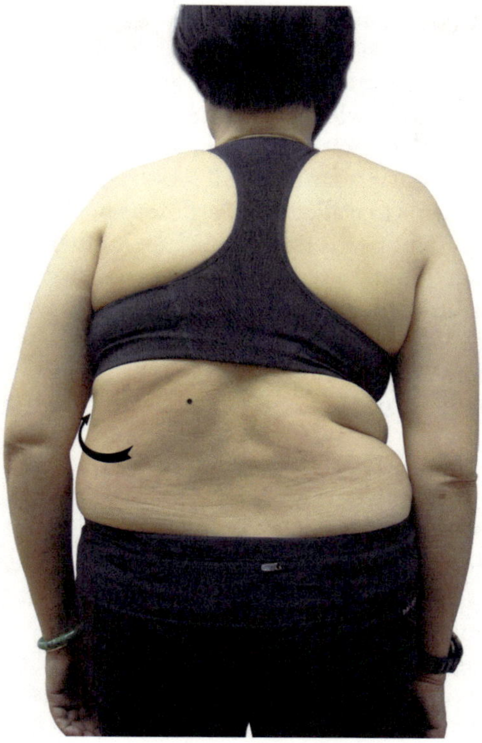

Figure 10.
This patient with left thoracolumbar scoliosis can derotate the left lumbar spine forward during daily activities.

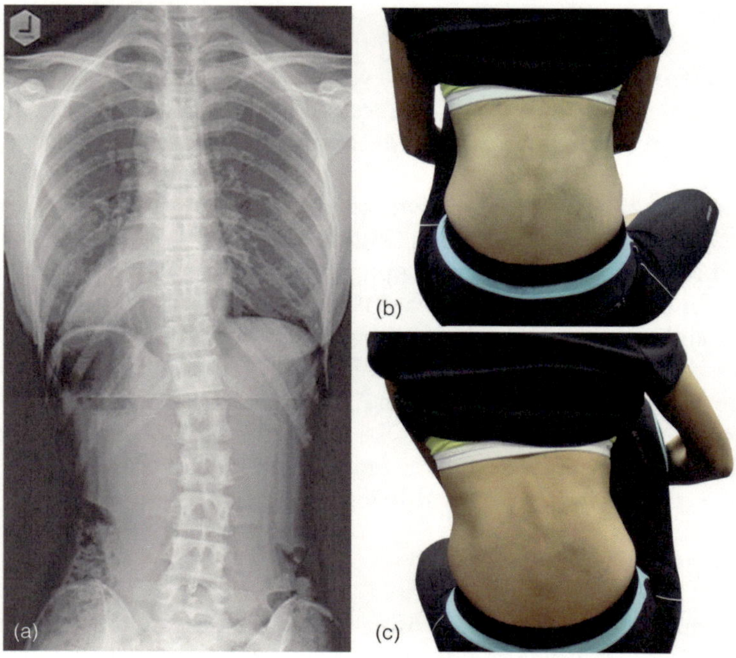

Figure 11.
Patient should refrain from faulty habitual postures, which would aggravate the scoliosis. (a) Frontal lumbar radiograph showed a right lumbar scoliosis, with apex at L2 in a female patient with ADIS. (b) When sitting on the floor, he habitually flexed her left hip and knee, increasing the right lumbar scoliosis. (c) When she flexed her right hip and knee, however, the lumbar curve reduced. Yet, the latter posture should also be discouraged, as lumbar lordosis was not maintained.

Yet, it is difficult to maintain the correct standing posture during ambulation, unless the patient learns how to level the pelvis. Patients with a left thoracolumbar or lumbar curve needs to contract the right hip abductor to bring the pelvis to the midline and level it (**Figure 9**) while derotating the left lumbar curve forward [51] (**Figure 10**). Similarly, patients with right thoracolumbar or lumbar curves need to derotate the right lumbar curve forward while contracting the left hip abductors [51]. The patient then learns to walk with the gluteus medius contracted.

When sitting, the patient needs to maintain the lumbar lordosis, as forced thoracolumbar lordosis was found to reduce double major curves [79]. In the presence of a loss of lumbar lordosis, the patient may be advised to wear a wearable lumbar cushion at all times, though its effects in single thoracolumbar or lumbar curve have not to date been investigated. It is also crucially important that the patient refrains from adopting postures or activities that reinforce the faulty scoliosis pattern (**Figure 11**).

8.2 Sole lift

Functional leg length discrepancy is common, as compensation in patients with DLS. Prescription of a sole lift, in the presence of an apparent LLD, but not anatomical LLD, may induce a compensatory lumbosacral hemicurve, instead of reducing the main lumbar curve [51]. Patients should preferably be advised to contract the gluteus medius on the side of higher pelvis to level the pelvis [51], to flex the knee on this side to lower the pelvis or to raise the heel of the leg ipsilateral to the convexity of the lumbar curve [78] to raise the pelvis.

8.3 Spinal bracing

Spinal bracing has been advocated in the management of adult scoliosis, to halt progression of curves, restore sagittal balance, and treat pain and disability. The effectiveness of braces, however, has been controversial [77, 80]. A number of studies opined that spinal braces do not halt curve progression. Any benefits of pain relief are offset by the deconditioning of the lumbar paraspinal muscles [80].

Recent studies, however, have shown that spinal bracing is effective in reducing pain and halting curve progression (**Figure 12**) [77, 80]. A study which used a lordosing bivalve polyethylene overlapping brace to treat 158 adults with spinal deformities for over 5 years showed that 24% of the curves improved by ≥5°, 56% of the curves stabilized, and 20% worsened by ≥5° [77]. The findings were supported by a long-term follow-up study of 22 years [80]. It was shown that brace wear reduced the progression of curves in both ADIS and DLS patients [80]. The yearly progression for curves in patients with DLS reduced from 1.47° to 0.24° per year [80]. de Mauroy [77] suggested that the brace treatment not only is palliative but also helps to stabilize the lumbar spine in lordosis [77].

8.4 Increase paraspinal muscle mass

Apart from SSE to reduce the scoliosis angles, patients should be encouraged to perform exercises to improve muscle mass, as sarcopenia is prevalent in patients with DLS [26].

Many studies have shown that physical exercises, proper nutrition, and optimal hormonal homeostasis are the three pillars to fight or treat (pre)-sarcopenia [81, 82]. Physical exercises should consist of resistance and endurance exercise training (50% resistance training and 50% endurance training). They should be

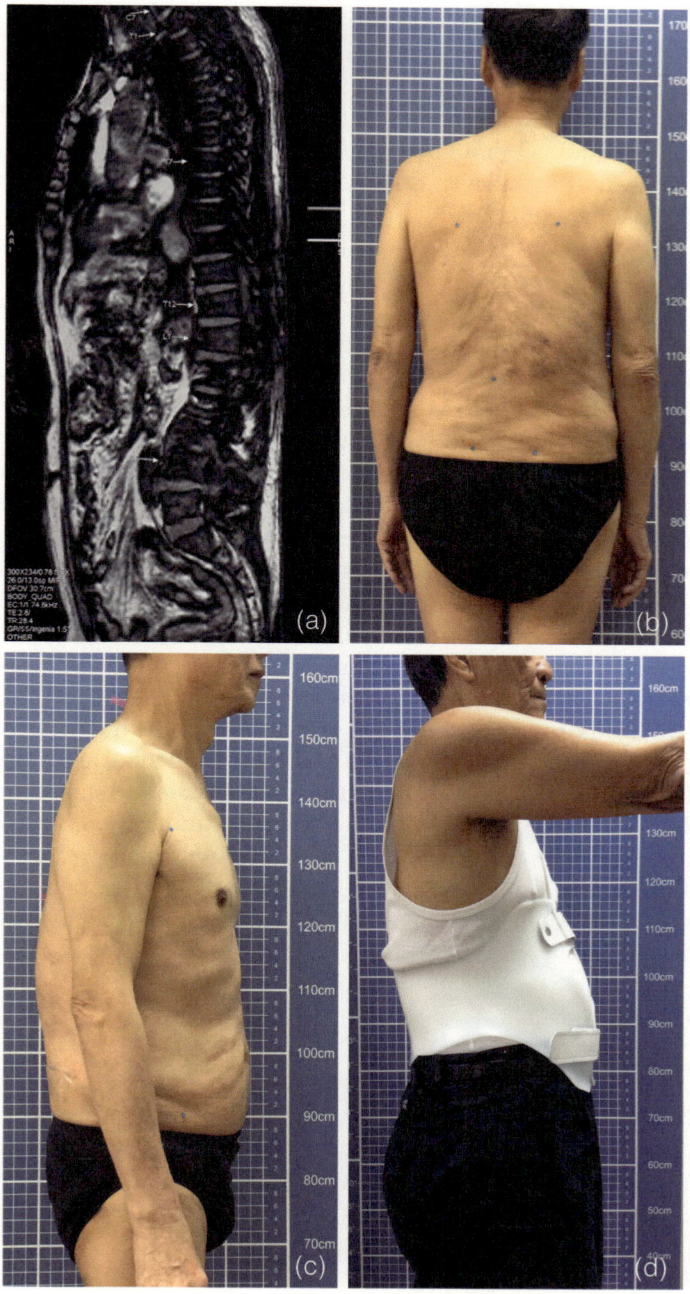

Figure 12.
The man aged 73 years of age complained of right anterior thigh pain with intermittent claudication. The lumbar radiograph and MRI (a) showed a right thoracolumbar scoliosis (b) with a reduction in thoracolumbar lordosis (c) and mild sagittal imbalance. The patient was treated by exercises that increased the thoracolumbar lordosis and a lordotic spinal brace. (d) Despite that the patient was non-compliant and wore the brace only at home for 4 hours daily, the brace treatment increased the walking distance from 10 minutes to around 30 minutes.

performed at least three times a week [83]. Resistance exercise training aims at improving muscle strength, muscle mass, and BMD and optimizing the hormonal milieu [81], whereas endurance exercise training targets at improving the cardiovascular function, increasing the insulin sensitivity and the anti-inflammatory effects, as well as maintaining the endocrine milieu [81, 83]. Thus patients with DLS should also be encouraged to take up a regular exercise program. Nourishment with optimal protein intake is also important. Patients should take 25–30 g of protein with essential amino acids daily [82]. Supplements should include long-chain omega 3 fatty acids and antioxidants (e.g., polyphenols such as hydroxytyrosol, resveratrol, epigallocatechin 3 gallate, curcumin, quercetin) and vitamin D [81, 84]. Ideally, vitamin D should be dosed to attain a serum level of 30 ng/L [82]. Depending on the hormonal level, testosterone and creatine may also be prescribed to treat the (pre)-sarcopenia [82].

8.5 Osteoporosis management

Reduction in BMD is common in patients with DLS. A study by Eguchi et al. [26] showed that trunk skeletal muscle mass correlated positively with BMD [26]. The presence of sarcopenia would thus be indicative of osteoporosis [26]. Depending on the BMD, treatment by medication and/or nutritional supplementation may be required. Pharmacological agents are indicated in the presence of a moderate or high risk of fracture. Common medications prescribed for postmenopausal osteoporosis include estrogen, estrogen + progestin, bisphosphonates, selective estrogen receptors modulators (SERMS), the denosumab, calcitonin, and teriparatide. Each of them has different indications and contraindications [85]. Whether these medications help stabilize or halt the progression of DLS has however not been studied to date. Clinically, however, the author has seen cases of rapidly progressing DLS controlled by administration of bisphosphonates.

Together with pharmacological agents, nutritional supplements such as calcium, vitamin D3, vitamin K2, and silica and abstinence from alcohol and smoking are indicated [86]. Recent studies have demonstrated that calcium supplementation is associated with a low bone calcium content with a parallel increase in vascular calcium content [86] and that low BMD is correlated with an increased cardiovascular mortality [87, 88]. The calcium paradox is speculated to be related to vitamin K2 deficiency [89]. It is thus prudent to advise patients with DLS and osteoporosis to take vitamin K2 along with a calcium supplement.

8.6 Surgery

When conservative treatment fails to provide pain relief or control the symptoms, the patient needs to be referred for surgery, particularly in the presence of neurological signs and symptoms [90], as the outcome of surgery has been reported to be superior to conservative treatment [48], albeit with a much higher risk of complications.

9. Conclusions

When treating patients with DLS, we should not only target symptomatic relief, but it is also necessary to address the underlying aggravating or risk factors of the condition. Physiotherapy, manipulation, and needling can be used to treat pain, together with spinal bracing. Scoliosis-specific exercises should be prescribed, and corrective postures should be encouraged during daily activities to improve the sagittal and coronal spinal imbalances. In the presence of sarcopenia and decreased BMD, resistance exercise training and nutritional supplements are also indicated.

Conflict of interest

The author declares no conflict of interest.

Author details

Shu Yan Ng
Hong Kong Chiropractic College Foundation, Hong Kong

*Address all correspondence to: ngshuyanhcc@gmail.com

References

[1] Aebi M. The adult scoliosis. European Spine Journal. 2005;**14**:925-948

[2] Hong JY, Suh SW, Modi HN, Hur CY, Song HR, Park JH. The prevalence and radiological findings in 1,347 elderly patients with scoliosis. Journal of Bone and Joint Surgery. British Volume (London). 2010;**92**:980-983

[3] Kebaish KM, Neubauer PR, Voros GD, Khoshnevisan MA, Skolasky RL. Scoliosis in adults aged 40 years and older: Prevalence and relationship to age, race, and gender. Spine (Phila Pa 1976). 2011;**36**(9):731-736

[4] Kobayashi T, Atsuta Y, Takemitsu M, Matsuno T, Takeda N. A prospective study of de novo scoliosis in a community based cohort. Spine (Phila Pa 1976). 2006;**31**:178-182

[5] Schwab F, Dubey A, Pagala M, Gamez L, Farcy JP. Adult scoliosis: A health assessment analysis by SF-36. Spine (Phila Pa 1976). 2003;**28**(6):602-606

[6] Kilshaw M, Baker RP, Gardner R, Charosky S, Harding I. Abnormalities of the lumbar spine in the coronal plane on plain abdominal radiographs. European Spine Journal. 2011;**20**:429-433

[7] Xu L, Sun X, Huang S, Zhu Z, Qiao J, Zhu F, et al. Degenerative lumbar scoliosis in Chinese Han population: Prevalence and relationship to age, gender, bone mineral density, and body mass index. European Spine Journal. 2013;**22**(6):1326-1331

[8] Murata Y, Takahashi K, Hanaoka E, Utsumi T, Yamagata M, Moriya H. Changes in scoliotic curvature and lordotic angle during the early phase of degenerative lumbar scoliosis. Spine. 2002;**27**(20):2268-2273

[9] Pritchett JW, Bortel DT. Degenerative symptomatic lumbar scoliosis. Spine (Phila Pa 1976). 1993;**18**(6):700-703

[10] Sun XY, Kong C, Lu SB, Wang W, Cheng YZ, Sun SY, et al. The parallelogram effect of degenerative structures around the apical vertebra in patients with adult degenerative scoliosis: The influence of asymmetric degeneration and diagonal degeneration on the severity of deformity. Medical Science Monitor. 2019;**25**:3435-3445

[11] Bao H, Zhu F, Liu Z, Bentley M, Mao S, Zhu Z, et al. Vertebral rotatory subluxation in degenerative scoliosis: Facet joint tropism is related. Spine (Phila Pa 1976). 2014;**39**(26 Spec No.):B45–B51

[12] Yagi M, Akilah KB, Boachie-Adjei O. Incidence, risk factors and classification of proximal junctional kyphosis: Surgical outcomes review of adult idiopathic scoliosis. Spine (Phila Pa 1976). 2011;**36**(1):E60-E68

[13] Shafaq N, Suzuki A, Matsumura A, Terai H, Toyoda H, Yasuda H, et al. Asymmetric degeneration of paravertebral muscles in patients with degenerative lumbar scoliosis. Spine. 2012;**37**(16):1398-1406

[14] Kim H, Lee CK, Yeom JS, Lee JH, Cho JH, Shin SI, et al. Asymmetry of the cross-sectional area of paravertebral and psoas muscle in patients with degenerative scoliosis. European Spine Journal. 2013;**22**(6):1332-1338

[15] Poureisa M, Behzadmehr R, Daghighi MH, Akhoondzadeh L, Fouladi DF. Orientation of the facet joints in degenerative rotatory lumbar scoliosis: An MR study on 52 patients. Acta Neurochirurgica. 2016;**158**(3):473-479

[16] Gao T, Lai Q, Zhou S, Liu X, Liu Y, Zhan P, et al. Correlation between facet tropism and lumbar degenerative disease: A retrospective analysis. BMC Musculoskeletal Disorders. 2017;**18**(1):483

[17] Hasegawa K, Shimoda H, Kitahara K, et al. What are the reliable radiological indicators of lumbar segmental instability? Journal of Bone and Joint Surgery. British Volume (London). 2011;**93**:650-657

[18] Kirkaldy-Willis WH, Wedge JH, Yong-Hing K, Reilly J. Pathology and pathogenesis of lumbar spondylosis and stenosis. Spine (Phila Pa 1976). 1978;**3**:319-328

[19] Kotwal S, Pumberger M, Hughes A, et al. Degenerative scoliosis: A review. HSS Journal. 2011;7:257-264

[20] Tempel ZJ, Gandhoke GS, Bonfield CM, et al. Radiographic and clinical outcomes following combined lateral lumbar interbody fusion and posterior segmental stabilization in patients with adult degenerative scoliosis. Neurosurgical Focus. 2014;**36**:E11

[21] Korovessis P, Piperos G, Sidiropoulos P, Diures A. Adult idiopathic lumbar scoliosis. A formula for prediction of progression and review of the literature. Spine. 1994;**19**(17):1926-1932

[22] Freedman BA, Horton WC, Rhee JM, et al. Reliability analysis for manual radiographic measures of rotatory subluxation or lateral listhesis in adult scoliosis. Spine (Phila Pa 1976). 2009;**34**:603-608

[23] Trammell TR, Schroeder RD, Reed DB. Rotatory olisthesis in idiopathic scoliosis. Spine (Phila Pa 1976). 1988;**13**:1378-1382

[24] Watanuki A, Yamada H, Tsutsui S, Enyo Y, Yoshida M, et al. Radiographic features and risk of curve progression of de-novo degenerative lumbar scoliosis in the elderly: A 15-year follow-up study in a community-based cohort. Journal of Orthopaedic Science. 2012;**17**(5):526-531

[25] Jimbo S, Kobayashi T, Aono K, Atsuta Y, Matsuno T. Epidemiology of degenerative lumbar scoliosis: A community-based cohort study. Spine (Phila Pa 1976). 2012;**37**(20):1763-1770

[26] Eguchi Y, Suzuki M, Yamanaka H, Tamai H, Kobayashi T, Orita S, et al. Associations between sarcopenia and degenerative lumbar scoliosis in older women. Scoliosis and Spinal Disorders. 2017;**12**:9

[27] Sanada K, Miyachi M, Tanimoto M, Yamamoto K, et al. A cross sectional study of sarcopenia in Japanese men and women reference values and association with cardiovascular risk factors. European Journal of Applied Physiology. 2010;**110**:57-65

[28] Liu W, Chen XS, Jia LS, Song DW. The clinical features and surgical treatment of degenerative lumbar scoliosis: A review of 112 patients. Orthopaedic Surgery. 2009;**1**(3):176-183

[29] Briard JL, Jegou D, Cauchoix J. Adult lumbar scoliosis. Spine. 1979;**4**(6):526-532

[30] Kostuik JP, Bentivoglio J. The incidence of low-back pain in adult scoliosis. Spine (Phila Pa 1976). 1981;**6**(3):268-273

[31] Simmons EH, Jackson RP. The management of nerve root entrapment syndromes associated with the collapsing scoliosis of idiopathic lumbar and thoracolumbar curves. Spine (Phila Pa 1976). 1979;**4**(6):533-541

[32] Glassman SD, Bridwell K, Dimar JR, Horton W, Berven S, Schwab F. The impact of positive sagittal balance in adult spinal deformity. Spine. 2005;**30**(18):2024-2029

[33] Jackson RP, Simmons EH, Stripinis D. Incidence and severity of back pain in adult idiopathic scoliosis. Spine (Phila Pa 1976). 1983;**8**(7):749-756

[34] Weinstein SL, Ponseti IV. Curve progression in idiopathic scoliosis. The Journal of Bone and Joint Surgery. American Volume. 1983;**65**(4):447-455

[35] Ploumis A, Liu H, Mehbod AA, Transfeldt EE, Winter RB. A correlation of radiographic and functional measurements in adult degenerative scoliosis. Spine (Phila Pa 1976). 2009;**34**(15):1581-1584

[36] Lafage V, Schwab F, Patel A, Hawkinson N, Farcy JP. Pelvic tilt and truncal inclination: Two key radiographic parameters in the setting of adults with spinal deformity. Spine (Phila Pa 1976). 2009;**34**(17):E599-E606

[37] Liu H, Ishihara H, Kanamori M, Kawaguchi Y, Ohmori K, Kimura T. Characteristics of nerve root compression caused by degenerative lumbar spinal stenosis with scoliosis. The Spine Journal. 2003;**3**(6):524-529

[38] Gardner RO, Torrie PA, Bertram W, Baker RP, Harding IJ. A radiological evaluation of lateral vertebral subluxation associated with spinal stenosis in the lumbar spine in degenerative scoliosis. Spinal Deformity. 2013;**1**(5):365-370

[39] Ferrero E, Khalif M, Marie-Hardy L, Regnard N, et al. Do curve characteristics influence stenosis location and occurrence of radicular pain in adult degenerative scoliosis? Spine Deformity. 2019;7:472-480

[40] Epstein JA, Epstein BS, Jones MD. Symptomatic lumbar scoliosis and degenerative changes in the elderly. Spine. 1979;**4**:542-547

[41] Grubb S, Lipscomb H. Diagnostic findings in painful adult scoliosis. Spine. 1992;**17**(5):518-527

[42] Vanderpool DW, James JI, Wynne-Davies R. Scoliosis in the elderly. The Journal of Bone and Joint Surgery. American Volume. 1969;**51**(3):446-455

[43] Amundsen T, Weber H, Nordal HJ, Magnaes B, Abdelnoor M, Lilleås F. Lumbar spinal stenosis: Conservative or surgical management? A prospective 10-year study. Spine. 2000;**25**(11):1424-1435

[44] Smith JS, Fu KM, Urban P, Shaffrey CI. Neurological symptoms and deficits in adults with scoliosis who present to a surgical clinic: Incidence and association with the choice of operative versus nonoperative management. Journal of Neurosurgery. Spine. 2008;**9**:326-331

[45] Fu KM, Rhagavan P, Shaffrey CI, Chernavvsky DR, Smith JS. Prevalence, severity, and impact of foraminal and canal stenosis among adults with degenerative scoliosis. Neurosurgery. 2011;**69**:1181-1187

[46] Marty-Poumarat C, Scattin L, Marpeau M, Garreau de Loubresse C, Aegerter P. Natural history of progressive adult scoliosis. Spine. 2007;**32**(11):1227-1234

[47] Faraj SS, Holewijn RM, van Hooff ML, de Kleuver M, Pellisé F, Haanstra TM. De novo degenerative lumbar scoliosis: A systematic review of prognostic factors for curve progression. European Spine Journal. 2016;**25**(8):2347-2358

[48] Buckland AJ, Vira S, Oren JH, Lafage R, Harris BY, et al. When is

compensation for lumbar spine stenosis a clinical sagittal plane deformity? The Spine Journal. 2016;**16**:971-981

[49] Stagnara P. Scoliosis in adults. Consequences of idiopathic scoliosis in adulthood. Chirurgie. 1982;**108**(4):356-363

[50] Radcliff KE, Orozco F, Molby N, Chen E, Sidhu GS, Vaccaro AR, et al. Is pelvic obliquity related to degenerative scoliosis? Orthopaedic Surgery. 2013;5(3):171-176

[51] Lehnert SC. Three-Dimensional Treatment for Scoliosis. A Physiotherapeutic Method for Deformities of the Spine. Palo Alto, CA: Martindale Press; 2007

[52] Acaroğlu RE, Dede O, Pellisé F, Güler UO, Domingo-Sàbat M, et al. Adult spinal deformity: A very heterogeneous population of patients with different needs. Acta Orthopaedica et Traumatologica Turcica. 2016;**50**(1):57-62

[53] Ames CP, Smith JS, Scheer JK, et al. Impact of spinopelvic alignment on decision making in deformity surgery in adults: a review. Journal of Neurosurgery: Spine. 2012;**16**(6):547-564

[54] Grubb SA, Lipscomb HJ, Coonrad RW. Degenerative adult onset scoliosis. Spine (Phila Pa 1976). 1988;**13**(3):241-245

[55] de Vries AAB, Mullender MG, Pluymakers WJ, Castelein RM, van Royen BJ. Spinal decompensation in degenerative lumbar scoliosis. European Spine Journal. 2010;**19**:1540-1544

[56] Schwab FJ, Blondel B, Bess S, Hostin R, Shaffrey CI, et al. Radiographical spinopelvic parameters and disability in the setting of adult spinal deformity: A prospective multicenter analysis. Spine (Phila Pa 1976). 2013;**38**(13):E803-E812

[57] Nakamae T, Kiyotaka Yamada K, Takuro Shimbo T, Toshikatsu Kanazawa T, et al. Bone marrow edema and low back pain in elderly degenerative lumbar scoliosis a cross-sectional study. Spine. 2016;**41**(10):885-892

[58] Buttermann GR, Mullin WJ. Pain and disability correlated with disc degeneration via magnetic resonance imaging in scoliosis patients. European Spine Journal. 2008;**17**(2):240-249

[59] Barker KL, Shamley DR, Jackson D. Changes in the cross-sectional area of multifidus and psoas in patients with unilateral back pain: The relationship to pain and disability. Spine. 2004;**29**(22):E515-E519

[60] Xie D, Zhang J, Ding W, Yang S, et al. Abnormal change of paravertebral muscle in adult degenerative scoliosis and its association with bony structural parameters. European Spine Journal. 2019;**28**(7):1626-1637

[61] Ding WY, Yang DL, Cao LZ, Sun YP, Zhang W, Xu JX, et al. Intervertebral disc degeneration and bone density in degenerative lumbar scoliosis: A comparative study between patients with degenerative lumbar scoliosis and patients with lumbar stenosis. Chinese Medical Journal. 2011;**124**(23):3875-3878

[62] Pappou IP, Girardi FP, Sandhu HS, Parvataneni HK, Cammisa FP Jr, Schneider R, et al. Discordantly high spinal bone mineral density values in patients with adult lumbar scoliosis. Spine (Phila Pa 1976). 2006;**31**(14):1614-1620

[63] Rand T, Seidl G, Kainberger F, et al. Impact of spinal degenerative changes on the evaluation of bone mineral density with dual energy X-ray

absorptiometry (DXA). Calcified Tissue International. 1997;**60**:430-433

[64] Casciaro S, Conversano F, Pisani F, Muratore M. New perspectives in echographic diagnosis of osteoporosis on hip and spine. Clinical Cases in Mineral and Bone Metabolism. 2015;**12**(2):142-150

[65] Cavalli L, Arioli G, Bianchi G, Caffarelli C. Radiofrequency echographic multi spectrometry (REMS) for the non-ionising diagnosis of osteoporosis at femoral neck: Results of a multicenter clinical study comparing rems and dxa. Annals of the Rheumatic Diseases. 2018;**77**(Suppl 2):811.1

[66] Everett CR, Patel RK. A systematic literature review of nonsurgical treatment in adult scoliosis. Spine (Phila Pa 1976). 2007;**32**(19 Suppl):S130-S134

[67] Kluba T, Dikmenli G, Dietz K, Giehl JP, Niemeyer T. Comparison of surgical and conservative treatment for degenerative lumbar scoliosis. Archives of Orthopaedic and Trauma Surgery. 2009;**129**:1-5

[68] Savage JW, Patel AA. Fixed sagittal plane imbalance. Global Spine Journal. 2014;**4**:287-296

[69] Ryan DJ, Protopsaltis TS, Ames CP, Hostin R, Klineberg E, Mundis GM, et al. T1 pelvic angle (TPA) effectively evaluates sagittal deformity and assesses radiographical surgical outcomes longitudinally. Spine (Phila Pa 1976). 2014;**39**(15):1203-1210

[70] Fishman M, Groessl EJ, Sherman KJ. Serial case reporting yoga for idiopathic and degenerative scoliosis. Global Advances in Health and Medicine. 2014;**3**(5):16-21

[71] Negrini A, Negrini MG, Donzelli S, Romano M, Zaina F, Negrini S. Scoliosis-specific exercises can reduce the progression of severe curves in adult idiopathic scoliosis: A long-term cohort study. Scoliosis. 2015;**10**:20

[72] Ng SY, Chan WY, Ho TK, Ng YL. A pilot study on the effect of outpatient Schroth exercises on thoracolumbar and lumbar curves in adult scoliosis patients. In: Bettany-Saltikov J, Schreiber S, editors. Innovations in Spinal Deformities and Postural Disorders. Rijeka: IntechOpen; 2017. pp. 93-112

[73] Monticone M, Ambrosini E, Cazzaniga D, Rocca B, Motta L, Cerri C, et al. Adults with idiopathic scoliosis improve disability after motor and cognitive rehabilitation: Results of a randomised controlled trial. European Spine Journal. 2016;**25**(10):3120-3129

[74] Barrios C, Lapuente JP, Sastre S. Treatment of chronic pain in adult scoliosis. Studies in Health Technology and Informatics. 2002;**88**:290-303

[75] Morningstar MW. Outcomes for adult scoliosis patients receiving chiropractic rehabilitation: A 24-month retrospective analysis. Journal of Chiropractic Medicine. 2011;**10**:179-184

[76] Harrison DE, Oakley PA. Scoliosis deformity reduction in adults: A CBP® Mirror Image case series incorporating the 'non-commutative property of finite rotation angles under addition' in five patients with lumbar and thoraco-lumbar scoliosis. Journal of Physical Therapy Science. 2017;**29**(11):2044-2050

[77] de Mauroy JC, Lecante C, Barral F, Pourret S. Prospective study of 158 adult scoliosis treated by a bivalve polyethylene overlapping brace and reviewed at least 5 years after brace fitting. Scoliosis and Spinal Disorders. 2016;**11**(Suppl 2):28

[78] Maruyama T, Kitagawal T, Takeshita K, Nakainura K. Side shift exercise for idiopathic scoliosis after skeletal maturity. Studies in Health Technology and Informatics. 2002;**91**:361-364

[79] van Loon PJ, Kühbauch BA, Thunnissen FB. Forced lordosis on the thoracolumbar junction can correct coronal plane deformity in adolescents with double major curve pattern idiopathic scoliosis. Spine (Phila Pa 1976). 2008;**33**(7):797-801

[80] Palazzo C, Montigny JP, Barbot F, Bussel B, Vaugier I, Fort D, et al. Effects of bracing in adult with scoliosis: A retrospective study. Archives of Physical Medicine and Rehabilitation. 2017;**98**:187-190

[81] Sgrò P, Sansone M, Sansone A, Sabatini S, Borrione P, Romanelli F, et al. Physical exercise, nutrition and hormones: Three pillars to fight sarcopenia. The Aging Male. 2019;**22**(2):75-88

[82] De Spiegeleer A, Petrovic M, Boeckxstaens P, Van Den Noortgate N. Treating sarcopenia in clinical practice: Where are we now? Acta Clinica Belgica. 2016;**71**(4):197-205

[83] Landi F, Marzetti E, Martone AM, Bernabei R, Onder G. Exercise as a remedy for sarcopenia. Current Opinion in Clinical Nutrition and Metabolic Care. 2014;**17**(1):25-31

[84] Driss F, El-Benna J. Chapter 143—Antioxidant effect of hydroxytyrosol, a polyphenol from olive oil by scavenging reactive oxygen species produced by human neutrophils. In: Olives and Olive Oil in Health and Disease Prevention. San Diego, USA: Acad Press; 2010. pp. 1289-1294

[85] Gallagher JC, Tella SH. Prevention and treatment of postmenopausal osteoporosis. The Journal of Steroid Biochemistry and Molecular Biology. 2014;**142**:155-170

[86] Persy V, D'Haese P. Vascular calcification and bone disease: The calcification paradox. Trends in Molecular Medicine. 2009;**15**:405-416

[87] Von der Recke P, Hansen MA, Hassager C. The association between low bone mass at the menopause and cardiovascular mortality. The American Journal of Medicine. 1999;**106**:273-278

[88] Farhat GN, Newman AB, Sutton-Tyrrell K, Matthews KA, Boudreau R, Schwartz AV, et al. The association of bone mineral density measures with incident cardiovascular disease in older adults. Osteoporosis International. 2007;**18**:999-1008

[89] Wasilewski GB, Vervloet MG, Schurgers LJ. The bone—Vasculature axis: Calcium supplementation and the role of vitamin K. Frontiers in Cardiovascular Medicine. 2019;**6**:6

[90] Neuman BJ, Baldus C, Zebala LP, Kelly MP, Shaffrey C, et al. Patient factors that influence decision making: Randomization versus observational nonoperative versus observational operative treatment for adult symptomatic lumbar scoliosis (ASLS). Spine (Phila Pa 1976). 2016;**41**(6):E349-E358

Chapter 8

Restoration of Cervical and Lumbar Lordosis: CBP® Methods Overview

Paul A. Oakley, Ibrahim M. Moustafa and Deed E. Harrison

Abstract

Low back and neck pain disorders are among the leading causes for work loss, suffering, and health care expenditures throughout the industrialized world. It has been extensively demonstrated that sagittal plane alignment of the cervical and lumbar spines impacts human health and well-being. Today there are reliable and predictable means through the application of extension spinal traction as part of comprehensive rehabilitation programs to restore the natural curvatures of the spine. High-quality evidence points to Chiropractic BioPhysics® (CBP®) methods offering superior long-term outcomes for treating patients with various craniocervical and lumbosacral disorders. CBP technique is a full spine and posture rehabilitation approach that incorporates mirror image® exercises, spinal and postural adjustments, and unique traction applications in the restoration of normal/ideal spinal alignment. Recent randomized controlled trials using CBP's unique extension traction methods in conjunction with various conventional physiotherapeutic methods have demonstrated those who restore normal lordosis (cervical or lumbar) get symptomatic relief that lasts up to 2 years after treatment. Comparative groups receiving various 'cookie-cutter' conventional treatments experience only temporary symptomatic relief that regresses as early as 3 months after treatment. The economic impact/benefit of CBPs newer sagittal spine rehabilitation treatments demand continued attention from clinicians and researchers alike.

Keywords: cervical lordosis, extension traction, lumbar lordosis, sagittal alignment, spinal subluxation, spine rehabilitation

1. Introduction

The Chiropractic BioPhysics® (CBP®) technique was invented in 1980 by Donald D. Harrison, a chiropractor who was also educated in engineering and mathematics [1]. After reading the 1974 paper by Panjabi [2] on the recommendation for the use of a Cartesian coordinate system to accurately describe the movement of body joints as rotations and translations around an origin, he applied this concept to upright human posture (**Figures 1** and **2**) [1, 3]. Instead of being applied to a single joint, Harrison presented the displacement of the head, thorax and pelvis as rotations and translations of the main masses of the body, with spinal coupling patterns that occur within the corresponding spinal junctions between the adjacent body masses for each particular movement/position.

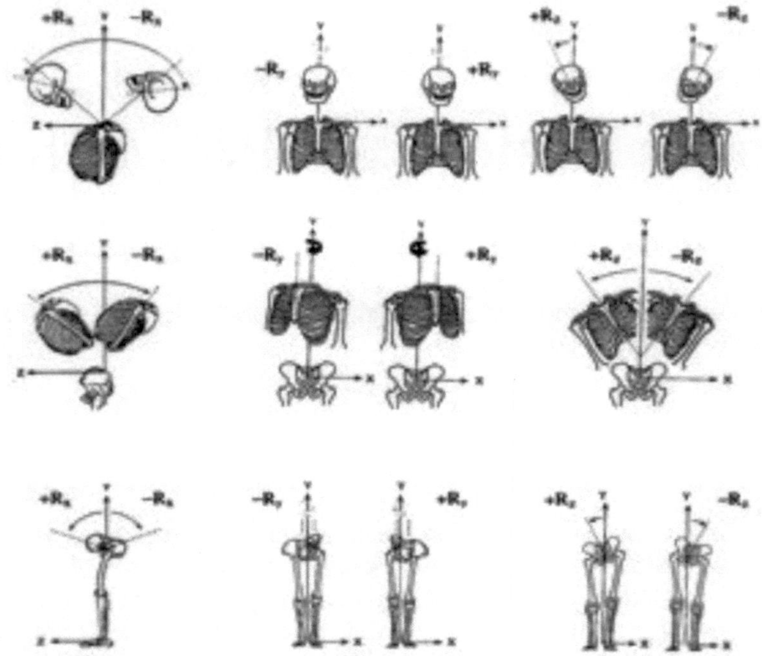

Figure 1.
Human posture described as rotations of the head, thorax, and pelvis about the x, y, and z-axes of the Cartesian coordinate system (Courtesy: CBP seminars).

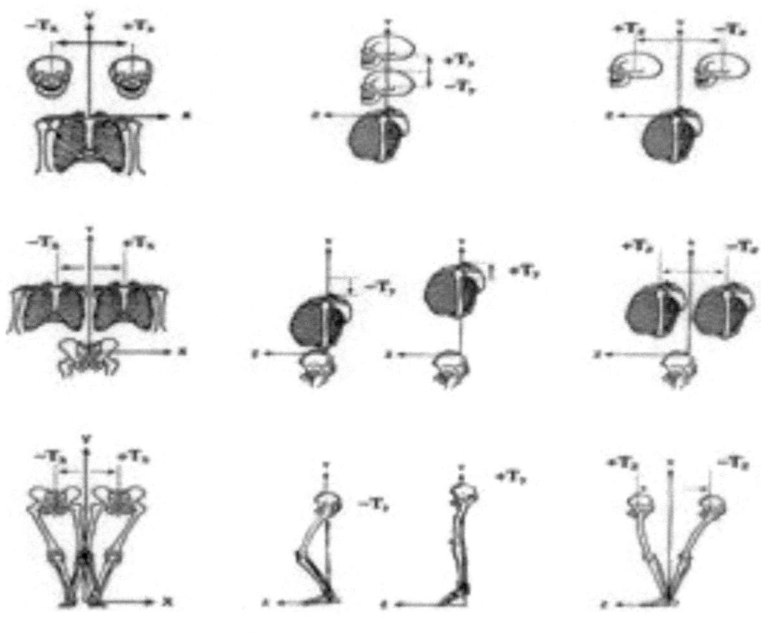

Figure 2.
Human posture described as translations of the head, thorax, and pelvis along the x, y, and z-axes of the Cartesian coordinate system (Courtesy: CBP seminars).

In an attempt to model the upright neutral sagittal spinal position, Don Harrison along with his son Deed Harrison and other colleagues performed a strategic set of studies. Although many research groups have attempted to model the shape of the normal human spine in the sagittal plane, few have done so as comprehensively and systematically as the Harrison group [4–11]. Elliptical shape modeling of the path of the posterior longitudinal ligament along the posterior vertebral body margins was chosen due to the ease of clear identification of these spine landmark points and for the ability to easily make measurements of spine segmental and total angle of curvature on patient radiographs to compare patient measurements to model predictions. Modeling was performed on radiographic samples of asymptomatic participants. Computer iterations of spinal shape modeling was applied to determine best-fit geometric spine shapes by fitting various ellipses of altering minor-to-major axes ratios to digitized posterior vertebral body corners on samples of radiographs of the cervical [4–6], thoracic [7, 8], and lumbar spinal regions [9–11] (**Figure 3**).

The Harrison normal spinal model (**Figure 3**) features a circular cervical lordosis, and portions of an elliptical curve for both the thoracic kyphosis (more curvature cephalad), and lumbar lordosis (more curvature caudad). Consequently, features of the normal human spine reveal that the opposite thoracic and lumbar curves meet together at the thoraco-lumbar junction being essentially straight; the upper, deeper curve of the upper thoracic spine reflects oppositely at the cervico-thoracic junction (between T1 and T2) and continues into the cervical lordosis; the lower lumbar spine increases its lordotic alignment having two-thirds of its curve between L4-S1 as it meets the forward tilted sacral base. The spine is modeled as vertical in the front view. The spine alignment is easily quantified by repeatable and reliable methods from measuring its position from standing X-rays [12–16] (**Figure 3**).

The Harrison normal spinal model has been validated in several ways. Simple analysis of alignment data on samples of the normal, asymptomatic population has been done [4–11]. Comparison studies between normal samples to symptomatic samples [4, 17]; as well as between normal samples to theoretical ideal models have been done [4, 5, 8, 10]. The statistical differentiation of asymptomatic subjects from symptomatic pain group patients based on alignment data has been performed [6, 11].

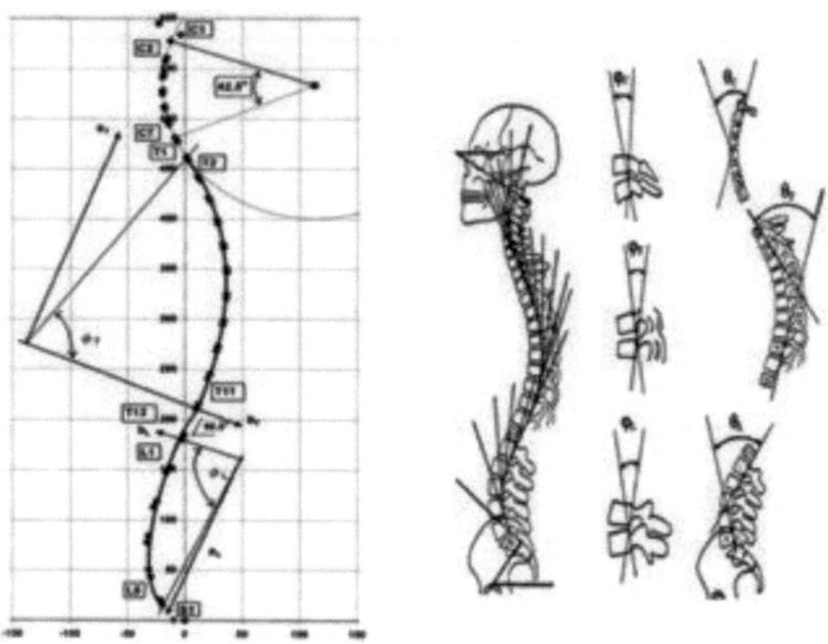

Figure 3.
Left: The Harrison normal spine model as the path of the posterior longitudinal ligament in the sagittal plane. Right: Harrison posterior tangent method are lines drawn contiguous with the posterior vertebral body margins used to quantify subluxation patterns (Courtesy: CBP seminars).

The demonstration of paralleled spine alignment improvements with reductions in pain and disability, versus no change in untreated control groups in pre-post clinical trials have been performed [18–23]. The demonstration in randomized clinical trials that only patient groups achieving lordosis and sagittal posture improvement (lumbar or cervical) achieve long-term improvements in various outcome measures versus comparative treatment groups not getting spine alignment improvement who experience regression in multiple outcome measures at follow-up have also been done [24–35].

CBP technique is a full-spine posture and spine rehabilitation method that incorporates mirror image® (MI) exercises, adjustments, and traction applications in the restoration of normal/ideal spine alignment [1, 36–38]. Chiropractors and other manual therapists practicing CBP structural rehabilitation techniques have used this spine model as a structural goal of care for over 20 years. It is noted that this model serves as the baseline for generalized patient comparison, however, specific patient comparisons must include patient-specific considerations related to thoracic inlet parameters [39] as well as pelvic morphology [40] as these may dictate a structural modification to the sagittal plane model for a given patient [37]. There are software programs (i.e., PostureRay Inc., Trinity, FL, USA) that aid in the ability for practitioners to assess spine alignment quickly in daily practice (**Figure 4**).

Today the evidence supporting the CBP approach to the correction of cervical lordosis and lumbar lordosis is substantial. There are now many randomized controlled clinical trials (RCT) documenting the reduction of anterior head translation

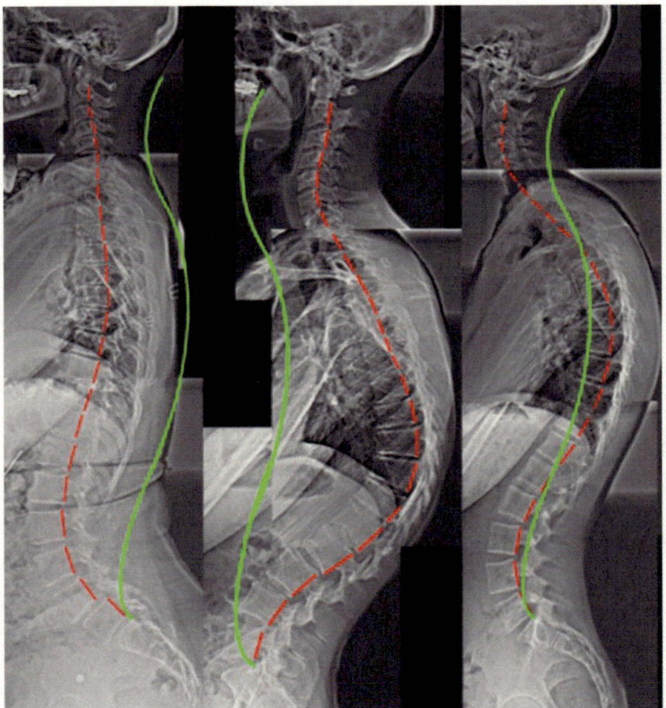

Figure 4.
Three patients demonstrating dramatically different spine alignment patterns. Left: Excessive lumbar hyperlordosis, L4 anterolisthesis, and excessive anterior sagittal balance in a mid-aged female with disabling low back pain; Middle: Excessive thoracolumbar kyphosis and early degenerative changes in a mid-aged male; Right: Excessive thoracic hyperkyphosis in a young male with Scheuermann's disease. Red line is contiguous with posterior vertebral body margins; green line represents Harrison normal spinal model. (Courtesy: PAO).

[24, 28–35], as well as the increase in cervical lordosis [24, 28–35], and the increase in lumbar lordosis [25–27] in patients presenting with hypolordosis in each of these spinal areas. These trials have also demonstrated that the postural and spinal improvements are associated with improvements in various patient outcomes, including: pain, disability, quality of life, range of motion as well as specific physiological measures such as improved neurological central conduction times—the ability of the brain to communicate with the body.

We will now address in different sections the CBP approach to the restoration of cervical lordosis and then the restoration of lumbar lordosis.

2. Restoration of cervical lordosis

The first clinical trial using CBP methods for the restoration of cervical lordosis was a non-randomized controlled trial (nRCT) published in 1994 [18]. This first trial substantiated two trends: (1) Sagittal cervical alignment could be changed routinely, in patient cohorts receiving extension traction; (2) Spine alignment does not improve following spinal manipulative therapy (SMT) as a comparative group receiving spinal manipulation had no improvement in lordosis. Two other nRCTs were published in 2002 [20] and 2003 [21] confirming the results in the first trial and demonstrated that follow-up of patients experiencing improvements in lordosis by extension traction showed these improvements were relatively stable (small or no loss) at 14 [21] or 15.5 [20] months follow-up. These two latter trials also documented pain reductions coinciding with the lordosis improvements [20, 21] versus no improvements in untreated control groups.

More recently, Moustafa et al. [24, 28–35] has performed multiple RCTs showing improvements in cervical lordosis with extension traction protocols as part of physiotherapeutic treatment programs. These trials have demonstrated superior long-term patient outcomes versus comparative patient groups who only receive the physiotherapy minus the extension traction. In fact, there is now good evidence substantiating CBP cervical extension traction protocols show long-term reduction of anterior head translation (**Figure 5**), long-term improvement in cervical lordosis (**Figure 6**), and long-term reduction in pain levels (**Figure 7**) versus treatments that are 'cookie-cutter' for the purpose of pain-relief.

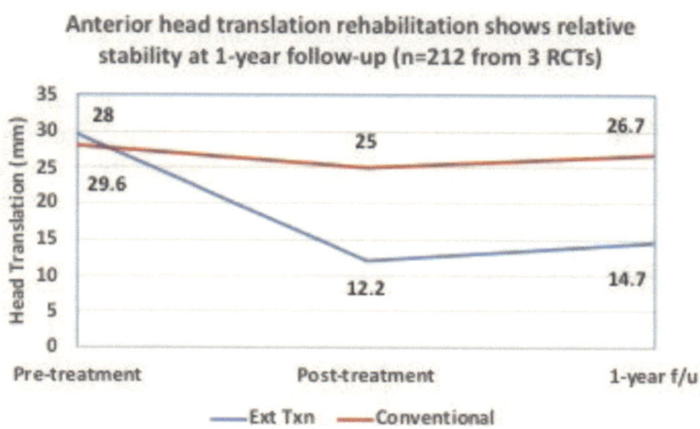

Figure 5.
Data from 3 RCTs demonstrates patients receiving cervical extension traction as well as conventional treatments have reduction of anterior head translation that is sustained for 1-year after stopping treatment versus the comparative groups (controls) remaining virtually unaffected by conventional treatments (Weighted averages from Moustafa et al. [28, 30, 31]).

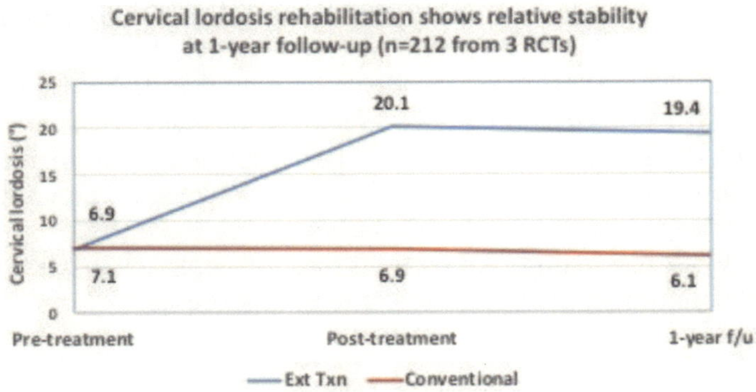

Figure 6.
Data from 3 RCTs demonstrates patients receiving cervical extension traction as well as conventional treatments have lordosis improvements that are sustained for 1-year after stopping treatment versus the cervical curve of comparative groups (controls) remaining unaffected by conventional treatments (Weighted averages from Moustafa et al. [28, 30, 31]).

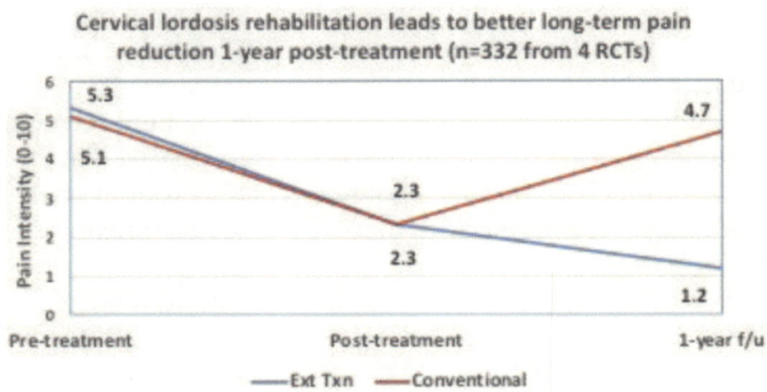

Figure 7.
Data from four RCTs demonstrates patients receiving cervical extension traction as well as conventional treatments have pain reductions that are sustained for 1-year after stopping treatment versus comparative groups (controls) who show a regression (increasing) of pain intensity towards baseline after stopping treatment (Weighted averages from Moustafa et al. [28, 30, 31, 33]).

Table 1 summarizes the main outcomes from eight separate RCTs on CBPs extension traction as part of physiotherapeutic treatment programs versus comparative groups only receiving the physiotherapy and not the extension traction. Notably, and as demonstrated in **Figures 5–7**, pain-relief treatment programs (i.e., stretching/strengthening exercises, infrared irradiation, spinal manipulation, myofascial release, TENS, mobilization, hot packs – not including extension traction) do not improve the spinal parameters and only provide short-term pain relief that regresses after the cessation of treatment.

2.1 CBP protocol for restoring cervical lordosis

The classic CBP "E-A-T" protocol includes Exercises, spinal Adjustments, and Traction in a MI application. Corrective exercises for a cervical spine that is hypolordotic/kyphotic includes cervical extension exercises (**Figure 8**). A new patient may begin with head extension exercises in mid-air, and then progress to using a resistance band placed at the mid/low neck at the apex of their curve abnormality. Repetitions may vary but may begin at 25 and increase to 50 or 100. The patient may be instructed to hold each repetition for 3–5 s [36, 37]. After the patient sufficiently demonstrates proficiency, prescription for home exercises should be made.

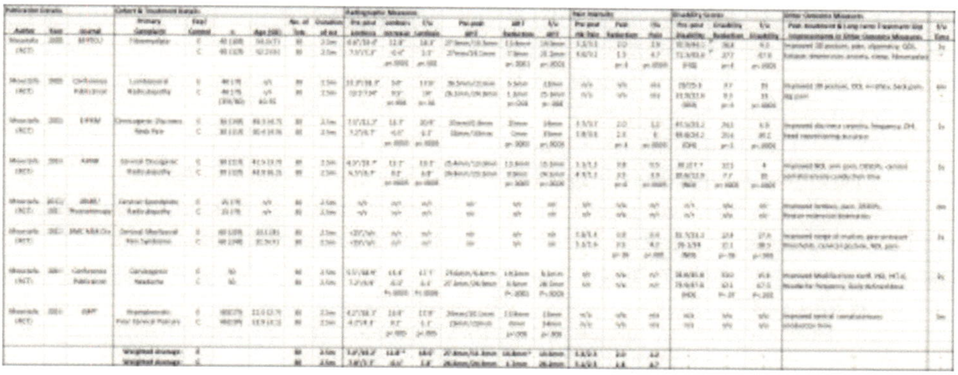

Table 1.
Summary of eight RCTs documenting results in cervical lordosis improvements and reduction of anterior head translation corresponding with various pain, disability, quality of life and physiological parameter improvements.

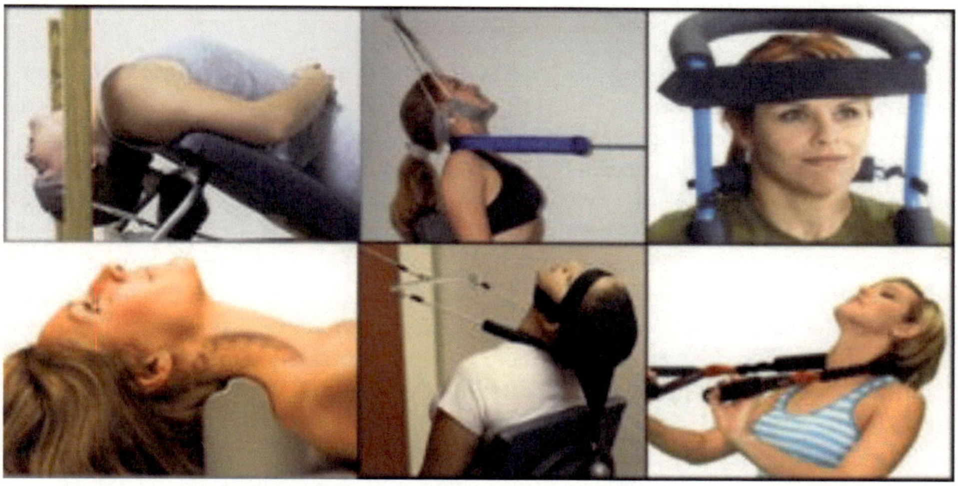

Figure 3.
Cervical extension traction. Bottom right: Cervical extension exercises with resistance band (Courtesy: CBP seminars).

The rationale for corrective exercises is to strengthen the weak muscles, and stretch the shortened muscles as presumably the patient has had the spinal misalignment for some time, usually many years, and the soft tissues will have, over time, adapted to the poor posture [41]. It is generally accepted that exercises alone will not lead to any substantial improvement in lordosis or decreased head translation, but are still important in order to provide stability to the spinal area as the patient is being simultaneously treated with passive spinal traction as part of the CBP rehabilitation program.

Although many CBP practitioners provide spinal manipulative therapy, the MI approach to treat a patient having cervical hypolordosis/kyphosis includes cervical hyperextension drop-table adjustments. The rationale for the application of these force vectors are to reset the tone of the postural muscles [42]. More often patients presenting with cervical spine hypolordosis or kyphosis have accompanying anterior head translation. For this reason, it is commonplace for the manual therapist to place the patient in the prone position and elevate the head support to position the patient in the MI. At the same time the patient can extend their neck backwards (i.e., look forward and place their chin on the head support) to further place the spine into a hyperextended position. The manual therapist would place their contact hand at the mid-neck and/or on the upper thoracic spine and provide a force downwards to engage the drop-piece on a "drop-table."

Spinal traction is applied to increase the cervical lordosis and the spine must be placed in a hyperextended position (**Figure 8**). There are several extension traction variations; each is specific to the actual cervical alignment. For example, a cervical kyphosis with evident anterior head translation requires a posterior head translation and a "2-way" extension traction set-up [20], while a kyphosis without significant anterior head translation could be sufficiently reduced using a "Pope 2-way" extension traction without posterior head translation [21]. A patient having significant AHT having hypolordosis (but no kyphosis) should have sufficient reduction of AHT and increase in lordosis receiving extension-compression extension traction [18]. Initially, traction should be performed for 3–5 min and progress to 10–20 min per treatment session.

3. Restoration of lumbar lordosis

The first clinical trial using CBP methods for the restoration of lumbar lordosis was a non-randomized trial in 2002 [19]. In this trial, 48 patients with chronic low back pain (CLBP) were treated with SMT and extension traction to the lumbar spine for an average of 36 treatment sessions over an average of 12 weeks. There was an average of an 11.3° increase in lumbar lordosis from L1-L5 ARA (9.1° increase from T12-S1 Cobb). A control group of 30 CLBP patients had no pain reduction and no improvement in spine parameters. This trial demonstrated, for the lumbar spine with CLBP patients having hypolordosis, that routine increases in lumbar curvature is achievable; patients who get no treatment have no increase in lumbar curve and remain in pain. Harrison et al. concluded: "This new method of lumbar extension traction is the first nonsurgical rehabilitative procedure to show increases in lumbar lordosis in chronic LBP subjects with hypolordosis."

Since the original trial outlining the CBP extension traction approach for lumbar hypolordosis, two more randomized controlled trials have documented that superior outcomes occur in mechanical LBP and sciatic patients receiving lumbar extension traction as part of comprehensive physiotherapeutic programs versus those who receive the physiotherapy without the extension traction (**Figures 9** and **10**) [25–27]. These results mirror the outcomes as found from the trials on the cervical spine by CBP extension traction methods [24, 28–35]. **Table 2** summarizes the two lumbar trials [25–27].

3.1 CBP protocol for restoring lumbar lordosis

Low back disorder patients who concurrently have lumbar hypolordosis require lumbar extension traction to increase their lumbar structural mal-alignment. **Figure 11** shows three different positions for the application of lumbar extension traction. Although there is not yet enough research to suggest one method over the other, the choice is up to the doctor/therapist. It is suggested that those having high intensity pain and/or those who are older and frail and/or those with balance and locomotor challenges perform lumbar traction in the supine position.

Similar to that discussed for the cervical spine, initial traction should be for 3–5 min and progress to 10–20 min per treatment session [19, 25–27]. Simultaneous physiotherapeutic treatments, including SMT, are in order to provide initial pain relief and improved mobility so that the patient is able to tolerate the traction [36–38].

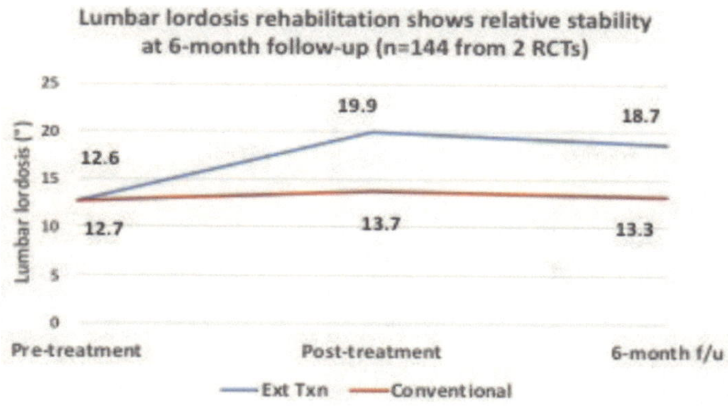

Figure 9.
Data from two RCTs demonstrates patients receiving lumbar extension traction as well as conventional treatments have lordosis improvements that are sustained for 6-months after stopping treatment versus the lumbar curve of comparative groups (controls) remaining unaffected by conventional treatments (Weighted averages from Moustafa et al. [26, 27]).

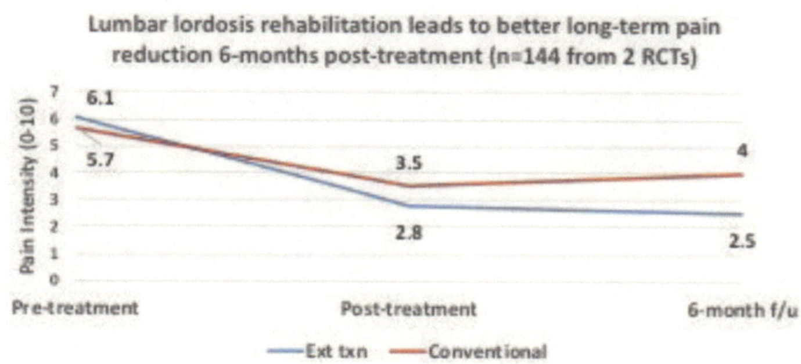

Figure 10.
Data from two RCTs demonstrates patients receiving lumbar extension traction as well as conventional treatments have pain reductions that are sustained for 6-months after stopping treatment versus comparative groups (controls) who show a regression (increasing) of pain intensity towards baseline after stopping treatment (Weighted averages from Moustafa et al. [26, 27]).

Publication Details			Cohort & Treatment Details						Radiographic Measures			Pain Intensity			Disability Scores			Other Outcome Measures	
Author	Year	Journal	Primary Complaint	Exp/Control	n	Age (SD)	No. Txts	Duration of txt	Pre-post Lordosis	Lordosis Increase	f/u Lordosis	Pre-post LBP	Pain Decrease	f/u LBP	Pre-post ODI	ODI Decrease	f/u ODI	Post-treatment & Long-term Treatment Gap Improvements in Other Outcome Measures	f/u Time
Diab/Diab (RCT)	2012/2013	JMPT/JEMR	Chronic LBP	E	40 (18M)	46.3 (12.0)	30	2.5m	13.8°/20.1°	6.2°	18.7°	6/3.2	2.8	2.6	31.4/21.0	10.6	13.8	Improved intervertebral movement, thoracic kyphosis, position of C7 plumbline	3/6m
				C	40 (17M)	45.9 (12.3)	30	2.5m	13.7°/15.2°	1.5°	14.7°	5.5/3.5	3.0	3.5	31.1/23.4	7.7	17.1		
										p=.0001	p=.0008		p=.28	p=.004		p=.3	p=.001		
Moustafa (RCT)	2018	Clin Rehab	Lumbosacral Radiculopathy	E	32 (13M)	41.9 (1.7)	40	2.5m	11°/19.7°	8.7°	18.1°	6.2/2.3	3.9	2.4	32.0/19.8	12.6	21.1	Improved leg pain, Modified Schober test, H-reflex, intersegmental movement	6m
			Radiculopathy	C	32 (15M)	41.2 (2.4)	40	2.5m	11.4°/11.8°	0.8°	11.0°	5.8/3.5	2.3	5.8	31.7/23.7	8.8	31.2		
										p=.001	p=.001		p=.086	p=.001		p=.001	p=.001		
			Weighted Average	E			30	2.5m	12.6°/19.9°	7.3°	18.7°	5.4/1.9	3.5	2.5	31.4/19.9	11.5	19.5	-	-
			Weighted Average	C			30	2.5m	12.7°/13.7°	1.1°	13.3°	5.3/3.5	2.2	4	31.4/23.5	7.8	19.5	-	-

Table 2.
Summary of two RCTs documenting results in lumbar lordosis improvements corresponding with various pain, disability, quality of life and physiological parameter improvements.

4. Extension traction mechanisms

Spinal traction has been around for literally hundreds of years. The unique aspect of CBP's traction for the purpose of increasing the physiologic lordosis whether for the cervical or lumbar spinal areas is performing traction in a hyper-extended position. The key to significant structural spine alignment changes lays in the viscoelastic creep properties of the intervertebral disk (and ligaments) and myofascial tissues under therapeutic conditions [43].

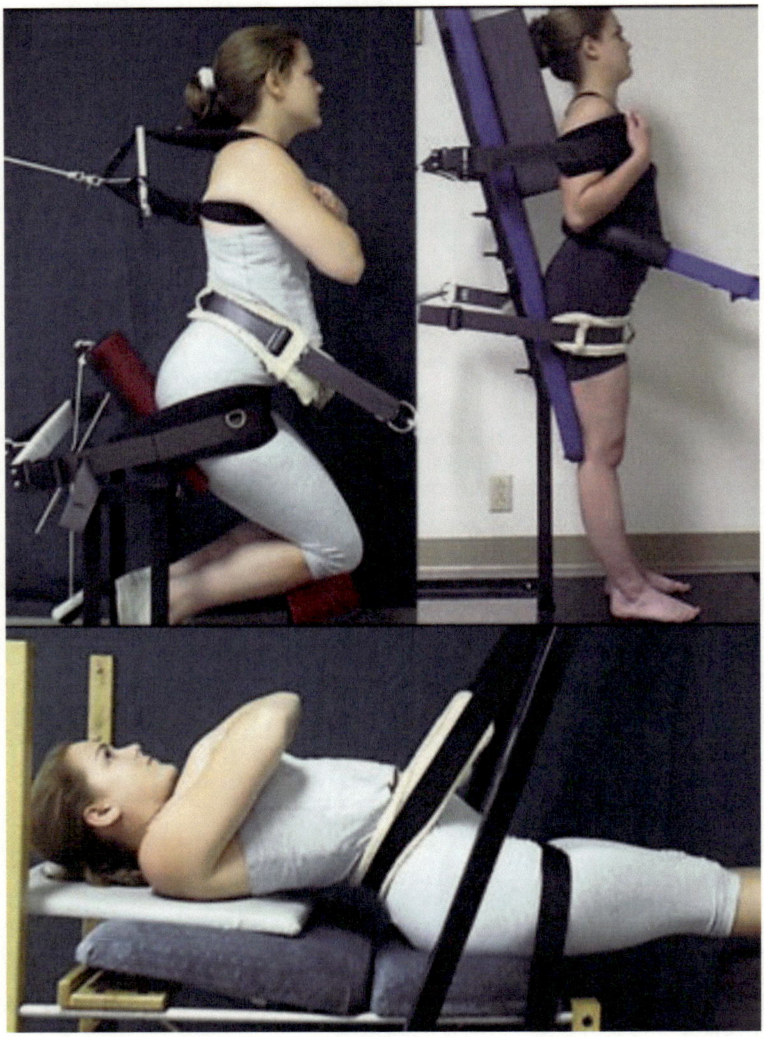

Figure 11.
Lumbar extension traction as preformed in the seated, standing and supine positions (Courtesy: CBP seminars).

Recently, Harrison and Oakley asked the question: *How does lumbar extension traction increase lordosis?* [44]. It was suggested that lumbar extension traction creates a sustained visco-elastic deformation in the soft tissues (muscles, ligaments, and discs) of the lumbar spine (or cervical spine). It is known that all soft tissues including tendons, ligaments, and discs display visco-elastic properties [45]. It is also known that when the soft tissues of the spine are subjected to a continuous load, the tissues will undergo three processes, "creep," "stress relaxation" and "hysteresis." Creep is the amount of deformation occurring in the tissues, stress relaxation is a reduction in the amount of the internal stress found in the tissues over time, and hysteresis is energy loss in the system from an exothermic reaction likely from the breaking of hydrogen-collagen bonds [45–49].

It is presumed that hyperextension traction targets the anterior portion of the discs, the anterior longitudinal ligament, and anterior column musculature specifically [36, 37]. Traction must be performed in a sustained and continuous manner for creep-relaxation and visco-elastic deformation to occur [45–49]. Thus, the biomechanical elongation of the anterior structures leads to a permanent structural tissue resting length change and when performed in a frequent manner (i.e., daily or three times per week), a steady and consistent change to the spine alignment will occur as has been demonstrated by CBP for increasing the cervical lordosis by an average of 10–18° [18, 20, 21, 24, 28–35] and lumbar lordosis by an average of 7–11° [19, 25–27, 44] over the duration of 10-14 weeks. Note that the amount of change in the cervical and lumbar lordosis were measured radiographically on follow-up spine X-rays using standardized, reliable, and valid measurement methods [18, 20, 21, 24, 28–35].

5. Extension traction protocols

Although strict CBP technique methods incorporate exercises, spinal adjustments and spinal traction (E-A-T), these protocols have been discussed elsewhere [1, 36–38]. We will outline the critical protocol parameters that apply specifically to extension traction.

A patient must be screened for the presence of spinal hypolordosis in the cervical or lumbar spine by standard standing X-ray. External (non-imaging methods) body measurements are not valid for the assessment of the magnitude, segmental contributions, and geometric shape of a patient's lumbar or cervical lordosis. Furthermore, only direct spine imaging allows the visualization and quantification of a patients pelvic and thoracic inlet morphologies which are known variables that influence the magnitude of sagittal curvature that should be present and can be achieved through rehabilitation [37, 39, 40]. In the majority of cases, all radiographs should be taken with the patient in a standardized position, standing freely without support, with arms fully flexed with the hands in the clavicle position [50, 51]. We recommend the feet to be positioned hip-widths apart without any shoes as well as the patient should have their eyes open and be staring straight ahead at eye level. Although full spine 36-inch lateral views may be used, it is recommended that a dedicated lateral cervical be taken to more accurately assess cervical subluxation as the 36-inch view projects the head more posteriorly and the cervical spine flatter [52, 53]. An obvious concern about routine X-rays is the exposure to radiation, we address this issue in the next section.

Although various measurement methods may be used, we recommend the Harrison posterior vertebral body tangent method as it is highly reliable (small standard error of measurement; i.e., <2° for regional measures of C2-7 and L1-5) [12–15]. Although C2-T1 absolute rotation angle (ARA) can be used, typically C2-C7 ARA is standard for measuring the cervical lordosis and L1-L5 ARA for the lumbar lordosis.

A patient may start traction for only 3–5 min initially. Increasing traction time may progress by 1–3 min on subsequent treatments pending their clinical tolerance and response. Total traction time should be between 10 to 20 min maximum. There is no significant benefit to performing traction longer than 20 min as the majority of visco-elastic creep deformation occurs in this time [48].

Typical treatment plans include seeing a patient three-times per week for 10–12 weeks prior to a repeat X-ray and analysis of structural improvement. As outlined in previous works [36–38], a patient may require several rounds of treatments to achieve a spinal alignment in the realm of normal/ideal; this is particularly true for patients having gross spinal deformities, high pain levels, and disability, as demonstrated in the treatment of non-iatrogenic flat back [44]. It is not untypical to treat a Patient three times per week, for 6–12 months in these cases.

6. Contraindications to extension traction

Generally, contraindications for extension traction protocols are the same as contraindications for SMT. Although traction protocols may be used in these cases, patients with a history of stroke, high blood pressure, bone spurring on the posterior aspect of the spine, spinal stenosis or other space occupying lesions represent potential high-risk, and therefore, extra caution should be taken to screen these patients for tolerance to this type of traction.

Patient screening for the ability to tolerate spinal extension traction should be performed for all patients. This typically includes assessing tolerance while laying supine on an extension traction device (e.g., Denneroll). The patient should be assessed for distress and/or an exacerbation of symptoms including the reporting of nausea, dizziness or increased pain. Those with rigid spine deformities and/or spinal osteoarthritis should have a stress view radiograph taken for flexion-extension as well as lying supine over an extension traction device.

The following represent absolute contraindications to the application of spinal extension traction [36, 37]:

- Pregnancy, especially in later stages nearing term;
- Infectious discitis and spinal tumors compromising vertebral stability;
- Abdominal aortic aneurysm;
- Severe osteoporosis and other bone diseases;
- Unstable vertebral fraction;
- Unstable segment under loading (verified by radiography) that cannot be reduced with extension traction loading;
- Multi-level spinal fusion;
- Recent spinal surgery;
- Abdominal hernias for lumbar traction;
- Other conditions that would be contraindicated for spinal manipulation;
- Patient having hyperlordosis of the cervical or lumbar spinal areas where extension traction is to be performed;
- Not having recent confirmatory standing X-rays of the spinal region to where the extension traction is to be applied.

The following represent relative contraindications to spinal extension traction that require diligent screening and clinical evaluation [36, 37]:

- Canal stenosis—although also proven useful for this [54];
- Spondylolisthesis—although also proven useful for this [55];
- Single-level fusions—to prevent hyperextension at the adjacent segment to the fusion;

- Hip replacement;
- Advanced osteoporosis;
- Locking (hyperextension) of the knees while in standing traction position—this may limit blood flow and induce syncope;
- Lack of food/nutrition and/or water several hours prior to treatment—may result in syncope;
- Extreme fatigue or illness or recently donating blood—may result in syncope;
- When pelvic morphology dictates a modification from ideal lumbar lordosis or thoracic inlet angle dictates a modification from ideal cervical lordosis such that the patient's actual lordosis is more or less than expected [36, 37, 39, 40];
- Kissing spinous's or Baastrup's disease will inhibit segmental extension from occurring.

When applying extension traction protocols, it is important to realize the obvious notion that this applies only to those presenting with hypolordosis, straightening, or kyphosis of the cervical or Lumbar spinal areas, not to those with hyperlordosis. In such cases, different CBP traction protocols apply which are beyond the scope of this brief review [39, 56]. Also, in the performance of assessing patient tolerance to extension traction, the slow progression of increasing time and transitioning to a more challenging extension stretch is found in the skill and art of the hands of the practitioner. Fortunately, extension traction protocols have been proven safe as no reports of deleterious outcomes have been reported in the multiple RCT's [24–35]. Further, this approach seems so safe that once thought of as contraindications, for example spondylolisthesis, have been shown to be able to be reduced by a special application of these methods [55]. Again, the experience and confidence of the practitioner will dictate whether this approach is selected for different candidate patients with their corresponding varying levels of difficult spinal conditions and case histories.

Concerns over radiation exposures during routine spinal X-ray imaging need discussion. Although this topic has been thoroughly discussed elsewhere [57–60], in brief, patient exposures from spinal X-rays are not harmful. First, the assumption that radiation exposures from low-doses are carcinogenic is false; low-doses of radiation (including X-rays and CT scans) stimulate the adaptive protection systems in the body to "over-repair" any genetic damage done, including DNA double strand breaks by imaging [61]. Second, because of point one, there is no cumulative effect; therefore, the only relative risk can be considered from a single session of X-rays (i.e., 1–3 mGy) [57, 58]. Third, due to point two, the amount of radiation from X-rays of 1–3 mGy is many times lower than the recognized dose threshold for leukemia of 1100 mGy (95% CI: 500–2600 mGy) [57, 62] and therefore cannot be carcinogenic.

7. Conclusions

Today there are reliable and predictable means through application of extension spinal traction as part of comprehensive rehabilitation programs to restore the natural curvatures of the spine. High-quality evidence points to CBP methods as offering superior long-term outcomes for treating patients with sagittal plane spine and posture deformities who present with various craniocervical and lumbosacral disorders.

Conflict of interest

PAO is a paid consultant to CBP; DEH sells products related to the treatment of spine deformity as depicted herein.

Nomenclature

AHT	anterior head translation
ARA	absolute rotation angle
CBP	chiropractic BioPhysics®
CLBP	chronic low back pain
E-A-T	exercises, adjustments, traction (mirror image)
LBP	low back pain
MI	mirror image®
nRCT	non-randomized controlled trial
RCT	randomized controlled trial
SMT	spinal manipulative therapy

Author details

Paul A. Oakley[1]*, Ibrahim M. Moustafa[2,3] and Deed E. Harrison[4]

1 Private Practice, Newmarket, Ontario, Canada

2 Department of Physiotherapy, College of Health Sciences, University of Sharjah, Sharjah, UAE

3 Basic science department, Faculty of Physical Therapy, Cairo University, Naser City, Cairo, Egypt

4 CBP NonProfit, Inc., Eagle, Idaho, USA

*Address all correspondence to: docoakley.icc@gmail.com

References

[1] Harrison DD, Janik TJ, Harrison GR, et al. Chiropractic Biophysics technique: A linear algebra approach to posture in chiropractic. Journal of Manipulative and Physiological Therapeutics. 1996;**19**:525-535

[2] Panjabi MM, White AA 3rd, Brand RA Jr. A note on defining body parts configurations. Journal of Biomechanics. 1974;7(4):385-387

[3] Harrison DD. Abnormal postural permutations calculated as rotations and translations from an ideal normal upright static posture. In: Sweere JJ, editor. Chiropractic Family Practice. Gaithersburg: Aspen Publishers; 1992. pp. 1-22. Chapter 6-1

[4] Harrison DD, Janik TJ, Troyanovich SJ, Holland B. Comparisons of Lordotic cervical spine curvatures to a theoretical ideal model of the static sagittal cervical spine. Spine. 1996;**21**(6):667-675

[5] Harrison DD, Janik TJ, Troyanovich SJ, Harrison DE, Colloca CJ. Evaluations of the assumptions used to derive an ideal normal cervical spine model. Journal of Manipulative and Physiological Therapeutics. 1997;**20**(4):246-256

[6] Harrison DD, Harrison DE, Janik TJ, Cailliet R, Haas JW, Ferrantelli J, et al. Modeling of the sagittal cervical spine as a method to discriminate hypo-lordosis: Results of elliptical and circular modeling in 72 asymptomatic subjects, 52 acute neck pain subjects, and 70 chronic neck pain subjects. Spine. 2004;**29**:2485-2492

[7] Harrison DE, Janik TJ, Harrison DD, Cailliet R, Harmon S. Can the thoracic kyphosis be modeled with a simple geometric shape? The results of circular and elliptical modeling in 80 asymptomatic subjects. Journal of Spinal Disorders. 2002;**15**(3):213-220

[8] Harrison DE, Harrison DD, Janik TJ, Cailliet R, Haas JW. Do alterations in vertebral and disc dimensions affect an elliptical model of the thoracic kyphosis? Spine. 2003;**28**(5):463-469

[9] Troyanovich SJ, Cailliet R, Janik TJ, Harrison DD, Harrison DE. Radiographic mensuration characteristics of the sagittal lumbar spine from a normal population with a method to synthesize prior studies of lordosis. Journal of Spinal Disorders. 1997;**10**(5):380-386

[10] Janik TJ, Harrison DD, Cailliet R, Troyanovich SJ, Harrison DE. Can the sagittal lumbar curvature be closely approximated by an ellipse? Journal of Orthopaedic Research. 1998;**16**(6):766-770

[11] Harrison DD, Cailliet R, Janik TJ, Troyanovich SJ, Harrison DE, Holland B. Elliptical modeling of the sagittal lumbar lordosis and segmental rotation angles as a method to discriminate between normal and low back pain subjects. Journal of Spinal Disorders. 1998;**11**(5):430-439

[12] Harrison DE, Harrison DD, Cailliet R, Troyanovich SJ, Janik TJ, Holland B. Cobb method or Harrison posterior tangent method: Which to choose for lateral cervical radiographic analysis. Spine. 2000;**25**(16):2072-2078

[13] Harrison DE, Cailliet R, Harrison DD, Janik TJ, Holland B. Centroid, Cobb or Harrison posterior tangents: Which to choose for analysis of thoracic kyphosis? Spine. 2001;**26**(11):E227-E234

[14] Harrison DE, Cailliet R, Harrison DD, Janik TJ, Holland B. Radiographic analysis of lumbar lordosis: Cobb method, centroidal method, TRALL or Harrison posterior tangents? Spine. 2001;**26**(11):E235-E242

[15] Harrison DE, Holland B, Harrison DD, Janik TJ. Further reliability analysis of the Harrison radiographic line drawing methods: Crossed ICCs for lateral posterior tangents and AP modified-riser Ferguson. Journal of Manipulative and Physiological Therapeutics. 2002;**25**:93-98

[16] Harrison DE, Harrison DD, Colloca CJ, et al. Repeatability over time of posture, radiograph positioning, and radiograph line drawing: An analysis of six control groups. Journal of Manipulative and Physiological Therapeutics. 2003;**26**:87-98

[17] McAviney J, Schulz D, Bock R, Harrison DE, Holland B. Determining the relationship between cervical lordosis and neck complaints. Journal of Manipulative and Physiological Therapeutics. 2005;**28**(3):187-193

[18] Harrison DD, Jackson BL, Troyanovich S, Robertson G, de George D, Barker WF. The efficacy of cervical extension-compression traction combined with diversified manipulation and drop table adjustments in the rehabilitation of cervical lordosis: A pilot study. Journal of Manipulative and Physiological Therapeutics. 1994;**17**(7):454-464

[19] Harrison DE, Harrison DD, Cailliet R, Janik TJ, Holland B. Changes in sagittal lumbar configuration with a new method of extension traction: Non-randomized clinical control trial. Archives of Physical Medicine and Rehabilitation. 2002;**83**(11):1585-1591

[20] Harrison DE, Cailliet R, Harrison DD, Janik TJ, Holland B. New 3-point bending traction method of restoring cervical lordosis combined with cervical manipulation: Non-randomized clinical control trial. Archives of Physical Medicine and Rehabilitation. 2002;**83**(4):447-453

[21] Harrison DE, Harrison DD, Betz J, Colloca CJ, Janik TJ, Holland B. Increasing the cervical lordosis with seated combined extension-compression and transverse load cervical traction with cervical manipulation: Non-randomized clinical control trial. Journal of Manipulative and Physiological Therapeutics. 2003;**26**(3):139-151

[22] Harrison DE, Harrison DD, Haas JW, Betz JW, Janik TJ, Holland B. Conservative methods to correct lateral translations of the head: A non-randomized clinical control trial. Journal of Rehabilitation Research and Development. 2004;**41**(4):631-640

[23] Harrison DE, Cailliet R, Betz JW, Harrison DD, Haas JW, Janik TJ, et al. Harrison mirror image methods for correcting trunk list: A non-randomized clinical control trial. European Spine Journal. 2005;**14**(2):155-162

[24] Moustafa IM, Diab AM, Ahmed A, Harrison DE. The efficacy of cervical lordosis rehabilitation for nerve root function, pain, and segmental motion in cervical spondylotic radiculopathy. Physical Therapy. 2011;**97**(Suppl):846-847

[25] Diab AA, Moustafa IM. Rehabilitation for pain and lumbar segmental motion in chronic mechanical low back pain: A randomized trial. Journal of Manipulative and Physiological Therapeutics. 2012;**35**(4):246-253

[26] Moustafa IM, Diab AA. Extension traction treatment for patients with discogenic lumbosacral radiculopathy: A randomized controlled trial. Clinical Rehabilitation. 2012;**27**(1):51-62

[27] Diab AA, Moustafa IM. The efficacy of lumbar extension traction for sagittal alignment in mechanical low back pain. A randomized trial. Journal of Back and Musculoskeletal Rehabilitation. 2013;**26**(2):213-222

[28] Moustafa IM. Does improvement towards a normal cervical configuration aid in the management of fibromyalgia. A randomized controlled trial. Bulletin of Faculty of Physical Therapy, Cairo University. 2013;**18**(2):29-41

[29] Moustafa IM, Diab AA, Harrison DE. Does improvement towards a normal cervical sagittal configuration aid in the management of lumbosacral radiculopathy: A randomized controlled trial. In: Proceedings of the 13th World Federation of Chiropractic Biennial Congress/ECU Convention; Athens, Greece; May 13-16, 2015. Paper #184 Mediterranean Region Award Winning Paper

[30] Moustafa IM, Diab AA, Taha S, Harrison DE. Addition of a sagittal cervical posture corrective orthotic device to a multimodal rehabilitation program improves short- and long-term outcomes in patients with discogenic cervical radiculopathy. Archives of Physical Medicine and Rehabilitation. 2016;**97**:2034-2044

[31] Moustafa IM, Diab AA, Harrison DE. The effect of normalizing the sagittal cervical configuration on dizziness, neck pain, and cervicocephalic kinesthetic sensibility: A 1-year randomized controlled study. European Journal of Physical and Rehabilitation Medicine. 2017;**53**:57-71

[32] Moustafa IM, Diab AAM, Hegazy FA, Harrison DE. Does rehabilitation of cervical lordosis influence sagittal cervical spine flexion extension kinematics in cervical spondylotic radiculopathy subjects? Journal of Back and Musculoskeletal Rehabilitation. 2017;**30**:937-941

[33] Moustafa IM, Diab AA, Hegazy F, Harrison DE. Does improvement towards a normal cervical sagittal configuration aid in the management of cervical myofascial pain syndrome: A 1- year randomized controlled trial. BMC Musculoskeletal Disorders. 2018;**19**:396

[34] Moustafa IM, Diab AA, Harrison DE. The effect of normalizing the sagittal cervical configuration for the management of cervicogenic headaches: A 2-year pilot randomized controlled trial. In: 15th World Federation of Chiropractic Biennial Congress/78th European Chiropractor's Union Convention; March 20-23, 2019. p. 142

[35] Moustafa IM, Diab AAM, Taha S, Harrison DE. Demonstration of central conduction time and neuroplastic changes after cervical lordosis rehabilitation in asymptomatic subjects: A randomized, placebo-controlled trial. Proceedings of the 14th biennial congress of the World Federation of Chiropractic, March 15-18, 2017.

[36] Harrison DE, Harrison DD, Haas JW. Structural Rehabilitation of the Cervical Spine. Evanston, WY: Harrison CBP® Seminars, Inc.; 2002

[37] Harrison DE, Betz JW, Harrison DD, et al. CBP Structural Rehabilitation of the Lumbar Spine. Eagle, ID, USA: Harrison Chiropractic Biophysics Seminars. 2007

[38] Oakley PA, Harrison DD, Harrison DE, Haas JW. Evidence-based protocol for structural rehabilitation of the spine and posture: Review of clinical biomechanics of posture (CBP®) publications. Journal of the Canadian Chiropractic Association. 2005;**49**:270-296

[39] Lee SH, Kim KT, Seo EM, Suk KS, Kwack YH, Son ES. The influence of thoracic inlet alignment on the craniocervical sagittal balance in asymptomatic adults. Journal of Spinal Disorders & Techniques. 2011;**25**(2):E41-E47

[40] Vrtovec T, Janssen MM, Likar B, Castelein RM, Viergever MA, Pernuš F. Evaluation of pelvic morphology in the sagittal plane. The Spine Journal. 2013;**13**(11):1500-1509

[41] Khayatzadeh S, Kalmanson OA, Schuit D, Havey RM, Voronov LI, Ghanayem AJ, et al. Cervical muscle-tendon unit length differences between neutral and forward head postures: Biomechanical study using human cadaveric specimens. Physical Therapy. 2017;**97**(7):756-766

[42] DeVocht JW, Pickar JG, Wilder DG. EMG activity levels of paraspinal muscles during spinal manipulation. In: Proceedings from the 29th annual meeting of ISSLS 2002; Vancouver, Canada; 2002

[43] Owens SC, Brismée JM, Pennell PN, Dedrick GS, Sizer PS, James CR. Changes in spinal height following sustained lumbar flexion and extension postures: A clinical measure of intervertebral disc hydration using stadiometry. Journal of Manipulative and Physiological Therapeutics. 2009;**32**:358-363

[44] Harrison DE, Oakley PA. Non-operative correction of flat back syndrome using lumbar extension traction: A CBP® case series of two. Journal of Physical Therapy Science. 2018;**30**:1131-1137

[45] Panjabi MM, White AA. Biomechanics in the Musculoskeletal System. Philadelphia, PA, USA: Churchill Livingstone; 2001

[46] Adams MA, Dolan P. Time-dependent changes in the lumbar spine's resistance to bending. Clinical Biomechanics. 1996;**11**:194-200

[47] Hukins DW, Kirby MC, Sikoryn TA, et al. Comparison of structure, mechanical properties, and functions of lumbar spinal ligaments. Spine. 1990;**15**:787-795

[48] Oliver MJ, Twomey LT. Extension creep in the lumbar spine. Clinical Biomechanics. 1995;**10**:363-368

[49] Woo S, Livesay GA, Runco TJ, et al. Structure and function of tendons and ligaments. In: Mow VC, Hayes WC, editors. Basics Orthopaedic Biomechanics. 2nd ed. Philadelphia: Lippincott-Raven; 1997. pp. 209-252

[50] Bess S, Protopsaltis TS, Lafage V, Lafage R, Ames CP, Errico T, et al. International spine study group. Clinical and radiographic evaluation of adult spinal deformity. Clinical Spine Surgery. 2016;**29**:6-16

[51] Horton WC, Brown CW, Bridwell KH, Glassman SD, Suk SI, Cha CW. Is there an optimal patient stance for obtaining a lateral 36″ radiograph? A critical comparison of three techniques. Spine. 2005;**30**:427-433

[52] Park SM, Song KS, Park SH, et al. Does whole-spine lateral radiograph with clavicle positioning reflect the correct cervical sagittal alignment? European Spine Journal. 2015;**24**:57-62

[53] Carreon LY, Smith CL, Dimar JR 2nd, Glassman SD. Correlation of cervical sagittal alignment parameters on full-length spine radiographs compared with dedicated cervical radiographs. Scoliosis and Spinal Disorders. 2016;**11**:12

[54] Weiner MT, Oakley PA, Dennis AK, Shapiro DA, Harrison DE. Increasing the cervical and lumbar lordosis is possible despite overt osteoarthritis and spinal stenosis using extension traction to relieve low back and leg pain in a 66-year-old surgical candidate: A CBP® case report. Journal of Physical Therapy Science. 2018;**30**:1364-1369

[55] Fedorchuk C, Lightstone DF, McRae C, Kaczor D. Correction of grade 2 spondylolisthesis following

a non-surgical structural spinal rehabilitation protocol using lumbar traction: A case study and selective review of literature. Journal of Radiology Case Reports. 2017;**11**:13-26

[56] Oakley PA, Ehsani NN, Harrison DE. Non-surgical reduction of lumbar hyperlordosis, forward sagittal balance and sacral tilt to relieve low back pain by Chiropractic BioPhysics® methods: A case report. Journal of Physical Therapy Science. 2019;**31**:860-864

[57] Oakley PA, Ehsani NN, Harrison DE. Repeat radiography in monitoring structural changes in the treatment of spinal disorders in chiropractic and manual medicine practice: Evidence and safety. Dose-Response. 2019;**17**(4):1559325819891043

[58] Oakley PA, Ehsani NN, Harrison DE. The scoliosis quandary: Are radiation exposures from repeated X-rays harmful? Dose-Response. 2019;**17**(2):1559325819852810

[59] Oakley PA, Cuttler JM, Harrison DE. X-ray imaging is essential for contemporary chiropractic and manual therapy spinal rehabilitation: Radiography increases benefits and reduces risks. Dose-Response. 2018;**16**(2):1559325818781437

[60] Oakley PA, Harrison DE. Radiophobia: 7 reasons why radiography used in spine and posture rehabilitation should not Be feared or avoided. Dose-Response. 2018;**16**(2):1559325818781445

[61] Löbrich M, Rief N, Kühne M, et al. In vivo formation and repair of DNA double-strand breaks after computed tomography examinations. Proceedings of the National Academy of Sciences of the United States of America. 2005;**102**:8984-8989

[62] Cuttler JM. Evidence of dose threshold for radiation-induced leukemia: Absorbed dose and uncertainty. Dose-Response. 2019;**17**(1):1559325818820973

Chapter 9

Brace Treatment for Children and Adolescents with Scoliosis

Hans-Rudolf Weiss and Deborah Turnbull

Abstract

The aim of brace treatment in patients with scoliosis during growth is (1) to stop curve progression and (2) to improve appearance/cosmesis. There is high quality evidence available supporting brace treatment. According to recent publications, the outcomes of different braces vary to a high extent. Although most of the scoliosis cases will not affect the patient's health, the impact of braces on the cosmetic outcome to date is not well determined. Standardised asymmetric braces (mainly Chêneau derivatives) have better outcomes than symmetric compression braces and may also lead to significant improvements of the deformity. For symmetric braces, no evidence exists that these could significantly change the deformity. Soft braces have no indication and the use of night-time braces should be largely restricted due to poor outcomes when compared to current standards of full-time bracing.

Keywords: scoliosis, deformity, progression, brace treatment

1. Introduction

Scoliosis is a three-dimensional deformity of the trunk and spine which may deteriorate quickly during phases of rapid growth [1–3]. Scoliosis may be caused by neuromuscular disorders and mesenchymal disorders, and it may be congenital and caused by other rare conditions, but for most cases (80–90%), it is referred to as idiopathic because no underlying cause has been identified [1–4]. Idiopathic scoliosis is further distinguished by the age at the onset of the condition. Infantile idiopathic scoliosis (IIS) is defined as starting at the age of 1.6–3 years, juvenile idiopathic scoliosis (JIS) at the age of 4–6 years and adolescent idiopathic scoliosis (AIS) at the age of 10–14 years old [1, 4]. The treatment of scoliosis consists of observation, exercises, brace treatment and spinal fusion surgery [1–3]. When considering surgery versus conservative treatment, high-quality evidence exists for the application of pattern specific exercises (PSE for example, Schroth) [5, 6] and spinal bracing [7–9]. No long-term evidence exists to support spinal fusion surgery [10–14]. Further comparisons are not possible when there is a lack of publicised surgical outcomes. High rates of complication have been reported in the mid and long terms [15–18], whilst no long-term complications have been publicised regarding PSE and brace treatment. AIS is a relatively benign disorder in most cases [19, 20] and therefore the long-term complications of spinal fusion surgery may outweigh the long-term consequences of the deformity [15–18, 21].

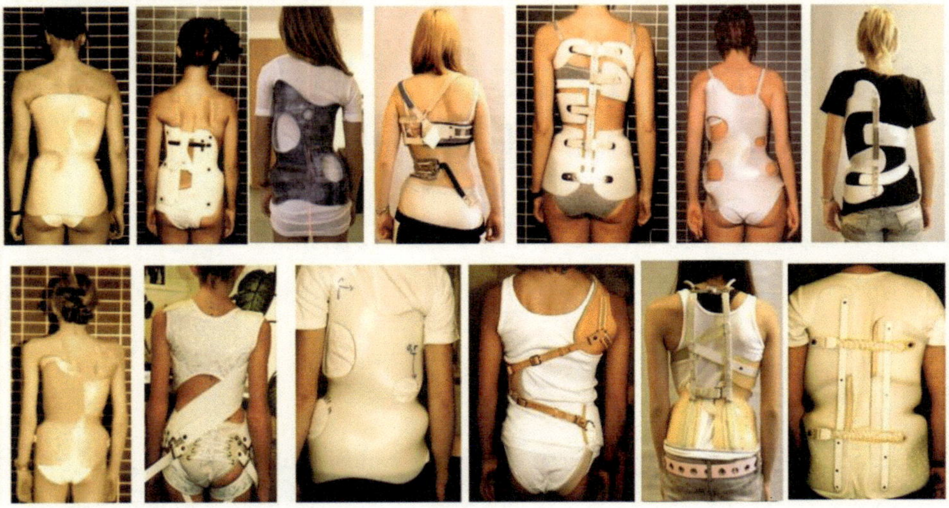

Figure 1.
Many different braces as still applied today for the treatment of scoliosis.

Consequently, the indication for spinal fusion surgery in patients with AIS is controversial [22] as is for most of the other scoliosis conditions [12, 23, 24]. When comparing surgery versus bracing and PSE, there is evidence for conservative treatment, but no published evidence for spinal fusion surgery for AIS.

It is well established in literature that pattern-based or pattern-specific exercises do have a positive impact on the course of the disease [5, 6, 25–27]. Obviously, general exercises or sport activities also reduce the incidence of progression in small curvatures [28] or in patients with a low risk for progression [29]. However, there is only one relevant randomised controlled trial (RCT) with an untreated control group [5], whilst other RCTs involving PSE have major flaws (amongst other things not providing an uncontrolled control group) and therefore would not contribute to high quality evidence [30, 31].

Brace treatment is supported by high-quality evidence as well [7–9]; however, the approach to bracing differs significantly in design (**Figure 1**). There are many types such as symmetrical braces [7, 9, 32–35], asymmetrical braces [8, 36–49], night-time braces [50–55] and soft braces [56, 57]. It has been shown that soft braces have no advantage over hard braces [8, 58–60]. The authors and company owners have published a body of literature [61], but independent high-quality papers have concluded that soft braces in patients at risk of progression, will not benefit from such treatment [8, 58–60]. Therefore, only hard braces should be used in patients at risk for progression.

Purpose of this review is to discuss the best possible approach for bracing scoliosis patients with respect to (1) rate of success and (2) impact on the deformity.

2. Materials and methods

A literature review has been undertaken using the Pub Med database on June 27th, 2019 and a hand search identifying outcome papers on the topic of bracing in adolescent idiopathic scoliosis containing data with respect to (1) rate of success and (2) impact on the deformity. Search terms used were (1) scoliosis, brace treatment, rate of success and (2) scoliosis, brace treatment, cosmetic outcome.

3. Results

The results of the search; (1) 31 items have been found of which 14 were found to be relevant reporting a rate of success [7, 9, 47, 52, 55, 62–70]; (2) 14 items were found of which 3 reported upon cosmetic outcomes [71–73]. In the hand search additional papers were revealed for search (1) [32–46, 48–51, 53–55, 74]. Hand search for search (2) revealed a narrative review on the topic [75].

Success rates between less than 50% and more than 90% were found [7–9, 32–55, 74]. In one study, there was a success rate of 100%; however, only small curves and only single curve patterns were included [42]. The latter study therefore cannot be regarded as being comparable to the content of the other studies found in literature.

More symmetrical braces (Boston style) have consistent success rates of just over 70% [7, 9, 32–35], whilst asymmetrical full-time braces show success rates between 50 and 95% [8, 36–49]. Night-time braces when compared to full-time braces seem to have poor results (57.1%) [55]. Standardised asymmetrical braces may have success rates exceeding 80% [8, 41, 46] even in curves of 40° and above [47, 74].

Most of the brace studies did not include any measures regarding the impact of the brace on the deformity of the trunk. Only in a few papers, the measurement of trunk deformity was reported [71–73] and in very few papers clinical and cosmetic improvements after brace treatment were documented [75].

4. Discussion

Symmetrical braces (Boston style with dorsal or ventral closures) provide success rates of 70% or little over [7, 9, 32–35] (**Figure 2**). Asymmetrical three-dimensional braces (mainly Chêneau style) may have success rates between less than 50 and more than 90% [8, 36–49]. There is a wide variety of outcomes used in research, which may be related to the differing qualities of asymmetrical brace adjustments and designs (**Figures 3–5**).

With a more or less symmetrical tube shape (**Figure 2**) brace construction is more simple, whilst asymmetrical braces can only be constructed and adjusted well

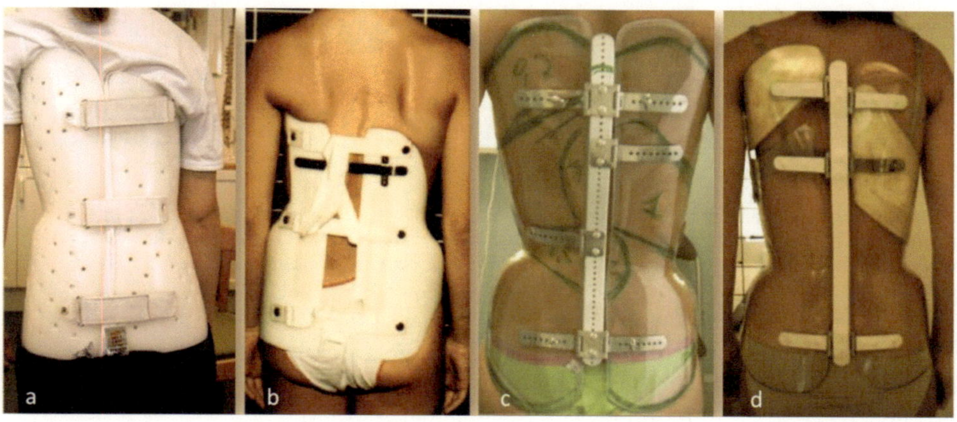

Figure 2.
Visually almost symmetrical braces mainly correcting via trunk compression. (a) Boston brace made with a little shift towards the thoracic concavity, (b) Boston brace from Denmark pushing the trunk into the main thoracic curve and (c and d) symmetrical compression braces from Italy [34, 35].

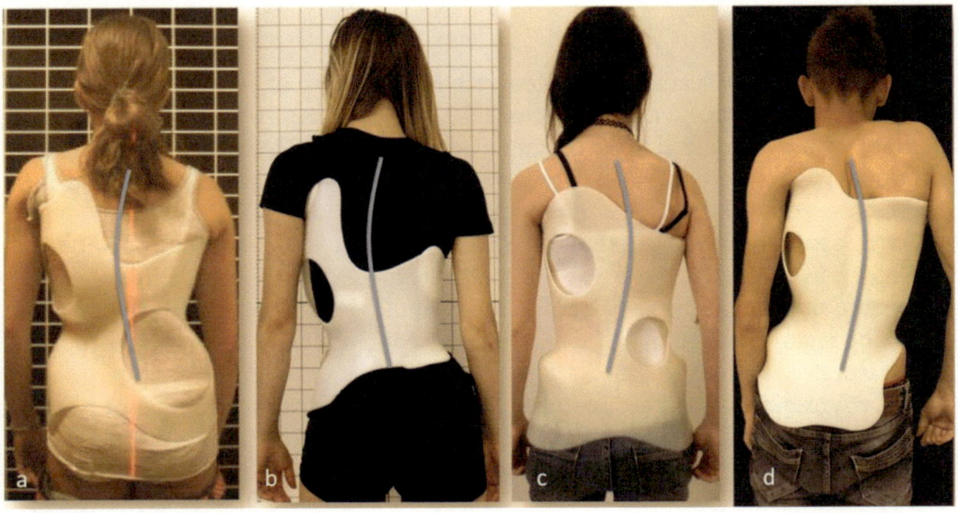

Figure 3.
Different Chêneau style braces all for a main thoracic curve to the right. (a) Rigo brace and (b) Gensingen (GBW) brace clearly mirroring the deformity shifting the thoracic part of the trunk to the left. (c and d) Hand-made Chêneau derivatives without obvious impact on the trunk deformity still decompensated to the right in the brace. In a good asymmetrical high correction brace mirroring of the deformity will always be visible (a and b).

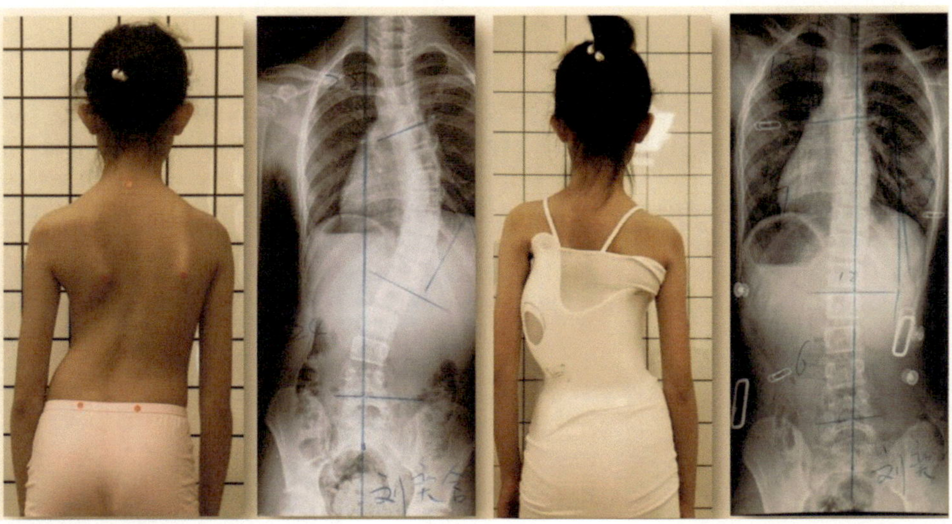

Figure 4.
Asymmetrical high correction brace (GBW) with a clear mirroring of the deformity in the brace and a reasonably successful cosmetic improvement along with the in-brace correction as shown on the right. GBW brace produced in May, 2019 with a thoracic curvature of 45°, lumbar curvature of 24°. In-brace X-ray, thoracic 7°, lumbar 7° Cobb (courtesy of Xiaofeng Nan, Xi'an, China).

with a very experienced and highly skilled technician/orthotist or by using well calibrated and reliable CAD (computer-aided design, see **Figures 3–5**) series based on certain classifications and proven reliable methods [76, 77].

It is not the name of the brace that ensures a good outcome; it is the brace manufacture and adjustments based on standardised algorithms [76, 77]. It is concerning that in many studies on brace treatment, an example of the brace design is not presented in a picture [55, 78]; sometimes the brace design is not even named [78].

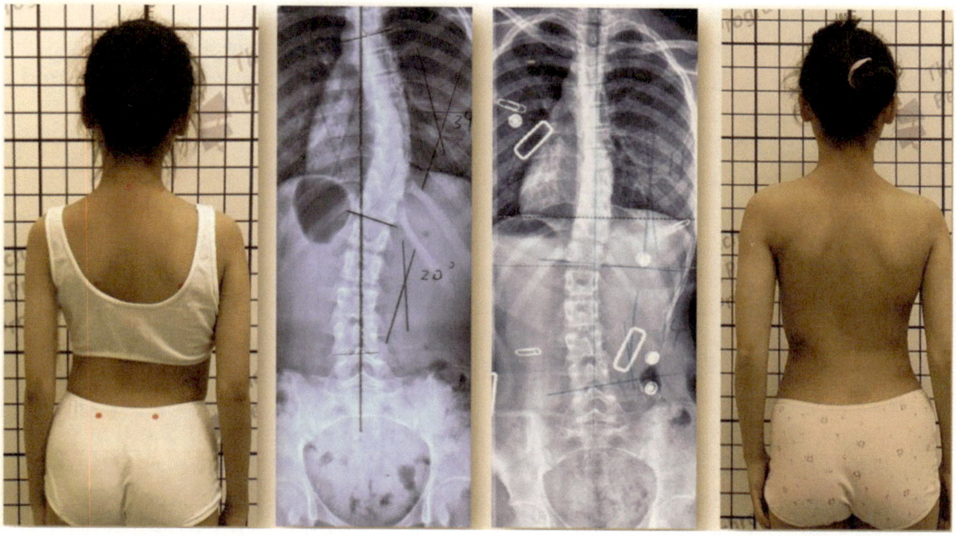

Figure 5.
Girl with a Risser stage of IV. The thoracic curve initially was 34° and the lumbar 20°. After wearing the GBW brace in-brace X-ray of the thoracic curve was 11° and lumbar 14°. Half a year later X-ray without the brace (for over 24 hours) is 24° and lumbar 20° with a reasonable clinical correction as seen on the right. This case shows that also in the more mature patient significant cosmetic improvements can be gained (courtesy of Xiaofeng Nan, Xi'an, China).

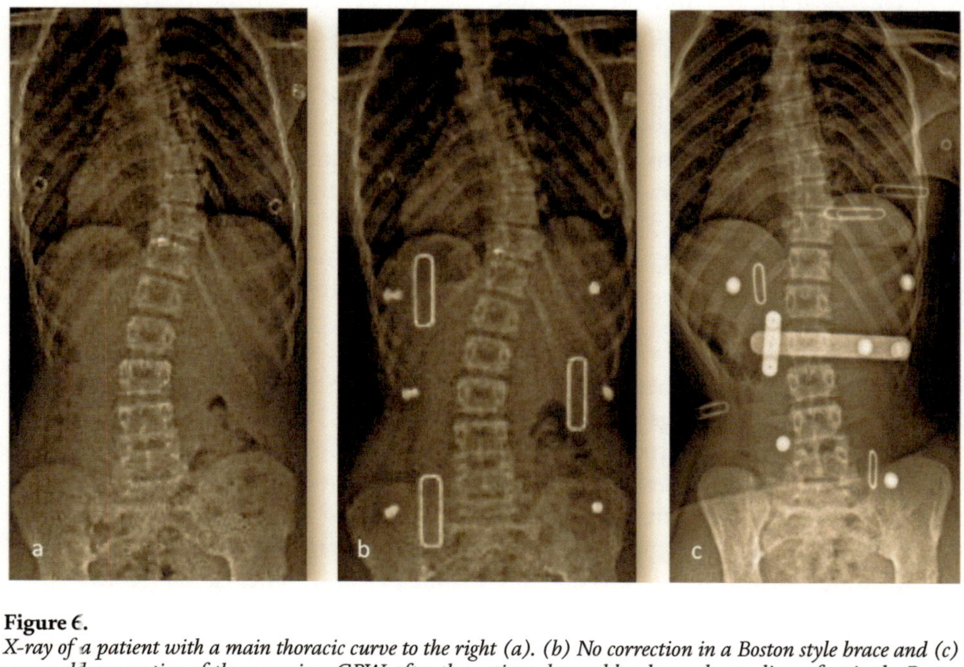

Figure 6.
X-ray of a patient with a main thoracic curve to the right (a). (b) No correction in a Boston style brace and (c) reasonable correction of the curve in a GBW, after the patient changed her brace due to discomfort in the Boston brace (courtesy of Dr Marc Moramarco, Scoliosis 3DC, Woburn, MA, US).

Outcomes with respect to Cobb angle: Landauer et al. in their retrospective study [37] examined 62 adolescent female patients with right thoracic scoliosis (20–40 Cobb degrees) treated with a Chêneau style brace. Initial correction improvements of >40% ($p < 0.002$) and satisfactory compliance ($p < 0.004$) gained a significantly successful outcome (**Figure 6**). There was an average improvement of 7° in Cobb angle, with patients with good compliance and with a significant initial correction.

The authors concluded that compliant patients with a high initial correction can expect a final correction of around 7°, whilst compliant patients with low initial correction may maintain the curve to some extent. Bad compliance was associated with curve progression.

Bullmann and colleagues in their study [38] had 52 patients with a Cobb angle of between 25 and 40°. Prior to starting brace treatment with the Chêneau-Toulouse-Muenster orthosis, skeletal age and flexibility of the curve (bending films) were evaluated. The average follow-up after weaning of the brace was 42 months (36–78 months). Three years after weaning there was an overall increase of the Cobb angle to 37° on average. The authors concluded that curve progression was prevented in 58%. Prognostic risk factors were a young age at the start of brace treatment, a thoracic curve, unsatisfactory curve correction in the brace and a male gender.

Zaborowska-Sapeta et al. presented a prospective study using SRS and SOSORT guidelines [40], including 79 progressive idiopathic patients (58 girls and 21 boys). The treatment included a Chêneau brace and physiotherapy. And the patient group included an initial Cobb angle between 20 and 45°, Risser 4 maturity at final assessment and no other or previous brace treatment. The follow up results were outlined that 25.3% improved, 22.8% were stable with no change in progression, 39.2% worsened and progressed but below the surgical indicated level of 50° Cobb angle and 12.7% worsened and progressed beyond 50°. Two patients out of the initial 79 patients progressed >60° Cobb angles. Progression concerned the younger and less skeletally mature patients. The results of this study may indicate that this Chêneau style and design of the brace used is more effective in reducing the incidence of surgery, even when it is compared to the natural history (without treatment) of this condition.

These are two studies with low quality Chêneau style braces. Both studies indicate that less skeletally mature patients had worse outcomes than the more mature patients. This seems the typical finding in low quality braces that patients more at risk for progression have worse outcomes than the more mature lower-risk patients [55, 70].

In studies with more high quality brace designs, the more immature patients seem easier to correct and preserve better outcomes than the more mature patients [45, 47, 74, 75, 79, 82].

Aulisa and colleagues reviewed 93 patients with adolescent idiopathic scoliosis (AIS) that implemented the PASB (Progressive Action Short Brace) and the Lyon method [46]. The age range was wide, ages from 10 to 35 years old. Two groups were separated according to their Cobb, less than 30° and more than 30°. The follow-up was long, at a mean age of 184.1 months (±72.60) after treatment was stopped. The pre-treatment mean Cobb angle was 32.28° (±9.4°), the post treatment mean was 19.35° and then increased to 22.12° in the 10 years after the end of treatment. No significant change was noted in the mean Cobb angle between the end of weaning and the later follow up ($p = 0.105$). Patients prescribed a brace from the beginning had reduced Cobb angles by 13° within the treatment period, which then worsened by 3° after treatment ended. The group with Cobb angles >30° showed a pre-brace mean curve of 41.15°; then at the end of treatment, the mean angle was 25.85° and had worsened with a mean of 29.73° at later follow-up. The group with ≤30° Cobb angle initially presented with a mean Cobb angle of 25.58° which then reduced to a mean of 14.24°, but then worsened after treatment to 16.38°. There was no significant change in the mean progression of Cobb angles between the two groups. This paper concluded that scoliosis did not progress in 15 years after treatment. The natural history of this pathology, at these levels of moderate severity, deems that normally a progressive but small increment will continue to worsen until skeletal maturity. High-quality bracing is a valuable and effective alternative treatment method, demonstrated by successful long-term follow-up outcomes, even with patients that initially present with moderate AIS.

In another paper with curves initially presenting at 40° and which included over fifty-five participants [47]. Just under half of the participants had a minimum follow-up of 18 months and an average of 30.4 months (SD 9.2).

The 25 patients had the following characteristics at their initial presentation: Cobb angle of 49° (SD 8.4; 40–71°); 12.4 years old (SD 0.82); Risser: 0.84 (SD 0.94; 0–2). A statistical z-test was used to compare the success rate in this cohort to the success rate in the prospective braced cohort from BrAIST (Bracing in Adolescent Idiopathic Scoliosis Trial).

At follow-up, the average Cobb angle was 44.2° (SD 12.9). Two patients progressed, 12 patients were able to halt progression, and 11 patients improved. Angle of trunk rotation (ATR), demonstrating cosmetic improvements, decreased from over 12° to just over 10° in the thoracic spine ($p = 0.11$) and from 4.7 to 3.6° ATR improvements noted in the lumbar spine ($p = 0.0074$). When comparing the success rate to the BrAIST cohort with the success rate of patients in this cohort, the difference was statistically significant ($z = -3.041$; $p = 0.01$). The Gensingen brace was successful in 92% of cases of patients with AIS, whose patient group initially presented with large curvatures and the improvements were significantly more effective when compared to the BrAIST study results of 72%, whose patient group initially had smaller curves comparatively.

Recently, a paper was published with the SRS inclusion criteria for studies on bracing (Girls only, Age 10–14 years, Risser 0–2, Cobb angle 25–40°), the range of Cobb angles was extended to curvatures of up to 45° in order to increase the amount of participants in the study [79]. Twenty-eight patients from their prospective cohort (12.5 years; Risser 0.8; Cobb 32.6°) were weaned off their CAD Chêneau style brace (Gensingen brace). The results of this cohort were compared with the BrAIST study by Weinstein et al. with the help of the z-test. Failure in both studies was defined as a Cobb angle reaching or exceeding 50° Cobb.

The in-brace correction was 51.4%. Two out of the 28 patients (7.1%) from this group reached or exceeded 50° Cobb angle at final follow-up making a success rate 92.9%. Comparative to the results of 72% in the BrAIST study, the improvement was highly significant in the z-test ($z = 2.58$, $t = -3,42$, $p = 0.01$).

The authors concluded that the results as achieved with the Gensingen brace were significantly better than the results as achieved with the Boston brace. Therefore, the standards should be adapted from symmetrical compression braces to asymmetrical high correction braces, maintaining improved standards by use of a classification-based corrective system for most of the possible curve patterns.

These results show the high variability of outcomes with different asymmetrical braces with very different qualities. Low quality asymmetrical braces seem to have outcomes with insignificant effects to natural history, and high-quality asymmetrical braces offer the advantage of improving Cobb angle and the cosmetic and postural issues of the deformity [45–47, 74, 75, 79–82].

4.1 Clinical outcomes

In patients with AIS (80–90% of all scoliosis patients) rarely suffer severe health problems [3, 19, 20]. The cosmetic outcome of brace treatment might be important rather than the Cobb angle which is visible on the X-ray only. However, there is only a small body of literature on brace treatment with a focus on cosmetic outcomes [75]. For more symmetrical braces mainly correcting the curve via trunk compression (**Figure 2**) no clinical evidence exists, that these would significantly influence the trunk deformity. In one paper on a modified Boston brace changes of lumbar ATR were detected, but in the thoracic region obviously no improvements were obtained [72]. For asymmetrical high-quality full-time braces, there is evidence that cosmetic improvements can be gained [46, 47, 73–75, 79–82].

Trunk deformity can be improved when using asymmetrical CAD libraries [46, 47, 73–75]. This has recently been confirmed in another end-result study [79]. It has also been shown that improvements of the trunk deformity may stay stable years after brace weaning [46, 82] (**Figure 7**).

In a study with more mature patients, cosmetic improvements have been reported [71]. The treatment indication for these patients was to improve aesthetic/cosmetic reasons and/or for curve reduction. Their Risser sign was 4–5 initially and by the end of treatment 34 females and 2 males, age 16.2 ± 1.6 years had a Cobb angle of 27.6° ± 8.9°. The Lyon or SPoRT (so called Symmetric, Patient oriented, Rigid, Three-dimensional, active) braces were used as treatment. A brace wearing prescription is of 18–24 hours daily, SEAS (Scientific Exercises Approach to Scoliosis) exercises, rapid weaning (2–3 hours every 6 months). 39% of this cohort improved and 46% of the group initially presented with curves over 30° cobb angle. Only one patient progressed 6°. Results were successful; statistically significant reductions of Cobb angle maximal (-4.4°), thoracic cobb angles (-6.0°), thoracolumbar cobb angles (-6.6°), and further statistically significant improvements for the Aesthetic Index outcome. The authors concluded that before 20 years of age, even in skeletally mature patients, it is possible to reach radiographic and aesthetic improvements, although it was not as significant as when during growth spurts. In a recent review, a case series is documented with obvious clinical corrections in patients treated with the Gensingen brace [75]. All patients from this case series had curvatures of 45° and over at the start of the treatment, whilst the patients were immature and were clearly recompensated after brace weaning (**Figures 8** and **9**).

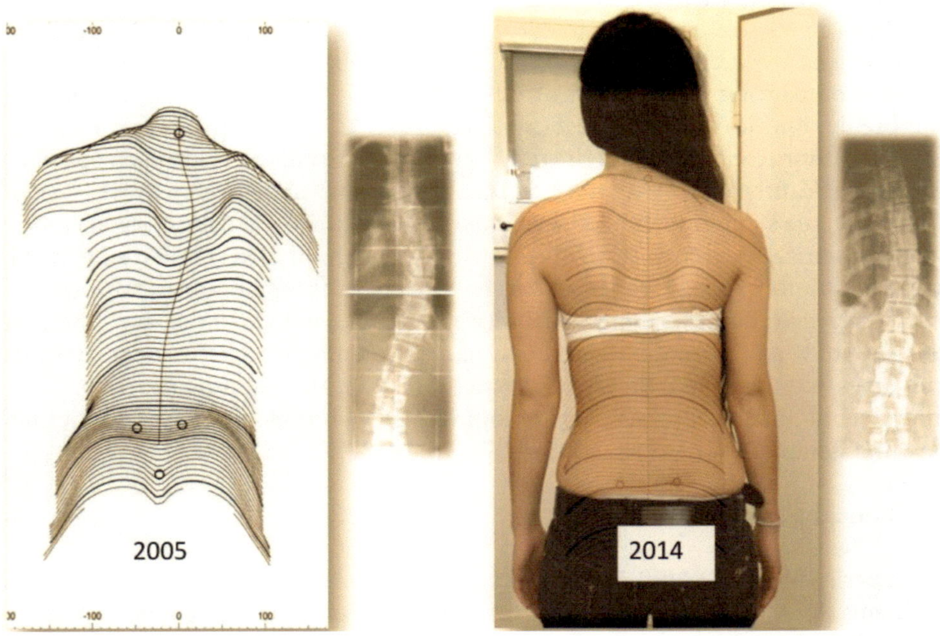

Figure 7.
Clinical and radiological improvement 5 years after weaning off a Chêneau light brace. Initially the patient had 38° and a significant decompensation of the trunk. Five years without the brace the patients' trunk seems recompensated and the residual curve is 19° [80].

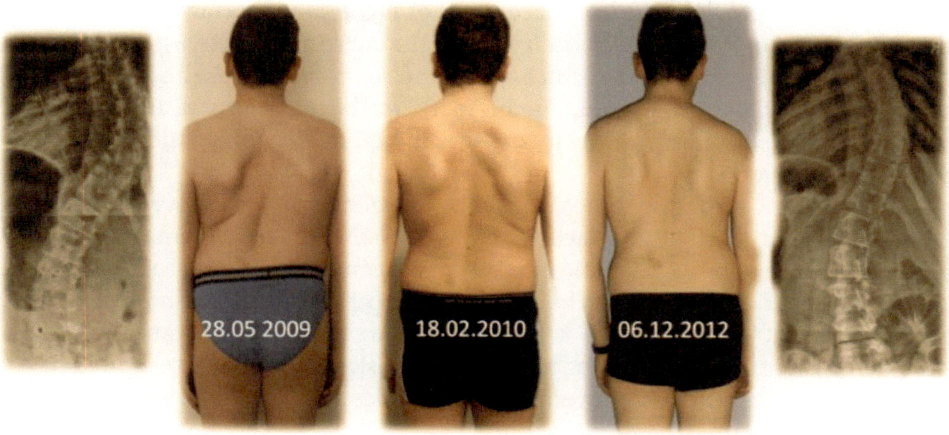

Figure 8.
Male patients with a decompensated thoracic curve of 56° to the right. Slightly recompensated 2010 as the intermediate result during the treatment with a GBW. Six months after brace weaning (2012), the posture and X-ray are clearly compensated. The patients' residual deformity is hardly visible although the Cobb angle is still 43° as shown on the right. This case shows that significant cosmetic improvements can be achieved with modern asymmetric high-quality braces [75].

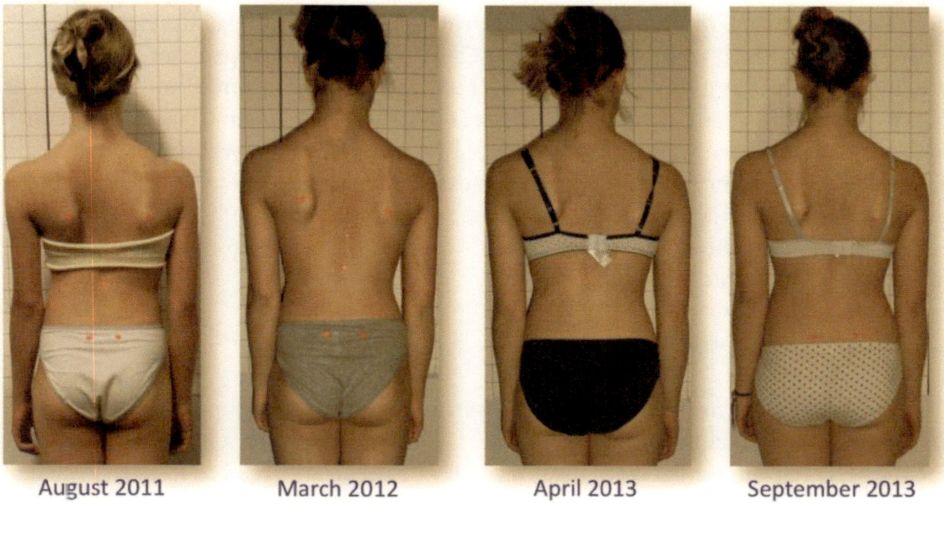

Figure 9.
Clinical changes from the start of treatment with a GBW (left) to 3 months after brace weaning (right). Initially, the patient is decompensated to the right and at the end a mature woman is visible with a well-compensated trunk [75].

In rare cases, it is possible that these braces can improve the trunk deformity significantly, whilst the Cobb angle stays unchanged [75] or even shows a progression [83]. Therefore, for patients with AIS, using CAD libraries and specialists should be preferred [46, 47, 73–75, 79–82].

4.2 Outcomes of part-time bracing

As early as in 1997 in a meta-analysis, it has been shown that part-time bracing is clearly inferior to full-time bracing [84]. Later, these findings have been confirmed [37, 85]. But night-time braces are still widely marketed [54, 55] despite of the fact that brace wearing time, along with in-brace correction determines the outcome of brace treatment [37, 84]. The low success rate of night-time bracing would not make this a beneficial option. In the contrary, when the curve gets worse with night-time bracing, the patient will lose trust in bracing and the compliance with full-time bracing will probably be reduced. Furthermore, the bigger the curve and the more mature the patient, the longer the treatment might last with less possibility of a cosmetic improvement.

On the other hand, when brace treatment in the immature adolescent with a moderate degree of curvature starts with a high-quality brace full-time in the most important phase of growth drastic improvements can be achieved (see **Figure 7**) and part-time brace wearing can be offered to the patients when the intermediate curve is below 20°. It is logical to start with full-time treatment with an asymmetrical high-quality brace in the immature patient at risk for curve progression as this will usually lead to a final improvement of cosmetics and to the shortest possible treatment duration.

With respect to patient compliance, the bracing service besides reliable in-brace corrections should also offer braces with the best possible comfort. This means the brace should be made as small as possible without compromising its corrective effect. Compression effects in the brace should be minimised, whilst the corrective movement (shift) should be maximised (**Figures 3–5**).

In patients at risk of progression and curvatures between 15 and 25°, however, night-time bracing may be of benefit. In a paper by Seifert and Selle [69], 22 children ranging from 5 to 12 years old were provided with a Chêneau derivate brace. Patients with a Cobb angle of 20–25° and 15–19° in cases of progression, bracing was indicated and provided in this study. Follow-up was 25 months and in the main curves, a successful correction of 82.2% was attained. The mean Cobb angle prior to brace treatment was 20.2°. At the end of brace treatment, it was 15.8° Cobb angle. Three cases experienced Cobb angle progression measuring over the 25° limit and then part-time bracing had to be re-adjusted to full-time bracing. In 86.4% patients, either improved Cobb angle measurements or their halted progression and spinal fusion operations were avoided.

4.3 The sagittal profile

AIS is a 3D deformity usually also compromising the sagittal profile of the spine and trunk. Structural thoracic curves lead to a flatback or even a hollow back in the thoracic region, whilst structural lumbar curves usually lead to loss of lumbar lordosis or to a lumbar kyphosis [1–3]. Whilst the long-term consequences of a thoracic flatback are yet to be determined, loss of lumbar lordosis is clearly correlated to non-specific chronic low back pain [86, 87]. Improvement of lumbar lordosis can also improve the frontal plane deformity (Cobb angle) [88–90]. A feature of a brace should also address the sagittal profile of the deformity [45, 47, 79, 91, 92]. It is concerning that braces are provided which reduce lumbar lordosis and increase thoracic flatback [32–35] (**Figure 10**).

4.4 Bracing in curves of 40° and over

There is some evidence that asymmetrical high-quality braces may stop curve progression in patients with Cobb angles exceeding 40° [47, 74]. In addition, significant clinical and radiological improvements have been documented [47, 75, 79, 82]. Considering that in patients with AIS, there is no long-term evidence supporting spinal fusion surgery [10–14], and in view of its significant long-term complications [15–18], brace treatment for curves exceeding 40° should be of importance. According to literature, asymmetrical high-quality braces offer success rates of about

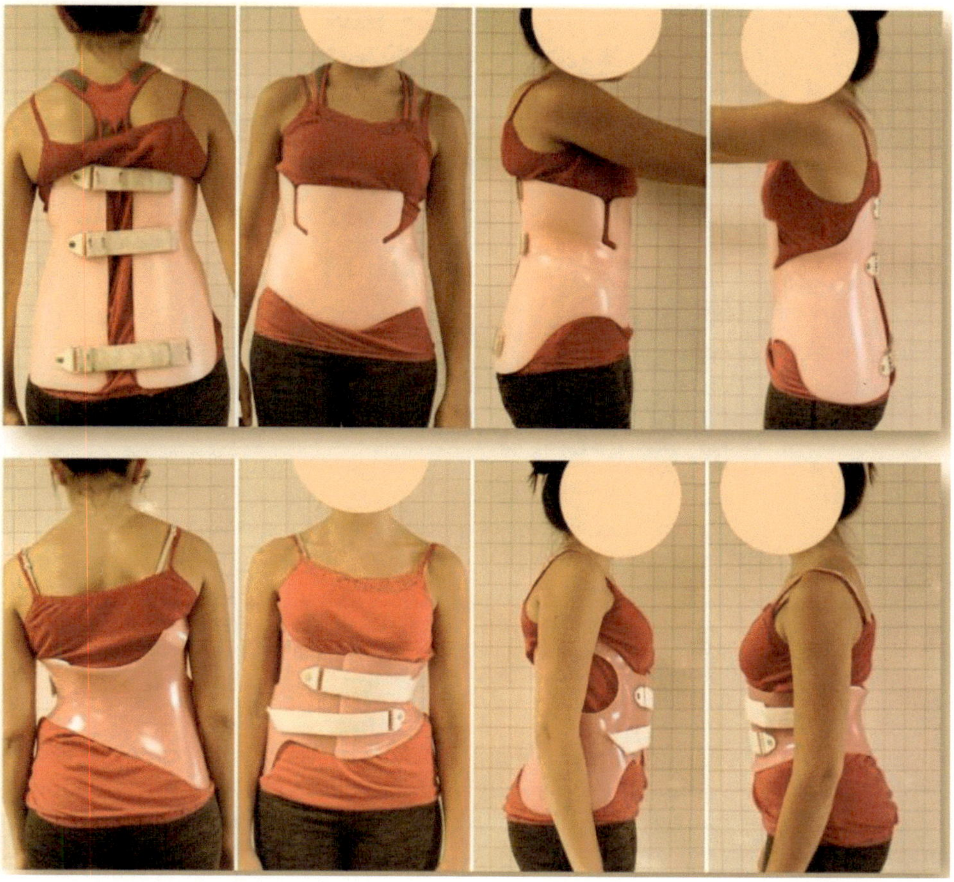

Figure 10.
Patient with a thoracolumbar curve pattern treated with a Boston brace (upper line of pictures) and later with a Gensingen brace (GBW, see lower line of pictures). For this curve pattern, the GBW is smaller compared to the Boston brace. It is also observed that the Boston brace reduces lumbar lordosis, whilst the GBW preserves lumbar lordosis (courtesy of Dr Marc Moramarco, Scoliosis 3DC, Woburn, MA, US).

90% in this group of patients and can be regarded as the safest bracing approach for curves exceeding 40° when worn full-time at the start of treatment (**Figure 11**).

4.5 Comparing outcomes symmetrical versus asymmetrical braces

There is a small body of literature comparing asymmetrical high-quality Chêneau style braces to symmetric Boston style braces [45, 47, 76, 79]. It has been shown that the outcome of Chêneau derivatives is significantly better with respect to the success rate [45, 47, 79]. Whilst in-brace corrections in the Rigo brace (RCO) were comparable to the in-brace corrections of the Boston brace [45], in-brace corrections in the Gensingen brace (GBW) at average have been significantly higher [47, 76, 79].

In research that implements the Rigo brace (RCO) and compares the outcome with a basic Boston-style TLSO brace (Thoraco-lumbar-orthosis) [45], a retrospective study was published over 15 years, up until 2014. The initial major curves included only those between 25 and 40° and included 108 patients (93 girls) with a mean (±standard deviation) age at brace initiation of 12.5 ± 1.3 years. Thirteen participants wore an RCO, and 95 participants wore a TLSO brace. Mean pre-bracing major curves were 32.7 ± 4.8° in the RCO group and 31.4 ± 4.4°, slightly lower in the TLSO patient group (p = 0.387). No RCO patient and 34% of TLSO patients progressed to spinal

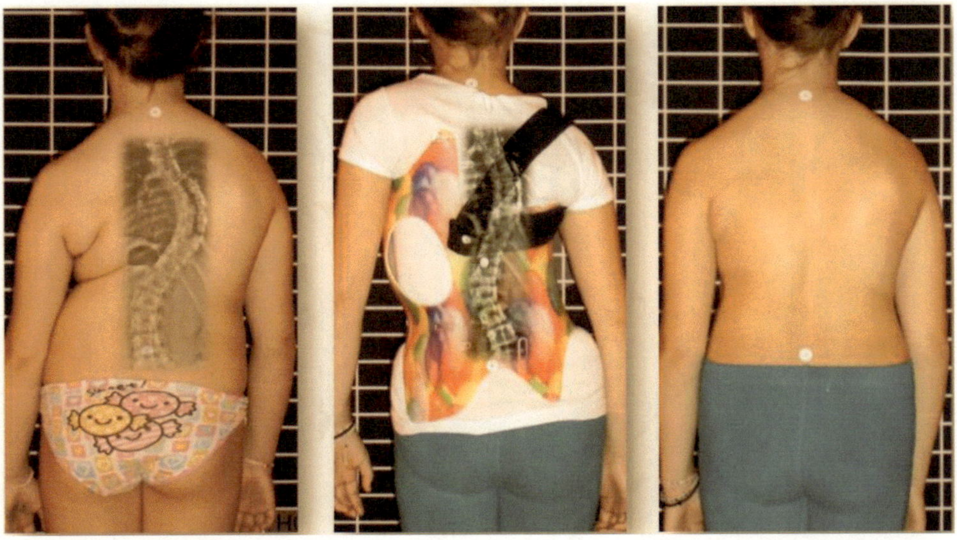

Figure 11.
Immature patient with a thoracic curve exceeding 70° treated with a GBW with an additional shoulder retraction strap. Clinically mirroring of the deformity is clearly visible whilst the patient is decompensated to the right without the brace on and an overcompensation to the left in the brace. After 9 months of full-time treatment, a clear improvement (re-compensation) has been achieved [47].

surgery ($p = 0.019$). After treatment ended, the main curves of patients improved by 6° or more in 31% of the RCO group and only 13% of the TLSO group ($p = 0.100$). Patients were comparatively similar at baseline and had similar compliance of in-brace time, but there was a significantly lower rate of spinal surgery in the RCO group [45].

5. Conclusions

Asymmetric high-quality braces provide the highest rate of success and the best documented cosmetic outcomes. Symmetric braces correcting via compression should be abandoned and their worldwide provision reconsidered.

There is no indication for soft braces.

There is no indication for night-time braces in the normal range of brace indications (curves of 25° and over).

Acknowledgements

Written informed consent for publication of the patient's information (X-rays, photos, records, etc.) has been obtained from both the patients and their parents. HRW provided the first draft and made the literature review. DT and JBS contributed to the improvement of the first draft and copyedited the final version.

Conflict of interest

HRW is receiving financial support for attending symposia and has received royalties from Koob GmbH & Co KG. The company is held by the spouse of HR Weiss. DT is employed by an orthotic company that supplies a wide range of orthotics, including spinal braces.

Author details

Hans-Rudolf Weiss[1]* and Deborah Turnbull[2]

1 Gesundheitsforum Nahetal, Germany

2 School of Health and Social Care, University of Teesside, Middlesbrough, UK

*Address all correspondence to: hr.weiss@skoliose-dr-weiss.com

References

[1] Lonstein JE. Idiopathic scoliosis. In: Lonstein J, Bradford D, Winter R, Ogilvie J, editors. Moe's Textbook of Scoliosis and Other Spinal Deformities. Philidelphia: WB Saunders; 1995. pp. 219-256

[2] Goldberg CJ, Moore DP, Fogarty EE, Dowling FE. Adolescent idiopathic scoliosis: Natural history and prognosis. Studies in Health Technology and Informatics. 2002;**91**:59-63

[3] Asher MA, Burton DC. Adolescent idiopathic scoliosis: Natural history and long-term treatment effects. Scoliosis. 2006;**1**(1):2

[4] Winter RB. Classification and terminology. In: Lonstein J, Bradford D, Winter R, Ogilvie J, editors. Moe's Textbook of Scoliosis and Other Spinal Deformities. Philadelphia: WB Saunders; 1995. pp. 39-44

[5] Kuru T, Yeldan I, Dereli EE, Ozdincler AR, Dikici F, Colak I. The efficacy of three-dimensional Schroth exercises in adolescent idiopathic scoliosis: A randomised controlled clinical trial. Clinical Rehabilitation. 2016;**30**(2):181-190

[6] Monticone M, Ambrosini E, Cazzaniga D, Rocca B, Ferrante S. Active self-correction and task-oriented exercises reduce spinal deformity and improve quality of life in subjects with mild adolescent idiopathic scoliosis. Results of a randomised controlled trial. European Spine Journal. 2014;**23**(6):1204-1214

[7] Nachemson AL, Peterson LE. Effectiveness of treatment with a brace in girls who have adolescent idiopathic scoliosis. A prospective, controlled study based on data from the brace study of the Scoliosis Research Society. The Journal of Bone and Joint Surgery. American Volume. 1995;**77**(6):815-822

[8] Weiss HR, Weiss GM. Brace treatment during pubertal growth spurt in girls with idiopathic scoliosis (IS): A prospective trial comparing two different concepts. Pediatric Rehabilitation. 2005;**8**(3):199-206

[9] Weinstein SL, Dolan LA, Wright JG, Dobbs MB. Effects of bracing in adolescents with idiopathic scoliosis. The New England Journal of Medicine. 2013;**369**(16):1512-1521

[10] Weiss HR. Adolescent idiopathic scoliosis (AIS) - An indication for surgery? A systematic review of the literature. Disability and Rehabilitation. 2008;**30**(10):799-807

[11] Bettany-Saltikov J, Weiss HR, Chockalingam N, et al. Surgical versus non-surgical interventions in people with adolescent idiopathic scoliosis. Cochrane Database of Systematic Reviews. 2015;**4**(4):CD010663

[12] Cheuk DK, Wong V, Wraige E, Baxter P, Cole A. Surgery for scoliosis in duchenne muscular dystrophy. Cochrane Database of Systematic Reviews. 2015;**10**(10):CD005375

[13] Bettany-Saltikov J, Weiss HR, Chockalingam N, Kandasamy G, Arnell T. A comparison of patient-reported outcome measures following different treatment approaches for adolescents with severe idiopathic scoliosis: A systematic review. Asian Spine Journal. 2016;**10**(6):1170-1194

[14] Ward WT, Friel NA, Kenkre TS, Brooks MM, Londino JA, Roach JW. SRS-22r scores in non-operated adolescent idiopathic scoliosis patients with curves greater than forty degrees. Spine (Phila Pa 1976). 2017;**42**(16):1233-1240

[15] Hawes M. Impact of spine surgery on signs and symptoms of spinal

deformity. Pediatric Rehabilitation. 2006;**9**(4):318-339

[16] Weiss HR, Goodall D. Rate of complications in scoliosis surgery - A systematic review of the Pub Med literature. Scoliosis. 2008;**3**:9

[17] Weiss HR, Moramarco M, Moramarco K. Risks and long-term complications of adolescent idiopathic scoliosis surgery vs. non-surgical and natural history outcomes. Hard Tissue. 2013;**2**(3):27

[18] Moramarco K. Least potential harm with treatment for adolescent idiopathic scoliosis patients. Hard Tissue. 2013;**2**(5):44. [http://www.oapublishinglondon.com/article/1011]

[19] Weinstein SL, Dolan LA, Spratt KF, Peterson KK, Spoonamore MJ, Ponseti IV. Health and function of patients with untreated idiopathic scoliosis: A 50-year natural history study. JAMA. 2003;**289**(5):559-567

[20] Weiss HR, Karavidas N, Moramarco M, Moramarco K. Long-term effects of untreated adolescent idiopathic scoliosis: A review of the literature. Asian Spine Journal. 2016;**10**(6):1163-1169

[21] Mueller FJ, Gluch H. Cotrel-dubousset instrumentation for the correction of adolescent idiopathic scoliosis. Long-term results with an unexpected high revision rate. Scoliosis. 2012;**7**(1):13

[22] Weiss HR, Moramarco M. Indication for surgical treatment in patients with adolescent idiopathic scoliosis - A critical appraisal. Patient Safety in Surgery. 2013;**7**(1):17

[23] Kaspiris A, Grivas TB, Weiss HR, Turnbull D. Surgical and conservative treatment of patients with congenital scoliosis: A search for long-term results. Scoliosis. 2011;**6**:12. DOI: 10.1186/1748-7161-6-12

[24] Weiss HR, Moramarco M. Congenital scoliosis (mini-review). Current Pediatric Reviews. 2016;**12**:43. DOI: 10.2174/1573396312666151117121011

[25] Weiss HR, Weiss G, Petermann F. Incidence of curvature progression in idiopathic scoliosis patients treated with scoliosis in-patient rehabilitation (SIR): An age- and sex-matched controlled study. Pediatric Rehabilitation. 2003;**6**(1):23-30

[26] Romano M, Minozzi S, Bettany-Saltikov J, Zaina F, Chockalingam N, Kotwicki T, et al. Exercises for adolescent idiopathic scoliosis. Cochrane Database of Systematic Reviews. 2012;**8**

[27] Anwer S, Alghadir A, Abu Shaphe M, Anwar D. Effects of exercise on spinal deformities and quality of life in patients with adolescent idiopathic scoliosis. BioMed Research International. 2015;**2015**:123848

[28] Weiss HR. Physical therapy intervention studies on idiopathic scoliosis-review with the focus on inclusion criteria1. Scoliosis. 2012;**7**(1):4

[29] Wan L, Wang GX, Bian R. Exercise therapy in treatment of essential S-shaped scoliosis: Evaluation of Cobb angle in breast and lumbar segment through a follow-up of half a year. Chinese Journal of Clinical Rehabilitation. 2005;**9**(34):82-84

[30] Schreiber S, Parent EC, Khodayari Moez E, et al. Schroth physiotherapeutic scoliosis-specific exercises added to the standard of care lead to better Cobb angle outcomes in adolescents with idiopathic scoliosis – An assessor and statistician blinded randomized controlled trial. PLoS One. 2016;**11**(12):e0168746

[31] Schreiber S, Parent EC, Khodayari Moez E, et al. The effect of Schroth exercises added to the standard of

care on the quality of life and muscle endurance in adolescents with idiopathic scoliosis—An assessor and statistician blinded randomized controlled trial: "SOSORT 2015 award winner". Scoliosis. 2015;**10**:24

[32] Emans J, Kaelin A, Bancel P, Hall J, Miller M. The Boston bracing system for idiopathic scoliosis: Follow-up results in 295 patients. Spine. 1986;**11**:792-801

[33] Danielsson AJ, Hasserius R, Ohlin A, Nachemson AL. A prospective study of brace treatment versus observation alone in adolescent idiopathic scoliosis: A follow-up mean of 16 years after maturity. Spine. 2007;**32**(20):2198-2207

[34] Negrini S, Marchini G, Tessadri F. Brace technology thematic series - The Sforzesco and Sibilla braces, and the SPoRT (symmetric, patient oriented, rigid, three-dimensional, active) concept. Scoliosis. 2011;**6**:8. DOI: 10.1186/1748-7161-6-8

[35] Donzelli S, Zaina F, Lusini M, Minnella S, Respizzi S, Balzarini L, et al. The three dimensional analysis of the Sforzesco brace correction. Scoliosis and Spinal Disorders. 2016;**11**(Suppl 2):34

[36] Hopf C, Heine J. Long-term results of the conservative treatment of scoliosis using the Chêneau brace. Zeitschrift für Orthopädie und Ihre Grenzgebiete. 1985;**123**(3):312-322

[37] Landauer F, Wimmer C, Behensky H. Estimating the final outcome of brace treatment for idiopathic thoracic scoliosis at 6-month follow-up. Pediatric Rehabilitation. 2003;**6**(3-4):201-207

[38] Bullmann V, Halm HF, Lerner T, Lepsien U, Hackenberg L, Liljenqvist U. Prospective evaluation of braces as treatment in idiopathic scoliosis. Zeitschrift für Orthopädie und Ihre Grenzgebiete. 2004;**142**(4):403-409

[39] Pham VM, Herbaux B, Schill A, Thevenon A. Evaluation of the Cheneau brace in adolescent idiopathic scoliosis. Annales de Réadaptation et de Médecine Physique. 2007;**50**(3):125-133

[40] Zaborowska-Sapeta K, Kowalski IM, Kotwicki T, Protasiewicz-Faldowska H, Kiebzak W. Effectiveness of Cheneau brace treatment for idiopathic scoliosis: Prospective study in 79 patients followed to skeletal maturity. Scoliosis. 2011;**6**(1):2

[41] Weiss HR, Werkmann M. Rate of surgery in a sample of patients fulfilling the SRS inclusion criteria treated with a Cheneau brace of actual standard. Studies in Health Technology and Informatics. 2012;**176**:407-410

[42] De Giorgi S, Piazzolla A, Tafuri S, Borracci C, Martucci A, De Giorgi G. Chêneau brace for adolescent idiopathic scoliosis: Long-term results. Can it prevent surgery? European Spine Journal. 2013;**22**(6):815-822

[43] Fang MQ, Wang C, Xiang GH, Lou C, Tian NF, Xu HZ. Long-term effects of the Chêneau brace on coronal and sagittal alignment in adolescent idiopathic scoliosis. Journal of Neurosurgery. Spine. 2015;**23**(4):505-509

[44] Matussek J, Dingeldey E, Benditz A, Rezai G, Nahr K. Conservative treatment of idiopathic scoliosis: Influence of archetypical Cheneau-Corsets on trunk asymmetry. Der Orthopäde. 2015;**44**(11):869-878

[45] Minsk MK, Venuti KD, Daumit GL, Sponseller PD. Effectiveness of the Rigo Chêneau versus Boston-style orthoses for adolescent idiopathicscoliosis: A retrospective study. Scoliosis and Spinal Disorders. 2017;**12**:7

[46] Aulisa AG, Guzzanti V, Falciglia F, Galli M, Pizzetti P, Aulisa L. Curve

progression after long-term brace treatment in adolescent idiopathic scoliosis: Comparative results between over and under 30 Cobb degrees - SOSORT 2017 award winner. Scoliosis and Spinal Disorders. 2017;**12**:36

[47] Weiss HR, Tournavitis N, Seibel S, Kleban A. A prospective cohort study of AIS patients with 40° and more treated with a Gensingen brace (GBW): Preliminary results. The Open Orthopaedics Journal. 2017;**11**:1558-1567

[48] Taghi Karimi M, Rabczuk T, Kavyani M. Evaluation of the efficiency of the Chêneau brace on scoliosis deformity: A systematic review of the literature. Der Orthopäde. 2018;**47**(3):198-204

[49] Korovessis P, Syrimpeis V, Tsekouras V, Vardakastanis K, Fennema P. Effect of the Chêneau brace in the natural history of moderate adolescent idiopathic scoliosis in girls: Cohort analysis of a selected homogenous population of 100 consecutive skeletally immature patients. Spine Deformity. 2018;**6**(5):514-522

[50] Price CT, Scott DS, Reed FR Jr, Sproul JT, Riddick MF. Nighttime bracing for adolescent idiopathic scoliosis with the Charleston bending brace: Long-term follow-up. Journal of Pediatric Orthopedics. 1997;**17**(6):703-707

[51] Yrjonen T, Ylikoski M, Schlenzka D, Kinnunen R, Poussa M. Effectiveness of the Providence nighttime bracing in adolescent idiopathic scoliosis: A comparative study of 36 female patients. European Spine Journal. 2006;**15**(7):1139-1143

[52] D'Amato CR, Griggs S, McCoy B. Nighttime bracing with the providence brace in adolescent girls with idiopathic scoliosis. Spine. 2001;**26**(18):2006-2012

[53] Janicki JA, Poe-Kochert C, Armstrong DG, Thompson GH. A comparison of the thoracolumbosacral orthoses and providence orthosis in the treatment of adolescent idiopathic scoliosis: Results using the new SRS inclusion and assessment criteria for bracing studies. Journal of Pediatric Orthopedics. 2007;**27**(4):369-374

[54] Bohl DD, Telles CJ, Golinvaux NS, Basques BA, DeLuca PA, Grauer JN. Effectiveness of Providence nighttime bracing in patients with adolescent idiopathic scoliosis. Orthopedics. 2014;**37**(12):e1085-e1090

[55] Davis L, Murphy JS, Shaw KA, Cash K, Devito DP, Schmitz ML. Nighttime bracing with the Providence thoracolumbosacral orthosis for treatment of adolescent idiopathic scoliosis: A retrospective consecutive clinical series. Prosthetics and Orthotics International. 2019;**43**(2):158-162. DOI: 10.1177/0309364618792727

[56] Coillard C, Circo AB, Rivard CH. SpineCor treatment for juvenile idiopathic scoliosis: SOSORT award 2010 winner. Scoliosis. 2010;**5**:25. DOI: 10.1186/1748-7161-5-25

[57] Weiss HR. History of soft brace treatment in patients with scoliosis: A critical appraisal. Hard Tissue. 2013;**2**(4):35

[58] Wong MS, Cheng JC, Lam TP, et al. The effect of rigid versus flexible spinal orthosis on the clinical efficacy and acceptance of the patients with adolescent idiopathic scoliosis. Spine. 2008;**33**(12):1360-1365

[59] Guo J, Lam TP, Wong MS, et al. A prospective randomized controlled study on the treatment outcome of SpineCor brace versus rigid brace for adolescent idiopathic scoliosis with follow-up according to the SRS standardized criteria. European Spine Journal. 2014;**23**(12):2650-2657

[60] Gutman G, Benoit M, Joncas J, Beauséjour M, Barchi S, Labelle H, et al. The effectiveness of the SpineCor brace for the conservative treatment of adolescent idiopathic scoliosis. Comparison with the Boston brace. The Spine Journal. 2016;**16**(5):626-631. DOI: 10.1016/j.spinee.2016.01.020

[61] Coillard C, Circo AB, Rivard CH. A prospective randomized controlled trial of the natural history of idiopathic scoliosisversus treatment with the SpineCor brace. Sosort Award 2011 winner. European Journal of Physical and Rehabilitation Medicine. 2014;**50**(5):479-487

[62] Harshavardhana NS, Lonstein JE. Results of bracing for juvenile idiopathic scoliosis. Spine Deformity. 2018;**6**(3):201-206. DOI: 10.1016/j.jspd.2017.10.009

[63] Thompson RM, Hubbard EW, Jo CH, Virostek D, Karol LA. Brace success is related to curve type in patients with adolescent idiopathic scoliosis. The Journal of Bone and Joint Surgery. American Volume. 2017;**99**(11):923-928. DOI: 10.2106/JBJS.16.01050

[64] Xu L, Qin X, Qiu Y, Zhu Z. Initial correction rate can be predictive of the outcome of brace treatment in patients with adolescent idiopathic scoliosis. Clinical Spine Surgery. 2017;**30**(4):E475-E479. DOI: 10.1097/BSD.0000000000000343

[65] Yamane K, Takigawa T, Tanaka M, Sugimoto Y, Arataki S, Ozaki T. Impact of rotation correction after brace treatment on prognosis in adolescent idiopathic scoliosis. Asian Spine Journal. 2016;**10**(5):893-900

[66] Kuroki H, Inomata N, Hamanaka H, Higa K, Chosa E, Tajima N. Efficacy of the Osaka Medical College (OMC) brace in the treatment of adolescent idiopathic scoliosis following Scoliosis Research Society brace studies criteria. Scoliosis. 2015;**10**:12. DOI: 10.1186/s13013-015-0036-9

[67] Moreau S, Lonjon G, Mazda K, Ilharreborde B. Detorsion night-time bracing for the treatment of early onset idiopathic scoliosis. Orthopaedics & Traumatology, Surgery & Research. 2014;**100**(8):935-939. DOI: 10.1016/j.otsr.2014.05.024

[68] Lee CS, Hwang CJ, Kim DJ, Kim JH, Kim YT, Lee MY, et al. Effectiveness of the Charleston night-time bending brace in the treatment of adolescent idiopathic scoliosis. Journal of Pediatric Orthopedics. 2012;**32**(4):368-372. DOI: 10.1097/BPO.0b013e3182561193

[69] Seifert J, Selle A. Is night-time bracing still appropriate in the treatment of idiopathic scoliosis? Der Orthopäde. 2009;**38**(2):146-150. DOI: 10.1007/s00132-008-1381-7

[70] Hanks GA, Zimmer B, Nogi J. TLSO treatment of idiopathic scoliosis. An analysis of the Wilmington jacket. Spine (Phila Pa 1976). 1988;**13**(6):626-629

[71] Negrini S, Donzelli S, Lusini M, Zaina F. Bracing can reduce high degree curves and improve aesthetics immediately after the end of growth. Final results of a retrospective case series. Studies in Health Technology and Informatics. 2012;**176**:393-396

[72] Grivas TB, Vasiliadis ES. Cosmetic outcome after conservative treatment of idiopathic scoliosis with a dynamic derotation brace. Studies in Health Technology and Informatics. 2008;**135**:387-392

[73] Rigo M. Radiological and cosmetic improvement 2 years after brace weaning--a case report. Pediatric Rehabilitation. 2003;**6**(3-4):195-199

[74] Aulisa AG, Guzzanti V, Falciglia F, Giordano M, Galli M, Aulisa L. Brace

treatment of idiopathic scoliosis is effective for a curve over 40 degrees, but is the evaluation of Cobb angle the only parameter for the indication of treatment? European Journal of Physical and Rehabilitation Medicine. 2019;**55**(2):231-240

[75] Weiss HR, Moramarco M. Remodelling of trunk and backshape deformities in patients with scoliosis using standardized asymmetric computer-aided design/computer-aided manufacturing braces. Hard Tissue. 2013;**2**(2):14

[76] Weiss HR, Kleban A. Development of CAD/CAM based brace models for the treatment of patients with scoliosis-classification based approach versus finite element modelling. Asian Spine Journal. 2015;**5**:661-667

[77] Weiss HR, Tournavitis T, Nan XF, Borysov M, Paul L. Workflow of CAD/CAM scoliosis brace adjustment in preparation using 3D printing. The Open Medical Informatics Journal. 2017;**11**:44-51

[78] Vergari C, Courtois I, Ebermeyer E, Pietton R, Bouloussa H, Vialle R. Skalli W (2019) head to pelvis alignment of adolescent idiopathic scoliosis patients both in and out of brace. European Spine Journal. 2019;**28**(6):1286-1295. DOI: 10.1007/s00586-019-05981-8

[79] Weiss HR, Turnbull D, Seibel S, Kleban A, Tournavitis N. First end result of a prospective cohort with AIS treated with the Gensingen brace. In: Proceedings of the 1st International Conference on Scoliosis Management on Behalf of the Turkish Scoliosis Society, April 12-13, Istanbul, Turkey. p. 20

[80] Rigo M. 3D correction of trunk deformity in patients with idiopathic scoliosis using Chêneau brace. Studies in Health Technology and Informatics. 1999;**59**:362-365

[81] Rigo M, Jelačić M. Brace technology thematic series: The 3D Rigo Chêneau-type brace. Scoliosis and Spinal Disorders. 2017;**12**:10. DOI: 10.1186/s13013-017-0114-2

[82] Weiss HR. Bracing can lead to a persistent correction in the treatment of adolescent idiopathic scoliosis: A case report. Hard Tissue. 2014;**3**(1):8

[83] Weiss HR. Clinical improvement and radiological progression in a girl with early onset scoliosis (EOS) treated conservatively--a case report. Scoliosis. 2006;**1**:13

[84] Rowe D, Bernstein S, Riddick M, Adler F, Emans J, Gardner-Bonneau D. A meta-analysis of the efficacy of non-operative treatments for idiopathic scoliosis. The Journal of Bone and Joint Surgery. American Volume. 1997;**79**(5):664-674

[85] Howard A, Wright JG, Hedden D. A comparative study of TLSO, Charleston, and Milwaukee braces for idiopathic scoliosis. Spine (Phila Pa 1976). 1998;**23**(22):2404-2411

[86] Glassman SD, Bridwell K, Dimar JR, Horton W, Berven SF. The impact of positive sagittal balance in adult spinal deformity. Spine. 2005;**30**:2024-2029

[87] Djurasovic M, Glassman SD. Correlation of radiographic and clinical findings in spinal deformities. Neurosurgery Clinics of North America. 2007;**18**(2):223-227

[88] Weiss HR. Das "Sagittal Realignment Brace" (physio-logic ® brace) in der Behandlung von erwachsenen Skoliosepatienten mit chronifiziertem Rückenschmerz. Medizinisch Orthopädische Technik. 2005;**125**:45-54

[89] Weiss HR, Dallmayer R, Gallo D. Sagittal counter forces (SCF) in the treatment of idiopathic scoliosis – A

preliminary report. Pediatric Rehabilitation. 2006;**9**:24-30

[90] van Loon PJ, Kühbauch BA, Thunnissen FB. Forced lordosis on the thoracolumbar junction can correct coronal plane deformity in adolescents with double major curve pattern idiopathic scoliosis. Spine. 2008;**33**(7):797-801

[91] Weiss HR, Lehnert-Schroth C, Moramarco M, Moramarco K. Schroth Therapy - Advancements in Conservative Scoliosis Treatment. 2nd ed. Saarbruecken: Lambert Academic Publishing (LAP); 2017

[92] Weiss HR, Turnbull D. Letter to the editor concerning "Head to pelvis alignment of adolescent idiopathic scoliosis patients both in and out of brace" by Vergari C, Courtois I, Ebermeyer E, Pietton R, Bouloussa H, Vialle R, Skalli W (Eur Spine J; 2019: DOI: 10.1007/s00586-019-05981-8). European Spine Journal. 2019;**28**(9):2225. DOI: 10.1007/s00586-019-06049-3

Chapter 10

Brace Treatment for Adults with Spinal Deformities

Hans-Rudolf Weiss and Deborah Turnbull

Abstract

The bracing indication for adults with spinal deformities is two-fold: (1) pain and (2) deformity. Although pain is more frequent in the adult population with scoliosis, there is no correlation between the angle of curvature and pain intensity. Pain is reportedly more frequent in patients who were operated. Non-specific pain can successfully be treated with stabilisation exercises; however, some patients may need brace treatment to improve their pain. Today, with the help of a simple clinical test, we can distinguish between different types of lower back pain allowing a differential approach to the symptom. There is some evidence that pain can successfully be reduced by these approaches mainly influencing the sagittal profile. In patients with bigger deformities and in patients aiming at reducing their deformity, pattern-specific scoliosis braces are a successful choice according to published research cases. The different specific brace types/designs along with the differential indication for these brace types will be described in this chapter.

Keywords: adult scoliosis, deformity, pain, brace treatment

1. Introduction

General remarks regarding chronic back pain have been reviewed in a previous study focussing on brace treatment for patients with spinal deformities [1]: within the adult population, certain complaints and diagnoses are increasing such as low back pain, degenerative scoliosis and spinal stenosis. The number of symptomatic patients with spinal stenosis complaints is not known but the main aims of interventions are to improve pain management, functional and lifestyle choices [2]. Spinal stenosis surgery is increasing, and in the 1980s and early 1990s, it is suggested by Ciol et al. [3] that the numbers increased eight-fold. It is controversial to assume that sedentary lifestyles contribute to back pain, but few discussions continue in this topic of research. It is hypothesised that there are negative consequences to this type of lifestyle, initially within muscles, which ultimately lead to compensation in the structure and function of connective tissue [4].

A sedentary choice in lifestyle may initially lead to a negative change in posture, such as a loss of lumbar lordosis. This postural position correlates significantly with a prevalence of lower back pain (LBP) and spinal claudication. In the adult population, lower back pain and spinal claudication can progress to degenerative, de novo scoliosis [5].

IntechOpen

Research focusing on younger adolescent female patients [6] demonstrated that non-specific LBP is reported even in this younger age group, especially those reporting a family member with lower back pain.

In 60% of secondary school pupils and 32% of students, lower back pain was a reported symptom. A correlation between lower back pain and displaying a sedentary position ($p < 0.001$ for pupils, and $p < 0.02$ for other students), and smoking ($p < 0.001$ for students and $p < 0.02$ for pupils) has shown to be statistical significant in analysis [7].

Furthermore, a beneficial consequence of an increase in physical activity and leisure time has shown to reduce musculoskeletal morbidity in patients of working age, specifically in those who have sedentary jobs [8].

Postmenopausal women who have sedentary lifestyles may benefit from regular weight-bearing exercise not only to reduce their back complaints but also to slow down the loss of bone mass.

Some studies argue the contrary and do not support the hypothesis that sedentary lifestyle contributes to lower back pain [9–11]. In one study, the lordotic angle seemed to have no influence on the prevalence of low back pain [9]. The presence of lordosis and the angle of lordosis alone may not be the only influential cause, but more specifically, it is the location of lordosis and shape of the posture, specifically the lordosis in the upper lumbar section of the spine that has the most effect upon reported pain levels [12, 13].

'Chronic low back pain' is an umbrella term and relates to patients reporting pain in the lumbar or sacral region or even in the sacroiliac pelvic joints. As the pelvis may be involved, the iliolumbar ligaments and even some radicular symptoms may also add to the complexity of the source of pain. With the presence of radicular symptoms, the nerve root affected would determine the origin of the lower back pain [14].

Without the presence of radicular symptoms, chronic lower back pain cannot be caused by a specific nerve root and may have a more complex cause involving L5/S1 or L4/5, and or the pelvis joints or ligaments [14].

Chronic low back pain without radicular symptoms and without any other specific clinical finding (for example, spondylolisthesis) is not classified and attributed in international research as being 'unspecific' or 'non-specific'. For bracing of this group of patients with chronic non-specific low back pain, simple physical tests have been published to predict the brace type the patient might benefit from. Based on the results of physical tests, a simple functional classification of 'non-specific' lower back pain has been developed [1].

In patients with scoliosis, besides the common cosmetics issues, pain is also a reported common issue [15]. Although back pain in patients with scoliosis is not related to the size of the curvature (Cobb angle) [16, 17], there is evidence that scoliosis patients experience statistically more back pain in later adulthood than age-matched controls [18–21]. This back pain is not always disabling [19–21] and can be treated conservatively with reasonable success [16, 17, 22, 23]. While low back pain increases after surgery [24], pain in patients with scoliosis without surgery can be reduced with exercises, be it core stabilisation exercises [22, 23] or pattern-specific exercises (for example, Schroth) [16, 17].

In rare cases, the pain cannot be reduced using the functional exercise approach. For these cases, bracing can be successful [1, 12, 13, 25–27].

As outlined above in patients with scoliosis, we distinguish between different kinds of chronic back pain [28]. Most complaints come from the lower back region. Specific chronic low back pain stems from the lumbosacral region and can usually be referred to an injured or inflamed nerve root. This type of pain mainly is caused by a disc prolapse with compression of a nerve root. Specific low back pain needs a

DOI: http://dx.doi.org/10.5772/intechopen.92321

specific treatment in order to reduce the nerve compression and, commonly, surgical decompression in case of significant impairment of the nerve [28].

But as already outlined, non-specific chronic low back pain cannot be referred to a single nerve root. In patients with chronic non-specific low back pain, there may be functional impairments of the sacroiliac joints, lumbar facet joints, overuse of the iliolumbar ligament and spinal stenosis, relative or absolute. Psychological issues also play a role in the development of chronic non-specific low back pain [14, 28]. This also applies to patients with spinal deformities.

Functionally, we may distinguish between postural low back pain (PLBP) and instability low back pain (ILBP) [1] (**Figure 1**). While PLBP mainly is related to loss of lumbar lordosis in later adulthood, ILBP is related to joint laxity or a definite instability like in patients with spondylolisthesis. Combinations of both entities are also possible [1].

In a study from 2009 [26], 130 patients presenting with spinal deformities (ranging from middle aged to older adults of 69 years old) and chronic unspecific low back pain were tested, using brace treatment for their chronic lower back pain. 16 of these patients presented with symptoms of spinal claudication. The sagittal re-alignment test (SRT) was applied (a lumbar hyperextension test) and a 'sagittal de-lordosation test' (SDT) to each participant. In addition, three female patients with spondylolisthesis were tested, including one female with symptoms of spinal claudication. 117 of the 130 patients reported a significant pain reduction when the SRT was applied. 13 patients, when applying the SDT also had significant reductions in pain. Three out of 130 patients had no significant change in their pain levels in either test. Pain intensity for all participants was high prior to the physical tests (VRS scale 0–5) and low while performing the physical test. These differences in pain scores were highly significant in analysis. There was an exception in three patients (2.3%): a clear distribution to one of the two classes was possible.

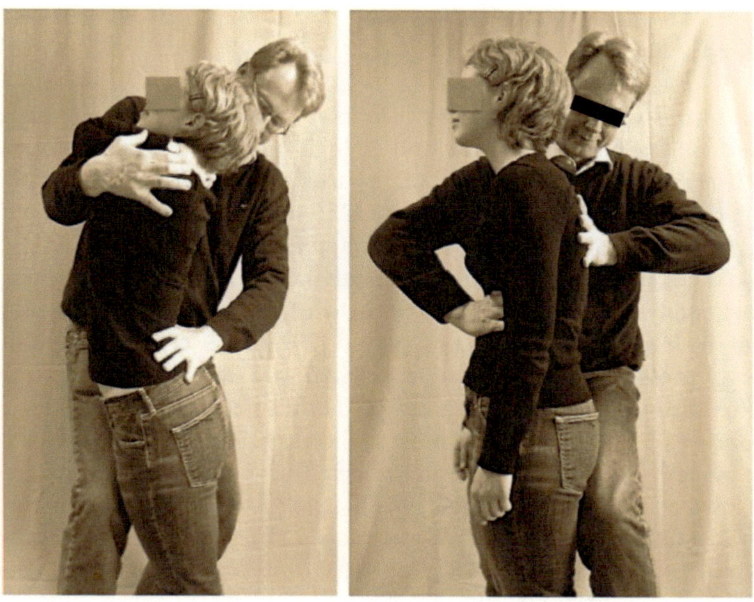

Figure 1.
The sagittal realignment test (SRT) seen on the left and the de-lordosation test (DT) with patient in the standing position. The sagittal realignment test (SRT)—a positive result in this test will present with an immediate reduction in chronic postural LBP (PLBP). The de-lordosation test (DT) pictured on the right—a positive result on this test will present with an immediate reduction in chronic LBP if this is due to instability low back pain (ILBP). Taken from [1] (Creative Commons Attribution Licence).

117 patients were supplied successfully with a sagittal realignment brace and 13 with a sagittal de-lordosing brace. A clear distribution of the patients from this sample to either chronic postural or chronic instability back pain was possible. In 2.3%, a combined chronic low back pain was found. The authors concluded that chronic non-specific low back pain may be classified physically. The functional classification described is necessary to decide which specific conservative approach (lordosation/de-lordosation of the lumbar spine) should be used [1]. However, the topic spinal deformities in conjunction with brace treatment is not well established in the international literature and research. Therefore, a systematic PubMed review has been undertaken in order to find more studies with the aim to establish a scientific basis for treatment suggestions for this group of patients [15].

2. Results from a recent review

A PubMed review was undertaken on the April 28, 2019, using the key words: (1) scoliosis, pain, brace treatment and (2) scoliosis, pain, orthotics [15]. From both searches, the studies were extracted containing patients with the diagnosis of a scoliosis with additional chronic non-specific low back pain who were treated with a brace [15].

142 items have been found for search (1) and 111 for search (2) [15]. Nine items have been identified to fulfil the inclusion criteria from search (1) and six from the search (2). As most of the items were found in both searches, the total number of different items as found in both searches was 10 [1, 12, 26, 27, 29–33]. There were two pilot studies [12, 29] six case reports/case series [13, 27, 30–33], one mid-term study [26] and one study containing a proposal for a simple classification allowing a specific approach for different types of low back pain as already outlined above [1].

3. Discussion

The authors discussed the findings as follows [15]: according to the papers found, there is little overall evidence and no high-quality research studies were found for bracing in relation to pain in this patient group. Only one study had a follow-up of more than 1 year (18 months) [26], allowing some initial conclusions that brace treatment might be effective in the treatment of chronic pain in patients with spinal deformities. In this mid-term study [26], a lumbar brace increasing lordosis was used with a successful outcome, while in a recent pilot investigation, a brace reducing lumbar lordosis was suggested [29]. In the latter study published in 2018, most of these earlier studies were not cited, nor was a differential indication of braces for chronic low back pain attempted or discussed [29].

Considering the facts that (1) in most scoliosis patients, a reduction of lumbar lordosis is evident [12, 25, 26, 34–36] and that (2) loss of lumbar lordosis is correlated to low back pain in adulthood [37, 38], the assumption that reducing lumbar lordosis is an appropriate approach, is not based upon any detailed reasoning or evidence, and even possibly worsen symptoms. Additionally, it has been shown that increasing lumbar lordosis stabilises or may even correct the three-dimensional scoliosis [25, 35]. Therefore, improving lumbar lordosis in this group of patients with scoliosis should be considered as an important issue to address in the initial stages of examination and related treatment. According to the findings within this review [1, 32], only in patients with chronic back pain due to vertebral instabilities, a brace reducing lumbar lordosis is indicated.

The success rate of brace treatment in patients with non-specific chronic low back pain in general does not appear to be significant, and compliance is generally described as moderate or poor [39–41]. A significant pain reduction has not been reported upon in most of the recent literature [41, 42].

In the mid-term follow-up of scoliosis patients treated with a sagittal re-alignment brace [26], there was a high compliance and a reasonable decrease of pain intensity and pain frequency (**Figures 2** and **3**). Patients who were able to feel the brace action and pain reduction before the start of brace treatment using clinical examination tests [1] may have resulted in an increase in compliance and success with treatment. In order to avoid costly brace treatment without any effect, it is suggested by the conclusions of this review, to test the patients for the most beneficial approach (lumbar lordosation/lumbar de-lordosation). When patients recognise that they can benefit from specific brace treatment, by an instant reduction in their pain symptoms, the matter of compliance may be vastly improved.

It seems important to note that true scoliosis is not easily correctable in adulthood, and therefore, specialists should be consulted when assessing these patients to ensure the examination and treatments are appropriate. In patients with an angle of trunk rotation (ATR) exceeding 10°, a pattern-specific brace is indicated [27, 31]. Symmetrical braces applied in patients with a significant rib hump/lumbar prominence will usually twist on the person's trunk according to the asymmetry and torsion effect and therefore will not remain in the correct position, hence the need for individual bespoke fit. There are case reports and a recent report on a cohort treated with a pattern specific Chêneau style brace showing that with specific braces for lower back pain can successfully be reduced [27, 43].

There is a case study of a 37-year-old female patient with late-onset idiopathic scoliosis [27]. The patient had chronic low back pain since the age of 23 and reported daily pain at a level of 5–7 on average on a Visual Analogue Scale of 0–10. She received a short scoliosis-specific Schroth exercise programme and was also fitted with a Gensingen brace (GBW) for part-time wear. At a 16-month follow-up, the patient no longer suffered from daily low back pain (with heavy lifting only)

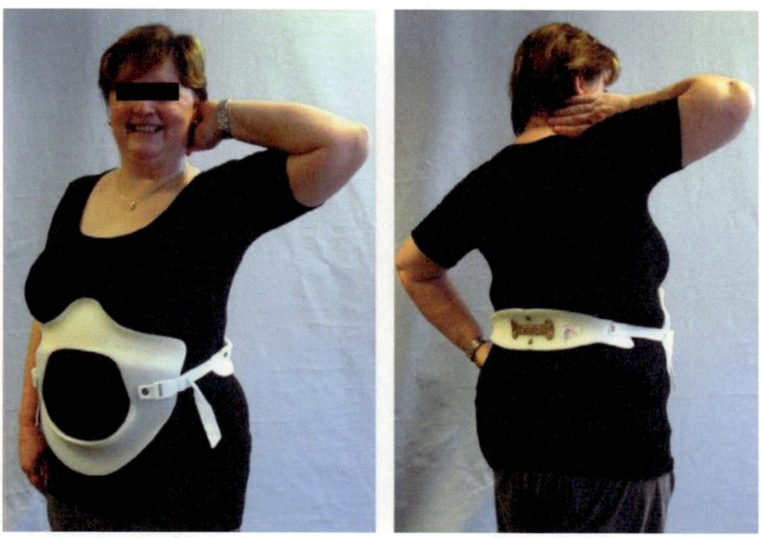

Figure 2.
Patient wearing a sagittal re-alignment brace. When the brace is adjusted to the patient, the main dorsal pressure should restore lordosis at the level of L2. Free space is necessary at the lower ribs while the pressure areas ventrally are located directly caudal of the pectoral region and cranial to the pubis. Taken from [26] (Creative Commons Attribution Licence).

and was fully active. Additionally, her lumbar Cobb angle and angle of trunk rotation improved. The authors concluded that patients with late-onset idiopathic scoliosis and may benefit from a pattern-specific conservative treatment approach (physiotherapy and bracing). In this population, surgical intervention should be regarded as the last resort, since there are many long-term unknowns with surgery in patients with scoliosis [44–51] (**Figure 4**).

Widjaja and Varani [43] investigated adolescent idiopathic scoliosis patients with a single lumbar curve pattern who wore a Gensingen Brace (GBW), which is a Chêneau style brace of standardised computer aided design (CAD). They included more mature or adult patients with a Risser sign of IV or V. The in-brace Cobb angle corrections were measured, and patients were monitored for 6 months after brace initiation in order to analyse the effects.

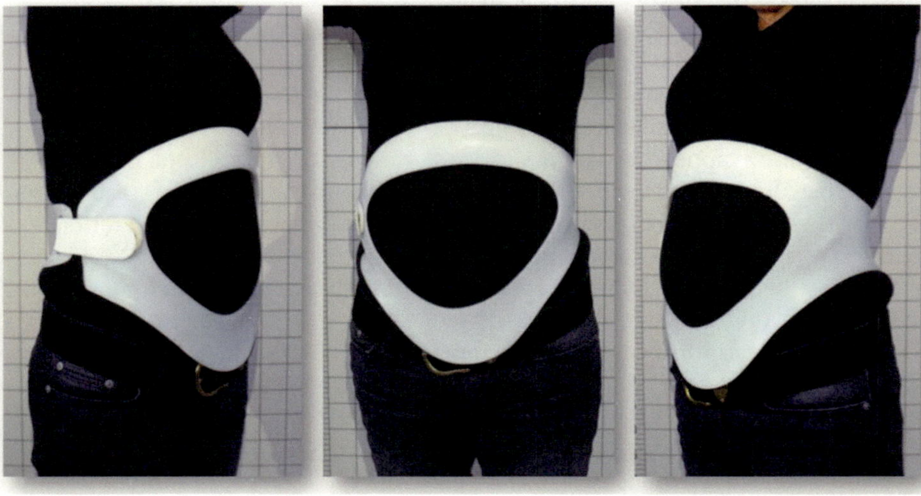

Figure 3.
Design of the sagittal re-alignment brace as applied currently.

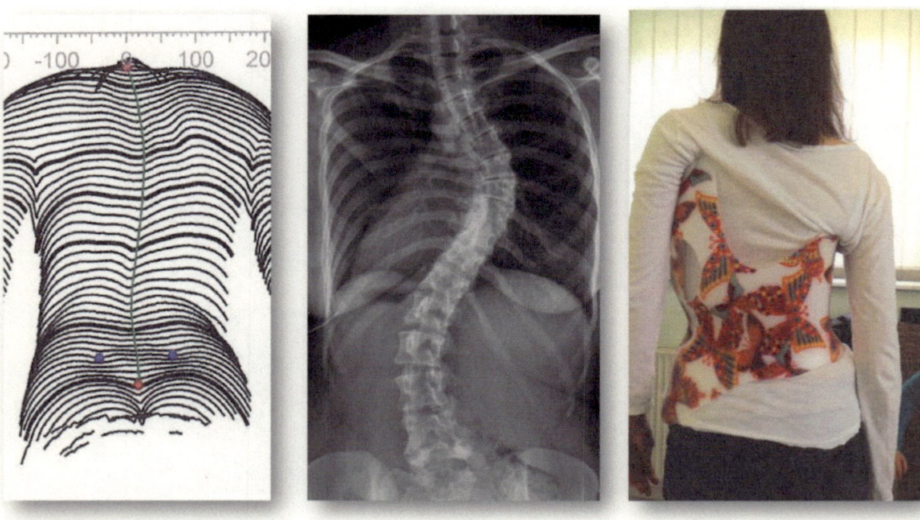

Figure 4.
Left: clinical appearance of the trunk at the start of treatment; middle: X-ray at the start of treatment and on the right: Gensingen brace (GBW) as constructed for the patient. Reproduced with permission of the Society of Physical Therapy Science from [27].

A total of 26 patients have been included. The average age was 17.7 years and the oldest patient from the study was 40 years. The average Cobb angle was 41.5° before treatment (20–72°). 19 patients from this study (73.1%) had chronic low back pain of various degrees before treatment and seven patients (26.9%) were asymptomatic but seeking treatment because of cosmetic reasons.

In-brace correction was 67%. At 6 months follow-up, correction without brace was 23% and the average Cobb angle was 33.2°. About 12 patients (54.5%) had a significant correction of >20%. After 6 months, all previously symptomatic patients reported that they no longer experienced low back pain.

As the GBW is a brace to increase lordosis of the lumbar spine from the results of this latter study [43], we may assume that in scoliosis patients with chronic low back pain, the re-alignment or increase of lumbar lordosis can be regarded as being highly effective with respect to pain reduction.

Although spinal claudication may arise from narrowing of the spinal canal, not all patients with narrowing develop symptoms [13]. The reason why some patients develop symptomatic stenosis and others do not is still unknown. Therefore, the term lumbar spinal stenosis refers to a clinical syndrome of lower extremity pain caused by mechanical compression on the neural elements or their blood supply [13]. A 47-year-old woman with a 55° lumbar scoliosis, 30° upper lumbar kyphosis, and highest pain levels under medication (Durogesic, 25 mg; Ibuprofen, 800 mg; and Mirtazapine, 15 mg) was treated with a sagittal re-alignment brace [13]. This patient is pictured in **Figure 2**. Self-reported walking distance was at around 800 m before the pain was referred to be 'unbearable' (since 5 years). Patient-reported walking distance was recorded in the brace 2 days and 10 days after adjustment. Walking distance increased to around 8000 m after 2 days and to around 12,000 after 10 days while pain intensity decreased only one point in the VRS, however now without any medication. The authors concluded: in contrary to current hypotheses about the aetiology of spinal claudication, augmentation of lordosis may lead to a significant improvement of symptoms associated with spinal stenosis and lumbar scoliosis. The brace used in this case was a physio-logic brace™ that increases lumbar lordosis [13].

In another case report, brace treatment for spinal claudication following severe spondylolisthesis has been described [32]: a 14-year-old girl with a 25° thoracic scoliosis (2 years post menarche), grade IV spondylolisthesis and spinal claudication underwent treatment with a spondylogic™ brace reducing lumbar lordosis (**Figure 5**). Walking distance without brace was at around 300 steps before intolerable pain was reported. Self-reported walking distance was recorded in the brace 14 days after adjustment. Walking distance increased to an unlimited number of steps after 14 days, while pain intensity decreased three points in the VRS. However, no correction effect of the orthosis on the degree of slippage was found. Although there is evidence that pain in patients with spondylolisthesis can be reduced using exercises and bracing in mild to moderate symptomatic cases, this case demonstrates that bracing can also improve signs and symptoms of spinal claudication in patients with spondylolisthesis of higher degrees [32].

These cases show that there is not a single brace covering the necessary principles of correction for all patients with scoliosis and chronic low back pain. Soft braces are insufficient in their action on the stiff deformity of adult scoliosis patients and therefore, cannot be regarded as effective tools for the treatment of chronic low back pain in scoliosis patients [15]. Hard braces have shown effectiveness and fulfil all possible treatment requirements [1, 26, 27, 43].

A simple clinical test enables the specialised physician to estimate the appropriate approach of bracing, increasing or decreasing lumbar lordosis [1]. In patients with more significant deformities and chronic low back pain, specific braces are indicated that allow a stable positioning of the brace on the patient's trunk [27, 43]. However, severely stiff and vast deformities may not be successfully treated by any type of brace (**Figure 6**). Therefore, mobility needs to be tested prior to bracing in order to avoid unnecessary treatment and costs.

In view of these findings, only pattern-specific braces or symmetric braces influencing the sagittal profile can be recommended. In general, however, braces without any visible effect on the deformity continue to be prescribed [52] obviously just immobilising the spine (**Figure 7**). This approach today should be regarded as being outdated.

Patients with thoracic kyphosis in later adulthood may suffer from chronic pain in the thoracic region related to facet joint degeneration and functional impairment of the adjacent ribs. When functional treatment including physiotherapy and spinal manipulation do not reduce the symptoms satisfactorily, brace treatment can also be trialled (**Figure 8**). When passive correction of a thoracic kyphosis leads to

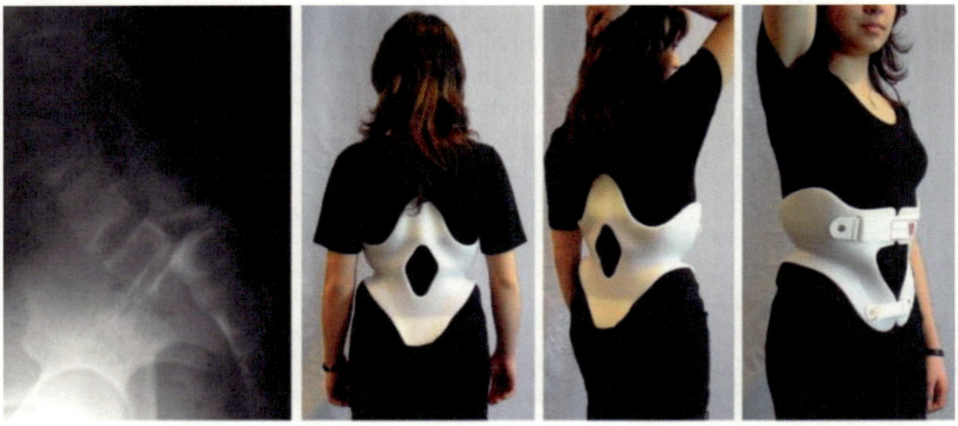

Figure 5.
The spondylogic® brace design. This 14-year-old patient has a scoliosis of <25° and a symptomatic (presenting with lower back pain) spondylolisthesis. Immediate in-brace pain relief was reported, and spinal stenosis symptoms also reduced. The patient wore the brace full-time when walking and standing to manage her pain. Further long-term effects from this brace design have not been researched at present. Taken from [1] (Creative Commons Attribution Licence).

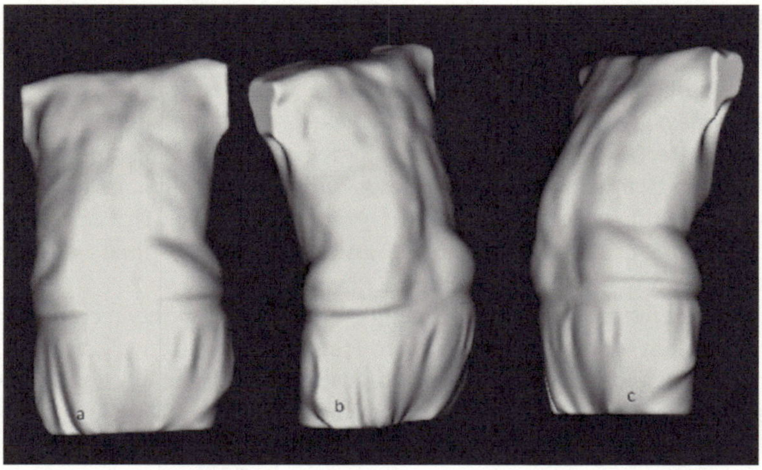

Figure 6.
Excessively stiff curves with huge complex deviations cannot be treated by specific bracing. Usually no correction is achievable: (a) view from the rear, (b) view from oblique left and (c) view from oblique right.

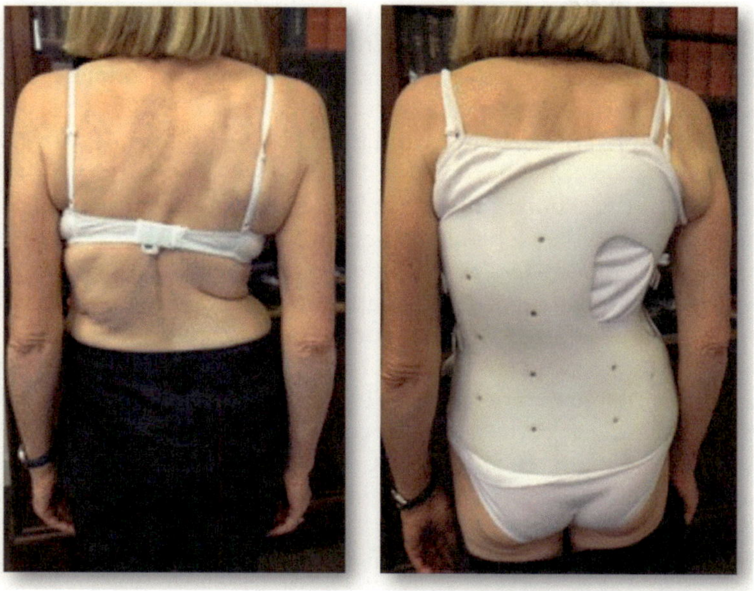

Figure 7.
Brace for an adult with pain. No correction visible, just immobilisation of the spine. This unspecific design could be regarded as outdated. Taken from [52] (Creative Commons Attribution Licence).

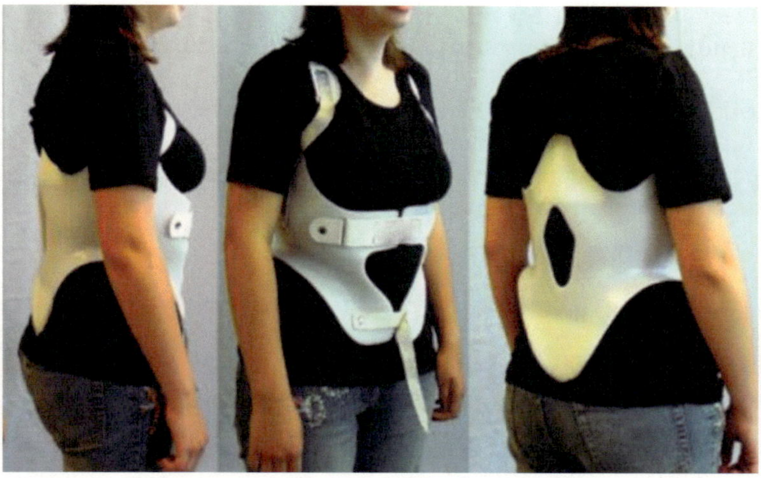

Figure 8.
Patient in a Kyphologic brace™ that may also be used in patients with chronic back pain in the thoracic area. Taken from [53] (Creative Commons Attribution Licence).

significant pain reduction, a brace to reduce thoracic kyphosis may be prescribed. A standardised bracing approach to correct a thoracic kyphosis has been described in literature [53].

Adult patients may experience deformity-related stress and lack of general participation in activities because of their deformity. This fact may be measured and monitored with health-related quality of life questionnaires [54–57].

Freidel et al. investigated women with idiopathic scoliosis with the help of age-appropriate health-related quality of life questionnaires (either the 36-Item Short-Form Health Status Survey, SF-36, or the Berner Questionnaire for Well-Being) [54]. The results from this sample were compared with general population norms.

In univariate and multivariate analyses, it was determined whether age, Cobb angle, and brace use had an impact on health-related quality of life.

Compared with the age-matched general population norm, adolescent patients with idiopathic scoliosis reported to be less happy ($P = 0.001$). They reported more physical complaints ($P < 0.001$) and had lower self-esteem ($P = 0.01$) and higher depression scores ($P = 0.021$). Adult patients reported more psychological ($P < 0.001$) and physical impairment than in the population norm ($P < 0.001$). These results were largely independent of age and Cobb angle.

The authors concluded as follows: the results show that health-related quality of life can be impaired in patients with idiopathic scoliosis. Therefore, the psychosocial situation should be considered in the treatment of these patients [54].

Patients who experienced less body asymmetry were more satisfied with treatment and had a better quality of life [56]. This fact might indicate that quality of life is also related to curve patterns. While combined patterns of curvature (double major) are more compensated and present with less body asymmetry, single curve patterns are more decompensated with significant body asymmetry possibly leading to decreased quality of life.

While there is some evidence that cosmetic improvements can be achieved with pattern specific braces in childhood and adolescence [58–61], there is no literature to be found in PubMed on adult patients with spinal deformities and improved trunk deformity after brace treatment. Nevertheless, there are case reports of adult patients showing a significant improvement of trunk asymmetry and balance (**Figures 9** and **10**). Therefore, high correction bracing should be tried in patients with reduced quality of life because of their trunk deformity. As to the experience of the first author, such improvements cannot be obtained in all adult scoliosis cases.

On the other hand, the cosmetic effects as achieved with the help of spinal fusion surgery are not stable in the mid- or long term [48–50]. Therefore, besides offering psychological support also pattern-specific brace treatment may be tried before a decision for invasive surgery is made.

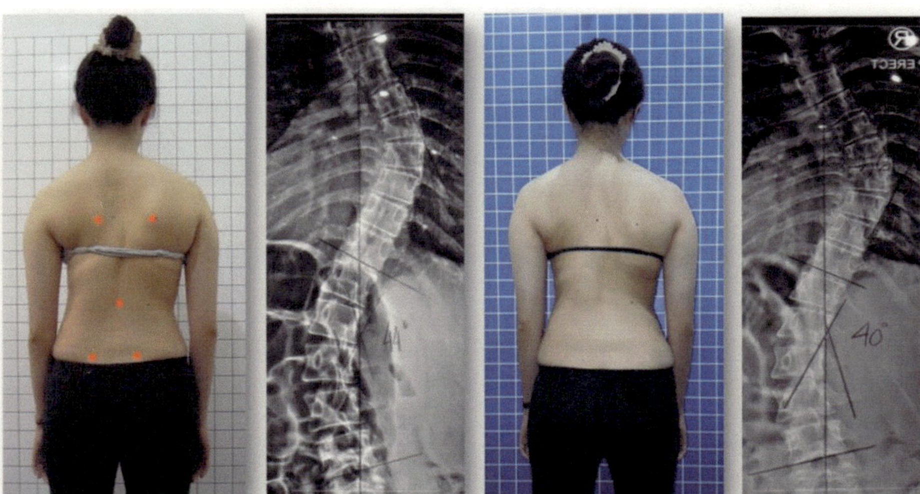

Figure 9.
A 23-year-old woman with a cobb angle of 60° at the start of treatment with a Gensingen brace without significant improvement of cobb angle, however with a clear cosmetic improvement showing a more balanced posture after 12 months of conservative treatment. With kind permission from Dr. Budi S. Widjaja, Jakarta, Indonesia.

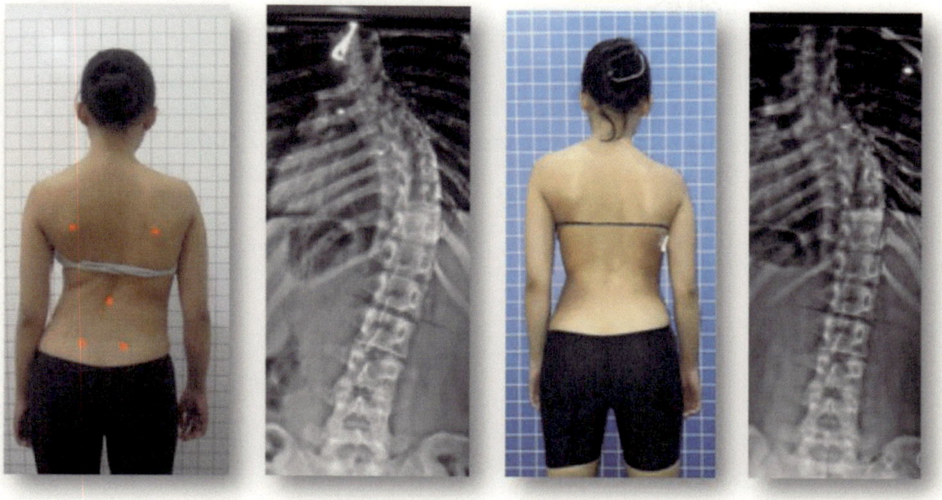

Figure 10.
An 18-month follow-up of a 20-year-old woman with a cobb angle of 52° at the start of the treatment with a Gensingen brace and a final cobb of 36°. A clear cosmetic improvement has been obtained. Courtesy of Dr. Budi S. Widjaja, Jakarta, Indonesia.

It is important to note that brace treatment in later adulthood must be accompanied by a specific daily physical exercise programme. It can be argued that brace wearing does not affect the postural muscles, when in the contrary postural muscle activity is increased while brace wearing [62, 63]. However, the reduction of mobility while wearing the brace may reduce bone mass, especially in postmenopausal women [64–66]. Therefore, regular trabecular loading should be preserved in order to keep bone mass. For patients wearing a brace for some hours per day a Qi Gong, Tai Chi or a Yoga programme involving exercises to mobilise and load the spine in all directions could be beneficial.

4. Conclusions

In adult patients with spinal deformities bracing may be indicated for pain and deformity. Soft braces are not useful for patients with stiff spinal deformities. The appropriate bracing approach can be tested before the brace is prescribed. There is some evidence that pain can successfully be reduced by these approaches mainly influencing the sagittal profile. In patients with bigger deformities and in patients aiming at reducing their deformity, pattern-specific scoliosis braces according to published cases have shown to be successful. There is no high-quality evidence supporting brace treatment for adult patients with spinal deformities; however, the existing evidence is promising.

Acknowledgements

Written informed consent for publication of the patient's information (X-rays, photos, records, etc.) has been obtained from the patients or their parents. HRW provided the first draft and made the literature review. DT contributed to the improvement of the first draft and copyedited the final version. Some parts of the text have been reproduced with permission of the Society of Physical Therapy Science from [15]. More comprehensive information may also be found in [67].

Conflict of interest

HRW is receiving financial support for attending symposia and has received royalties from Koob GmbH & Co KG. The company is held by the spouse of HRW. HRW holds a patent on a sagittal realignment brace (EP 1604624 A1). DT is employed by an orthotic company who make orthotics, including spinal bracing.

Author details

Hans-Rudolf Weiss[1]* and Deborah Turnbull[2,3]

1 Schroth Best Practice Academy, Abtweiler, Germany

2 The London Orthotic Consultancy, Kingston upon Thames, UK

3 School of Health and Social Care, University of Teesside, Middlesbrough, UK

*Address all correspondence to: hr.weiss@skoliose-dr-weiss.com

References

[1] Weiss HR, Werkmann M. Unspecific chronic low back pain—A simple functional classification tested in a case series of patients with spinal deformities. Scoliosis. 2009;**4**:02

[2] Ploumis A, Transfledt EE, Denis F. Degenerative lumbar scoliosis associated with spinal stenosis. The Spine Journal. 2007;7(4):428-436. DOI: 10.1016/j.spinee.2006.07.015

[3] Ciol MA, Deyo RA, Howell E, Kreif S. An assessment of surgery for spinal stenosis: Time trends, geographic variations, complications, and reoperations. Journal of the American Geriatrics Society. 1996;**44**:285-290

[4] Gordon GA. A molecular basis for low back pain in western industrialized cultures. Medical Hypotheses. 1990;**33**(4):251-256. DOI: 10.1016/0306-9877(90)90137-4

[5] Ploumis A, Liu H, Mehbod A, Transfeldt E. Can radiographic measurement of degenerative lumbar scoliosis predict clinical symptoms? In: Proceedings of the 5th International Conference on Conservative Management of Spinal Deformities, Athens, April 2-5, 2008. 2008

[6] Masiero S, Carraro E, Celia A, Sarto D, Ermani M. Prevalence of nonspecific low back pain in schoolchildren aged between 13 and 15 years. Acta Paediatrica. 2008;**97**(2):212-216. DOI: 10.1111/j.1651-2227.2007.00603.x

[7] Lebkowski WJ. "Back pain" in teenagers and young adults. Polski Merkuriusz Lekarski. 1997;**2**(8):111-112

[8] Hildebrandt VH, Bongers PM, Dul J, van Dijk FJ, Kemper HC. The relationship between leisure time, physical activities and musculoskeletal symptoms and disability in worker populations. International Archives of Occupational and Environmental Health. 2000;**73**(8):507-518. DOI: 10.1007/s004200000167

[9] Nourbakhsh MR, Moussavi SJ, Salavati M. Effects of lifestyle and work-related physical activity on the degree of lumbar lordosis and chronic low back pain in a Middle East population. Journal of Spinal Disorders. 2001;**14**(4):283-292. DOI: 10.1097/00002517-200108000-00002

[10] Leboeuf-Yde C. Back pain—Individual and genetic factors. Journal of Electromyography and Kinesiology. 2004;**14**(1):129-136. DOI: 10.1016/j.jelekin.2003.09.019

[11] Yip VY. New low back pain in nurses: Work activities, work stress and sedentary lifestyle. Journal of Advanced Nursing. 2004;**46**(4):430-440. DOI: 10.1111/j.1365-2648.2004.03009.x

[12] Weiss HR, Dallmayer R, Stephan C. First results of pain treatment in scoliosis patients using a sagittal realignment brace. Studies in Health Technology and Informatics. 2006;**123**:582-585

[13] Weiss HR, Dallmayer R. Brace treatment of spinal claudication in an adult with lumbar scoliosis—A case report. Studies in Health Technology and Informatics. 2006;**123**:586-589

[14] Weiss HR. Epidemiologie und Risikofaktoren des chronischen Kreuzschmerzes. Orthopädische Praxis. 1999;**35**(8):469-477

[15] Weiss HR, Turnbull D. Non-specific chronic low back pain in patients with scoliosis—An overview of the literature on patients undergoing brace treatment. Journal of Physical Therapy Science. 2019;**31**(11):960-964

[16] Weiss HR. Scoliosis-related pain in adults - treatment influences. European Journal of Physical and Rehabilitation Medicine. 1993;**31**:91-94

[17] Weiss HR, Verres C, Steffan K, Heckel I. Scoliosis and pain—Is there any relationship? In: IAF S, editor. Research into Spinal Deformities 2. Amsterdam: IOS Press; 1999. pp. 293-296

[18] Danielsson AJ, Wiklund I, Pehrsson K, Nachemson AL. Health-related quality of life in patients with adolescent idiopathic scoliosis: A matched follow-up at least 20 years after treatment with brace or surgery. European Spine Journal. 2001;**10**(4):278-288

[19] Weinstein SL, Dolan LA, Spratt KF, Peterson KK, Spoonamore MJ, Ponseti IV. Health and function of patients with untreated idiopathic scoliosis: A 50-year natural history study. JAMA. 2003;**289**(5):559-567

[20] Grauers A, Topalis C, Moller H, Normelli H, Karlsson M, Danielsson A, et al. Prevalence of back problems in 1069 adults with idiopathic scoliosis and 158 adults without scoliosis. Spine (Phila Pa 1976). 2014;**39**(11):886-892

[21] Weiss HR, Karavidas N, Moramarco M, Moramarco K. Long-term effects of untreated adolescent idiopathic scoliosis: A review of the literature. Asian Spine Journal. 2016;**10**(6):1163-1169

[22] Zapata KA, Wang-Price SS, Sucato DJ, Thompson M, Trudelle-Jackson E, Lovelace-Chandler V. Spinal stabilization exercise effectiveness for low back pain in adolescent idiopathic scoliosis: A randomized trial. Pediatric Physical Therapy. 2015;**27**(4):396-402

[23] Yagci G, Yakut Y. Core stabilization exercises versus scoliosis-specific exercises in moderate idiopathic scoliosis treatment. Prosthetics and Orthotics International. 2019;**43**(3):301-308

[24] Upasani VV, Caltoum C, Petcharaporn M, Bastrom TP, Pawelek JB, Betz RR, et al. Adolescent idiopathic scoliosis patients report increased pain at five years compared with two years after surgical treatment. Spine (Phila Pa 1976). 2008;**33**(10):1107-1112

[25] Weiss HR. Das "Sagittal Realignment Brace" (physio-logic ® brace) in der Behandlung von erwachsenen Skoliosepatienten mit chronifiziertem Rückenschmerz. MOT. 2005;**125**:45-54

[26] Weiss HR, Werkmann M. Treatment of chronic low back pain in patients with spinal deformities using a sagittal re-alignment brace. Scoliosis. 2009;**4**:03

[27] Weiss HR, Moramarco K, Moramarco M. Scoliosis bracing and exercise for pain management in adults-a case report. Journal of Physical Therapy Science. 2016;**28**(8):2404-2407

[28] Dewitte V, De Pauw R, De Meulemeester K, Peersman W, Danneels L, Bouche K, et al. Clinical classification criteria for nonspecific low back pain: A Delphi-survey of clinical experts. Musculoskeletal Science & Practice. 2018 Apr;**34**:66-76

[29] Zaina F, Poggio M, Donzelli S, Negrini S. Can bracing help adults with chronic back pain and scoliosis? Short-term results from a pilot study. Prosthetics and Orthotics International. 2018;**42**(4):410-414

[30] Polastri M, Romano M. Lumbar scoliosis: Reducing lower back pain and improving function in adulthood. A case report with a 2-year follow-up. Journal of Bodywork and Movement Therapies. 2017;**21**(1):81-85

[31] Gallo D. Case reports: Orthotic treatment of adult scoliosis patients with chronic back pain. Scoliosis. 2014;**9**:18

[32] Weiss HR, Dallmayer R. Brace treatment of spinal claudication in an adolescent with a grade IV spondylosisthesis—A case report. Studies in Health Technology and Informatics. 2006;**123**:590-593

[33] Brubaker ML, Sinaki M. Successful management of iliocostal impingement syndrome: A case series. Prosthetics and Orthotics International. 2016;**40**(3):384-387

[34] Asher MA, Burton DC. Adolescent idiopathic scoliosis: Natural history and long-term treatment effects. Scoliosis. 2006;**1**(1):2

[35] van Loon PJ, Kühbauch BA, Thunnissen FB. Forced lordosis on the thoracolumbar junction can correct coronal plane deformity in adolescents with double major curve pattern idiopathic scoliosis. Spine. 2008;**33**(7):797-801

[36] Burwell RG. Aetiology of idiopathic scoliosis: Current concepts. Pediatric Rehabilitation. 2003;**6**(3-4):137-170

[37] Glassman SD, Bridwell K, Dimar JR, Horton W, Berven SF. The impact of positive sagittal balance in adult spinal deformity. Spine. 2005;**30**:2024-2029

[38] Djurasovic M, Glassman SD. Correlation of radiographic and clinical findings in spinal deformities. Neurosurgery Clinics of North America. 2007;**18**(2):223-227

[39] Jellema P, Bierma-Zeinstra SM, van Poppel MN, Bernsen RM, Koes BW. Feasibility of lumbar supports for home care workers with low back pain. Occupational Medicine (London). 2002;**52**(6):317-323

[40] van Poppel MN, Koes BW, van der Ploeg T, Smid T, Bouter LM. Lumbar supports and education for the prevention of low back pain in industry: A randomized controlled trial. JAMA. 1998;**279**:1789-1794

[41] Alaranta H, Hurri H. Compliance and subjective relief by corset treatment in chronic low back pain. Scandinavian Journal of Rehabilitation Medicine. 1988;**20**:133-136

[42] Jellema P, van Tulder MW, van Poppel MN, Nachemson AL, Bouter LM. Lumbar supports for prevention and treatment of low back pain: A systematic review within the framework of the Cochrane Back review group. Spine. 2001;**26**:377-386

[43] Widjaja BS, Varani R. Single lumbar curvatures are treated effectively with Gensingen brace (GBW) in late adolescent and adult scoliosis patients. In: Proceedings of the 1st. International Conference on Scoliosis Management on Behalf of the Turkish Scoliosis Society, April 12-13. Istanbul, Turkey; 2018. p. 19

[44] Bettany-Saltikov J, Weiss HR, Chockalingam N, et al. Surgical versus non-surgical interventions in people with adolescent idiopathic scoliosis. Cochrane Database of Systematic Reviews. 2015;**4**(4):CD010663

[45] Cheuk DK, Wong V, Wraige E, Baxter P, Cole A. Surgery for scoliosis in duchenne muscular dystrophy. Cochrane Database of Systematic Reviews. 2015;**10**(10):CD005375

[46] Bettany-Saltikov J, Weiss HR, Chockalingam N, Kandasamy G, Arnell T. A comparison of patient-reported outcome measures following different treatment approaches for adolescents with severe idiopathic scoliosis: A systematic review. Asian Spine Journal. 2016;**10**(6):1170-1194

[47] Ward WT, Friel NA, Kenkre TS, Brooks MM, Londino JA, Roach JW.

SRS-22r scores in non-operated adolescent idiopathic scoliosis patients with curves greater than forty degrees. Spine (Phila Pa 1976). 2017;**42**(16):1233-1240

[48] Hawes M. Impact of spine surgery on signs and symptoms of spinal deformity. Pediatric Rehabilitation. 2006;**9**(4):318-339

[49] Weiss HR, Goodall D. Rate of complications in scoliosis surgery—A systematic review of the PubMed literature. Scoliosis. 2008;**3**:9

[50] Weiss HR, Moramarco M, Moramarco K. Risks and long-term complications of adolescent idiopathic scoliosis surgery vs. non-surgical and natural history outcomes. Hard Tissue. 2013;**2**(3):27

[51] Moramarco K. Least potential harm with treatment for adolescent idiopathic scoliosis patients. Hard Tissue. 2013;**2**(5):44. Available from: http://www.oapublishinglondon.com/article/1011

[52] de Mauroy JC, Lecante C, Barral F, Pourret S. Bracing in adult with scoliosis: Experience in diagnosis and classification from a 15 year prospective study of 739 patients. Scoliosis and Spinal Disorders. 2016;**11**(Suppl 2):29. DOI: 10.1186/s13013-016-0090 y

[53] Weiss HR, Turnbull D, Bohr S. Brace treatment for patients with Scheuermann's disease—A review of the literature and first experiences with a new brace design. Scoliosis. 2009;**4**:09

[54] Freidel K, Petermann F, Reichel D, Steiner A, Warschburger P, Weiss HR. Quality of life in women with idiopathic. Spine (Phila Pa 1976). 2002;**27**(4):E87-E91

[55] Weiss HR, Seibel S, Kleban A. Deformity-related stress in a sample of patients with adolescent idiopathic scoliosis after brace weaning: A cross-sectional investigation. OA Musculoskeletal Medicine. 2014;**2**(1):5

[56] Danielsson AJ, Hasserius R, Ohlin A, Nachemson AL. Body appearance and quality of life in adult patients with adolescent idiopathic scoliosis treated with a brace or under observation alone during adolescence. Spine (Phila Pa 1976). 2012;**37**(9):755-762. DOI: 10.1097/BRS.0b013e318231493c

[57] Diarbakerli E, Grauers A, Danielsson A, Gerdhem P. Health-related quality of life in adulthood in untreated and treated individuals with adolescent or juvenile idiopathic scoliosis. The Journal of Bone and Joint Surgery. American Volume. 2018;**100**(10):811-817. DOI: 10.2106/JBJS.17.00822

[58] Rigo M. Radiological and cosmetic improvement 2 years after brace weaning—A case report. Pediatric Rehabilitation. 2003;**6**(3-4):195-199

[59] Weiss HR, Moramarco M. Remodelling of trunk and backshape deformities in patients with scoliosis using standardized asymmetric computer-aided design/computer-aided manufacturing braces. Hard Tissue. 2013;**2**(2):14

[60] Weiss HR. Bracing can lead to a persistent correction in the treatment of adolescent idiopathic scoliosis: A case report. Hard Tissue. 2014;**3**(1):8

[61] Weiss HR, Tournavitis N, Seibel S, Kleban A. A prospective cohort study of AIS patients with 40° and more treated with a Gensingen brace (GBW): Preliminary results. The Open Orthopaedics Journal. 2017;**11**:1558-1567

[62] Güth V, Abbink F, Götze HG, Heinrichs W. Kinesiologic and electromyographic studies on the effects of the Milwaukee corset. Zeitschrift

für Orthopädie und Ihre Grenzgebiete. 1976;**114**(4):480-483

[63] Güth V, Abbink F, Götze HG, Heinrichs W. Investigation of gait of patients with idiopathic scoliosis and the influence of the Milwaukee brace on gait (author's transl). Zeitschrift für Orthopädie und Ihre Grenzgebiete. 1978;**116**(5):631-640

[64] Schmitt NM, Schmitt J, Doren M. The role of physical activity in the prevention of osteoporosis in postmenopausal women-an update. Maturitas. 2009;**63**:34-38

[65] Yu PA, Hsu WH, Hsu WB, et al. The effects of high impact exercise intervention on bone mineral density, physical fitness, and quality of life in postmenopausal women with osteopenia: A retrospective cohort study. Medicine (Baltimore). 2019;**98**(11):e14898. DOI: 10.1097/MD.0000000000014898

[66] Gonzalo-Encabo P, McNeil J, Boyne DJ, Courneya KS, Friedenreich CM. Dose-response effects of exercise on bone mineral density and content in post-menopausal women. Scandinavian Journal of Medicine & Science in Sports. 2019;**29**(8):1121-1129. DOI: 10.1111/sms.13443

[67] Weiss HR. Pain and deformity. In: Moramarco M, Borysov M, Ng SY, Weiss HR, editors. Schroth's Textbook of Scoliosis and Other Spinal Deformities. Newcastle Upon Tyne, UK: Cambridge Scholars Publishing Ltd; 2020. pp. 613-628. ISBN: 978-1527538290

Chapter 11

The Functional Effects of Adult Spinal Deformity and the Effectiveness of Surgery

David Christopher Kieser and Michael Charles Wyatt

Abstract

The prevalence of adult spinal deformity (ASD) is increasing worldwide, driven by changing patient demographics, as well as an increased capacity to diagnose and treat this condition. ASD carries the worst healthcare burden of all chronic conditions including arthritis, chronic lung disease, congestive heart failure, diabetes and ischaemic heart disease. Recent advances in diagnostic and treatment modalities have resulted in an increase in surgical intervention for this condition. To be successful, however, a comprehensive understanding of the functional deficits caused by ASD must be recognised by those clinicians managing such patients. This chapter provides an overview of the functional deficits caused by ASD and its treatment.

Keywords: spine, function, deformity

1. Introduction

Spinal conditions are some of the most common health conditions affecting adults [1]. Many spinal conditions do not affect spinal alignment, whilst others induce spinal deformity. Adult spinal deformity (ASD) is an umbrella term for a complex spectrum of spinal conditions causing spinal deformity [2]. The most common causes of ASD are degenerative disease and idiopathic (**Figure 1**). Other causes of ASD include oncologic, traumatic, neuromuscular and iatrogenic. Whilst the exact incidence of ASD is unknown, the rate of ASD increases with age with a reported prevalence of 32% of patients aged over 50 years and 68% of patients aged over 70 years [3].

Despite this prevalence, many patients have mild deformities and little or no symptoms. Conversely some patients have marked spinal deformity with global spinal imbalance causing severe disability [4]. The predominant reason for this disability is that spinal imbalance prevents the normal economic resting posture of the spine, whereby the centre of gravity runs in close proximity to the spine and the head is centred over the hips. This therefore requires an increase in the physiological demands of the spine and peri-spinal musculature which subsequently causes pain, fatigue and disability. It is therefore perhaps unsurprising that the extent of spinal imbalance directly relates to the degree of disability [5–8].

It is now recognised that the consequences of an imbalanced spine on a patient's function and quality of life (QoL) can be devastating [3, 5, 6, 8, 9]. In fact, compared to all other common long-term disorders, such as arthritis, chronic lung disease, congestive heart failure, diabetes and ischaemic heart disease, ASD has the worst patient reported QoL [10] (**Figure 2**). Furthermore, because of its increasing

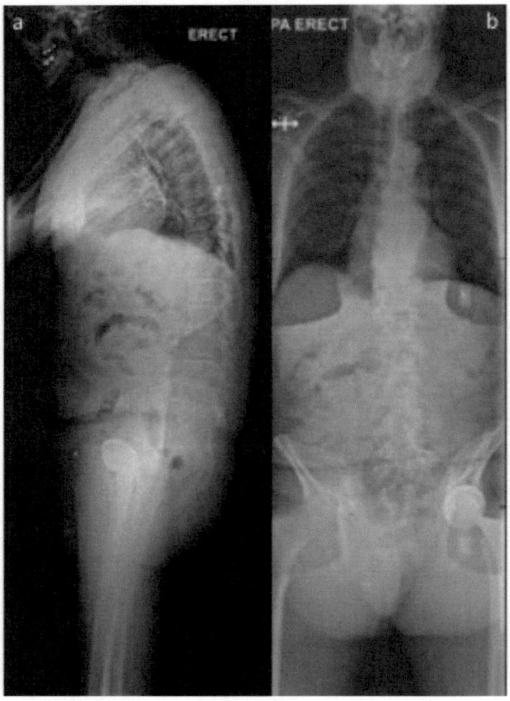

Figure 1.
Lateral (a) and postero-anterior (b) standing X-rays of a 70-year old male with adult spinal deformity predominantly affecting the sagittal plane. Note the compensatory mechanisms for his lack of lumbar lordosis, notably thoracic hypokyphosis and pelvic retroversion, which results in a typical flat-back deformity.

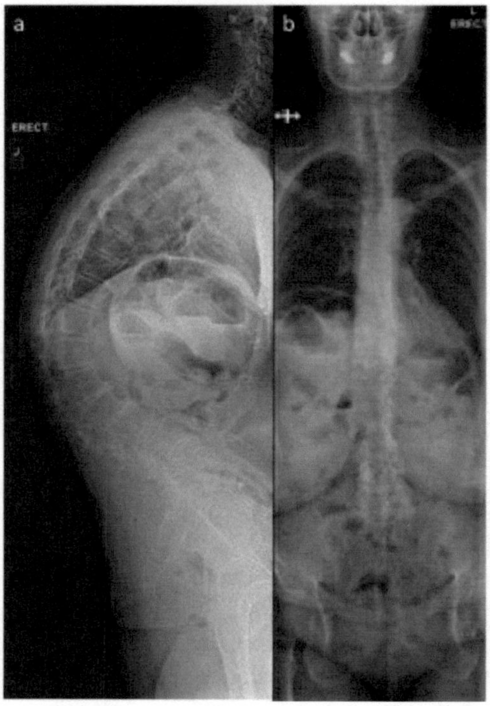

Figure 2.
Lateral (a) and postero-anterior (b) standing X-rays of a 55-year old female previous athlete who is now house-bound due to severe axial pain caused by her degenerative thoraco-lumbar spine, causing severe local kyphosis. Note her attempted spinal compensation for the thoraco-lumbar kyphosis, notably pelvic retroversion, lower lumbar hyperlordosis, thoracic hypokyphosis and cervical hyperlordosis.

incidence, driven by multiple factors, ASD is the highest ranked disorder in estimates of global disease burden [10].

In order to quantify the degree of disability and effect on a patient's well-being from ASD, multiple functional scores have been employed [11]. Some scores have been specifically developed to assess spinal conditions, whilst others have been developed for other conditions but offer a proxy for "well-being" in patients with ASD. The most useful parameters available to understand the effect of ASD on a patient's well-being are pain, function and QoL. Thus, scores assessing these factors are commonly used to report outcomes in patients with ASD.

In general, pain scores numerically rate a patient's degree of pain (numeric rating scale (NRS)) in specific anatomical locations through a visual analogue score (VAS). For ASD, pain is usually separated into back and leg pain. In contrast, functional outcome scores attempt to understand what specific functions or activities are inhibited by a condition. In ASD, the most commonly used functional outcome score is the Oswestry Disability Index (ODI) [12]. This score was initially described to evaluate low back pain in a general population rather than evaluate the functional outcome of patients with ASD [12]. However, it is now widely used to evaluate the functional deficits induced by ASD and the response to treatment.

The ODI is a questionnaire that evaluates activities of daily living (ADL) that offers a subjective score of the respondent's level of disability. This index specifically assesses pain, personal care, lifting, walking, sitting, standing, sleeping, sexual life, social life and travelling [12]. For each domain the total achievable score is 5, with zero being no disability and 5 being severe disability. The scores for each domain are then summed and an overall percentage of disability is calculated. Whilst the overall disability value is one of the most commonly reported values in the literature, within each domain of the ODI the degree of disability can be scored and used to determine the effect of ASD treatment on specific ADLs.

QoL scores attempt to quantify the global effect that a condition has on the patient's life. The two most commonly reported QoL scores in ASD are the Scoliosis Research Society 22 (SRS-22) and Short Form 36 (SF36). The SRS-22 is a composite questionnaire of 22 questions developed specifically to determine the pain, function, self-image, mental health, and satisfaction of patients with spinal deformity [13]. In contrast, the SF36, which comprises 36 questions, was not specifically developed for spinal conditions, but does determine a patient's physical function, pain, vitality, social function, emotional effect, mental health and general health [14].

2. Discussion

To date a complete understanding of which factors independently affect patient pain, function and QoL in patients with ASD remains unclear. In the general population affected by back pain a number of factors are reported to affect pain, function and QoL, with most factors contributing a variable amount to the disability. Because of this multi-factorial affect a biopsychosocial approach to understand the interconnected importance of each factor is appropriate. Biologically, the more sinister the cause and the more severe the condition, the more likely the patients are to be symptomatic. Similarly, the greater the spinal load, particularly increased body mass index (BMI), but also physical workload, as well as the more medical conditions affecting the patient the more likely they are to experience back pain [5, 15–17].

Psychologically, the psychological profile and capacity to cope influence the degree of back pain and dysfunction experienced by patients as does the patient's locus of control. A patient with an intrinsic locus of control (a patient who takes personal responsibility for their own outcome) as opposed to a patient with an extrinsic locus of control (a patient who relies on others for their outcome) is likely to experience less pain and dysfunction. From a social perspective, those with a higher socio-economic status, greater supports, current employment and non-smokers experience less pain and disability. It is also known that other factors including geographic, and genetic factors influence back pain, function and QoL in the general population [18–22].

Similar to that of the general population, it is likely that multiple factors affect the pain, function and QoL of patients with ASD. However, only relatively few of these factors have been analysed in depth. The most well recognised correlation is that of sagittal imbalance. Sagittal balance can be described clinically as one's sagittal position of the skull relative to the hips, however, it is most accurately defined

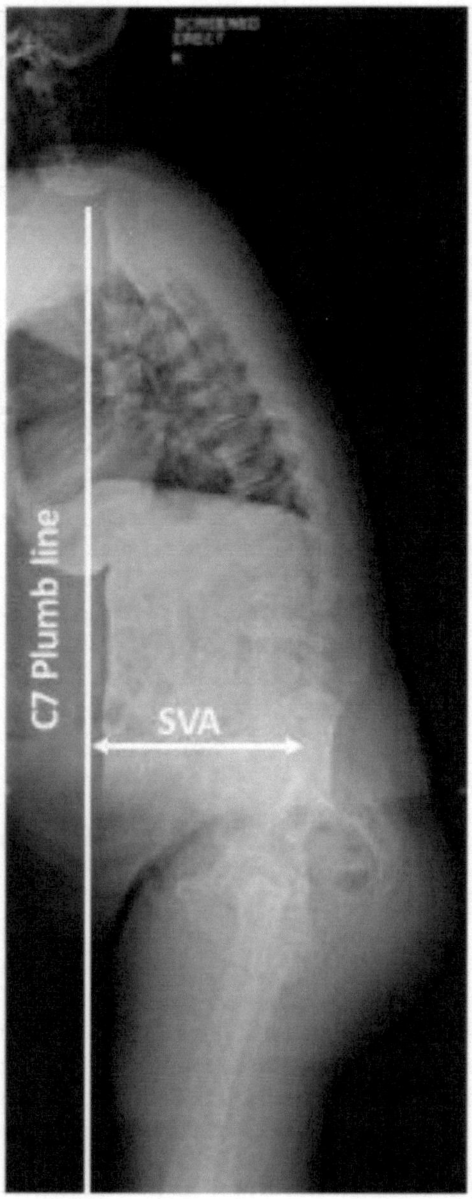

Figure 3.
Representative standing lateral X-ray demonstrating the measurement of the sagittal vertical axis (SVA).

radiologically as the sagittal vertical axis (SVA) which is the distance from the posterior superior aspect of the first sacral vertebral body to a line drawn perpendicular to the floor that runs through the middle of the C7 vertebra (C7 plumb line) in a standing patient (**Figure 3**).

Glassman and colleagues were the first to study this parameter and its effect on functional outcomes and found that an increase in sagittal balance directly affects functional outcomes in patients with ASD [5]. This finding has been confirmed in a number of subsequent publications [6–8].

Obesity has also been studied and shown to affect pain, function and QoL in patients with ASD. Intuitively an increased load on a compromised spine would affect a patient's well-being, however, the exact mechanism by which obesity affects these patients remains unproven. Furthermore, the effect of weight loss on the improvement of symptoms is yet to be determined. That said, the fact that obesity negatively affects the pain, function and QoL in these patients is of significant concern considering the rate of obesity is increasing internationally [23, 24].

Despite the paucity of data on other factors affecting the disability profile of patients with ASD, it is likely that there are multifactorial contributors that are yet to be studied. These include the patient's baseline requirements and ADLs, often driven by age, occupation and social activities; the patient's locus of control; the location and cause of the spinal deformity as well as the severity and number of levels affected; the degree of stiffness of the spine and hips and capacity to compensate for the deformity, the degree of coronal imbalance and global tilt. The contribution that each plays towards the patient's disability is likely varied, but on-going research into this area is warranted.

Similarly, the specific functional limitations induced by ASD have a likely multifactorial basis, which makes specific treatments for specific functional deficits limited. However, it is recognised that severe ASD can affect all ADL and severely affect QoL [3, 6, 8]. Since Glassman's correlation between the ODI and SVA, the use of health-related quality of life scores (HRQLs) to assess the success of treatments in ASD has become routine [5, 25]. Unfortunately, there is a lack of published material on the specific disabilities induced by ASD. In contrast, some information is available on the specific functional benefits of the treatment of ASD.

The treatment of ASD is challenging. To date, non-operative treatment, although used extensively, has not been shown to improve long term outcomes for these patients, especially when significant anatomical abnormality and spinal imbalance is present [26, 27]. However, core strengthening, aerobic exercise and weight loss strategies are useful in the treatment of LBP in the general population and are relatively cheap, easy, safe with patients gaining a degree of self-control over their condition and gaining multiple other health benefits of such lifestyle modifications. Pain management offers symptom control to alleviate pain which may improve function, but often at the effect of sedation. Furthermore, long-term symptom control is required with the development of medication tolerance and reliance, with the associated expense and complications of long-term medical treatment. Injection therapy with epidurals, nerve blocks and facet injections may offer some temporary benefit. Bracing may offer short term benefit but defunctions the paraspinal musculature which often worsens symptoms when the brace is removed. Glassman and colleagues analysed the non-operative resource utilisation and cost benefit of non-operative treatment in ASD. They identified a large resource utilisation and cost for patients with ASD, particularly those with severe symptoms, but no improvement in the health status at 2-year follow-ups with non-operative treatment [26, 27].

In contrast to non-operative care, operative intervention has shown long-term improvements in pain, function and QoL in symptomatic patients, and this has fuelled the increased number of complex ASD surgeries being performed worldwide [2, 28–31]. In the last decade the number of complex operations being performed for ASD has doubled in many countries, including the USA and UK, which contrasts with the 20% increase in all other spinal surgeries [2, 29].

The surgery for this condition can vary from a single level neural decompression to global deformity correction. However, there is growing evidence that most patients with symptomatic ASD benefit from a restoration of their spinal balance [7, 32, 33]. But, procedures to restore spinal balance are far more complex than simple decompressive procedures. Furthermore, spinal realignment surgery is expensive with the demands of a single case and impact on health services being disproportionately greater than those of other elective procedures, such as total hip joint replacement [28, 30, 31]. The average total hospital cost for a primary procedure is estimated at US$103,143, and therefore the improvement in pain, function and QoL needs to be justified [34].

Furthermore, despite the evidence that spino-pelvic fusion is associated with excellent patient satisfaction and improvements in overall function, patients increasingly require information on the specific functional benefits and limitations induced by ASD treatment in order to make informed decisions and avoid inaccurate patient expectations [14]. Kieser and colleagues reviewed the effect of primary spino-pelvic fusion on the specific functional outcomes of ASD in a retrospective review of 45 consecutive patients enrolled in the European Spine Study Group database with a minimum 2-year follow-up [35]. Their study confirms that spino-pelvic fusion significantly improves the overall ODI score at a 2-year follow-up for patients with ASD. They identified a mean 13.5% overall improvement in disability, with a reduction in pain and improvement in function and QoL.

When assessing the effect of ASD surgery on specific ADLs, Kieser and colleagues reported a variable degree of benefit for each ODI domain. Large improvements were found for pain and sexual function, moderate improvements for walking, sitting, standing, social life and travelling and minimal improvements for sleeping, personal care and lifting [35]. No domains were found to worsen after surgery at a 2-year follow-up. These results suggest that the pain relief, spinal stability and balance offered by these procedures improve ADLs such as walking, sitting, standing, travelling, social life and sexual function. However, the rigidity imparted by the fusion limits the improvement in personal care and lifting, which often relies on spinal mobility.

Conceptually, long-segment fusions should worsen certain ADLs such as personal care. Yet the study by Kieser and colleagues revealed an improvement in these functions but commented that this improvement was not statistically or clinically significant [35]. They suggested that the pre-operative spinal mobility of patients with ASD is usually poor, either from stiffness or pain, and therefore fusion carries a less significant functional effect in this condition than in conditions with normal spinal mobility. In addition, the minimal improvement in sleep has been postulated to be due to the effect of gravity driving disability in the upright position being non-influential when lying down [35]. However, the study was limited by only assessing the ODI without including other outcome scores and by the variance in underlying cause, curve type, extent of deformity and preoperative symptoms of included patients.

Recognising that spino-pelvic fusion reduces the overall level of disability in patients with ASD allows the surgeon to advocate for such procedures, but understanding the large improvement in pain and sexual function, moderate improvement in walking, sitting, standing, social life and travelling and limited improvement in sleeping, personal care and lifting allows patients to make informed decisions with clear expectations, that empowers them to make the right personal decision.

Although the only study assessing the effect of ASD surgery on specific ADLs, the study by Kieser and colleagues only assessed primary procedures [35]. To date, no comparable study has been undertaken on revision procedures. However, Scheer and colleagues previously identified that patients requiring revision deformity correction have a worse longer-term outcome than those who do not require revision [36]. This is important to recognise because ASD surgery carries a high complication rate, with a reported major complication rate of 20% and 30-day mortality of 2.4% [25, 37]. Therefore, when contemplating the first procedure, despite the potential increased initial expense and risk involved in a comprehensive deformity correction, it is in a patient's and institution's best interests to optimise the first procedure, to optimise outcome and reduce the longer-term costs associated with revision surgery. An approach to "getting it right first time" is therefore warranted [38].

3. Conclusion

Within the current literature there remain significant deficits in our understanding of the functional effects of ASD and its treatments. It is clear that this condition causes severe disability with significant pain, functional limitations with most ADLs and poor QoL. Non-operative management options do not resolve the spinal imbalance which appears to be the biggest determinant of improved patient outcome and therefore little evidence exists for its efficacy. In contrast, operative intervention has improved patient outcomes, but with high expense and complication rates. Future treatment strategies should therefore focus on enhancing functional outcomes, whilst limiting risk and expense. Furthermore, a holistic biopsychosocial approach should be provided if all factors influencing outcome are to be addressed.

Author details

David Christopher Kieser* and Michael Charles Wyatt
Department of Orthopaedic Surgery and Musculoskeletal Medicine, University of Otago, Christchurch, New Zealand

*Address all correspondence to: kieserdavid@gmail.com

References

[1] Salomon JA, Haagsma JA, Davis A, de Noordhout CM, Polinder S, Havelaar AH, et al. Disability weights for the global burden of disease 2013 study. The Lancet Global Health. 2015;**3**(11):e712-e723

[2] Good CR, Auerbach JD, O'Leary PT, Schuler TC. Adult spine deformity. Current Reviews in Musculoskeletal Medicine. 2011;**4**(4):159-167

[3] Schwab F, Dubey A, Gamez L, El Fegoun AB, Hwang K, Pagala M, et al. Adult scoliosis: Prevalence, SF-36, and nutritional parameters in an elderly volunteer population. Spine (Phila Pa 1976). 2005;**30**(9):1082-1085

[4] Acaroglu E, Yavuz AC, Guler UO, et al. A decision analysis to identify the ideal treatment for adult spinal deformity: Is surgery better than non-surgical treatment in improving health-related quality of life and decreasing the disease burden? European Spine Journal. 2016;**25**(8):2390-2400

[5] Glassman SD, Bridwell K, Dimar JR, Horton W, Berven S, Schwab F. The impact of positive sagittal balance in adult spinal deformity. Spine (Phila Pa 1976). 2005;**30**(18):2024-2029

[6] Lafage V, Schwab F, Patel A, Hawkinson N, Farcy JP. Pelvic tilt and truncal inclination: Two key radiographic parameters in the setting of adults with spinal deformity. Spine (Phila Pa 1976). 2009;**34**(17):E599-E606

[7] Schwab F, Patel A, Ungar B, Farcy JP, Lafage V. Adult spinal deformity-postoperative standing imbalance: How much can you tolerate? An overview of key parameters in assessing alignment and planning corrective surgery. Spine (Phila Pa 1976). 2010;**35**(25):2224-2231

[8] Schwab FJ, Blondel B, Bess S, Hostin R, Shaffrey CI, Smith JS, et al. Radiographical spinopelvic parameters and disability in the setting of adult spinal deformity: A prospective multicenter analysis. Spine (Phila Pa 1976). 2013;**38**(13):E803-E812

[9] Schwab F, Dubey A, Pagala M, Gamez L, Farcy JP. Adult scoliosis: A health assessment analysis by SF-36. Spine (Phila Pa 1976). 2003;**28**(6):602-606

[10] Pellise F, Vila-Casademunt A, Ferrer M, Domingo-Sabat M, Bago J, Perez-Grueso FJ, et al. Impact on health related quality of life of adult spinal deformity (ASD) compared with other chronic conditions. European Spine Journal. 2015;**24**(1):3-11

[11] Cawley DT, Larrieu D, Fujishiro T, Kieser D, Boissiere L, Acaroglu E, et al. NRS20: combined back and leg pain score: A simple and effective assessment of adult spinal deformity. Spine. 2018;**43**(17):1184-1192

[12] Fairbank JC, Couper J, Davies JB, O'Brien JP. The Oswestry low back pain disability questionnaire. Physiotherapy. 1980;**66**(8):271-273

[13] Asher M, Min Lai S, Burton D, Manna B. The reliability and concurrent validity of the scoliosis research society-22 patient questionnaire for idiopathic scoliosis. Spine (Phila Pa 1976). 2003;**28**(1):63-69

[14] Ware JE Jr, Sherbourne CD. The MOS 36-item short-form health survey (SF-36). I. Conceptual framework and item selection. Medical Care. 1992;**30**(6):473-483

[15] Heuch I, Hagen K, Heuch I, Nygaard O, Zwart JA. The impact of body mass index on the prevalence of

low back pain: The HUNT study. Spine. 2010;**35**(7):764-768

[16] Heuch I, Heuch I, Hagen K, Zwart JA. Body mass index as a risk factor for developing chronic low back pain: A follow-up in the Nord-Trondelag Health Study. Spine. 2013;**38**(2):133-139

[17] Boissière L, Takemoto M, Bourghli A, Vital JM, Pellisé F, Alanay A, et al. Global tilt and lumbar lordosis index: Two parameters correlating with health-related quality of life scores—But how do they truly impact disability? The Spine Journal. 2017;**17**(4):480-488

[18] Lackner JM, Carosella AM. The relative influence of perceived pain control, anxiety, and functional self efficacy on spinal function among patients with chronic low back pain. Spine. 1999;**24**(21):2255-2260

[19] Goldberg MS, Scott SC, Mayo NE. A review of the association between cigarette smoking and the development of nonspecific back pain and related outcomes. Spine. 2000;**25**(8):995-1014

[20] Freburger JK, Holmes GM, Agans RP, Jackman AM, Darter JD, Wallace AS, et al. The rising prevalence of chronic low back pain. Archives of Internal Medicine. 2009;**169**(3):251-258

[21] Lake JK, Power C, Cole TJ. Back pain and obesity in the 1958 British birth cohort: Cause or effect? Journal of Clinical Epidemiology. 2000;**53**(3):245-250

[22] Livshits G, Popham M, Maliin I, Sambrook PN, MacGregor AJ, Spector T, et al. Lumbar disc degeneration and genetic factors are the main risk factors for low back pain in women: The UK Twin Spine Study. Annals of the Rheumatic Diseases. 2011;**70**(10):1740-1745

[23] Muller-Riemenschneider F, Reinhold T, Berghofer A, et al. Health-economic burden of obesity in Europe. European Journal of Epidemiology. 2008;**23**(8):499-509

[24] Sturm R, Hattori A. Morbid obesity rates continue to rise rapidly in the United States. International Journal of Obesity. 2013;**37**(6):889-891

[25] Daubs MD, Lenke LG, Cheh G, Stobbs G, Bridwell KH. Adult spinal deformity surgery: Complications and outcomes in patients over age 60. Spine (Phila Pa 1976). 2007;**32**(20):2238-2244

[26] Glassman SD, Berven S, Kostuik J, Dimar JR, Horton WC, Bridwell K. Nonsurgical resource utilization in adult spinal deformity. Spine (Phila Pa 1976). 2006;**31**(8):941-947

[27] Glassman SD, Carreon LY, Shaffrey CI, Polly DW, Ondra SL, Berven SH, et al. The costs and benefits of nonoperative management for adult scoliosis. Spine (Phila Pa 1976). 2010;**35**(5):578-582

[28] Liu S, Schwab F, Smith JS, Klineberg E, Ames CP, Mundis G, et al. Likelihood of reaching minimal clinically important difference in adult spinal deformity: A comparison of operative and nonoperative treatment. The Ochsner Journal. 2014;**14**(1):67-77

[29] McCarthy I, O'Brien M, Ames C, Robinson C, Errico T, Polly DW Jr, et al. Incremental cost-effectiveness of adult spinal deformity surgery: Observed quality-adjusted life years with surgery compared with predicted quality-adjusted life years without surgery. Neurosurgical Focus. 2014;**36**(5):E3

[30] Smith JS, Shaffrey CI, Fu KM, Scheer JK, Bess S, Lafage V, et al. Clinical and radiographic evaluation of the adult spinal deformity patient.

Neurosurgery Clinics of North America. 2013;**24**(2):143-156

[31] Smith JS, Klineberg E, Lafage V, Shaffrey CI, Schwab F, Lafage R, et al. Prospective multicenter assessment of perioperative and minimum 2-year postoperative complication rates associated with adult spinal deformity surgery. Journal of Neurosurgery. Spine. 2016;**25**(1):1-14

[32] Bridwell KH, Glassman S, Horton W, Shaffrey C, Schwab F, Zebala LP, et al. Does treatment (nonoperative and operative) improve the two-year quality of life in patients with adult symptomatic lumbar scoliosis: A prospective multicenter evidence-based medicine study. Spine (Phila Pa 1976). 2009;**34**(20):2171-2178

[33] Scheer JK, Smith JS, Clark AJ, Lafage V, Kim HJ, Rolston JD, et al. Comprehensive study of back and leg pain improvements after adult spinal deformity surgery: Analysis of 421 patients with 2-year follow-up and of the impact of the surgery on treatment satisfaction. Journal of Neurosurgery. Spine. 2015;**22**(5):540-553

[34] McCarthy IM, Hostin RA, Ames CP, Kim HJ, Smith JS, Boachie-Adjei O, et al. Total hospital costs of surgical treatment for adult spinal deformity: An extended follow-up study. The Spine Journal. 2014;**14**(10):2326-2333

[35] Kieser D, Boissière L, Ghailane S, Larrieu D, Bourghli A, Yilgor C, et al. Adult spinal deformity (ASD) surgery: Understanding the true impact on specific activities of daily living. Lebanese Medical Journal. 2018;**66**(4):193-196

[36] Scheer JK, Tang JA, Smith JS, Klineberg E, Hart RA, Mundis GM Jr, et al. Reoperation rates and impact on outcome in a large, prospective, multicenter, adult spinal deformity database: Clinical article. Journal of Neurosurgery. Spine. 2013;**19**(4):464-470

[37] Pateder DB, Gonzales RA, Kebaish KM, Cohen DB, Chang JY, Kostuik JP. Short-term mortality and its association with independent risk factors in adult spinal deformity surgery. Spine. 2008;**33**(11):1224-1228

[38] Soroceanu A, Burton DC, Diebo BG, Smith JS, Hostin R, Shaffrey CI, et al. Impact of obesity on complications, infection, and patient-reported outcomes in adult spinal deformity surgery. Journal of Neurosurgery. Spine. 2015;**23**(5):656-664